MAKING MENTAL MIGHT:

HOW TO LOOK TEN TIMES SMARTER THAN YOU ARE

•••

BERNAND MICHAEL PATTEN, M.D.

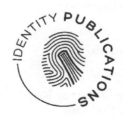

MAKING MENTAL MIGHT:

HOW TO LOOK TEN TIMES SMARTER THAN YOU ARE

For permission requests, write to the publisher at:
contact@identitypublications.com.

Ordering Information:
Quantity sales. Special discounts are available on quantity purchases by corporations, associations, and others. For details, contact the publisher at the address above.

Orders by U.S. trade bookstores and wholesalers.
Please contact Identity Publications:

Tel: (805) 259-3724 or visit www.IdentityPublications.com.

ISBN-13: 978-1-945884-18-4 (paperback)
ISBN-13: 978-1-945884-19-1 (hardcover)

First Edition
Publishing by Identity Publications.
www.IdentityPublications.com

Cover and Interior Formatting Design by Resa Embutin
Interior Formatting by Sheena Embutin

Fellow of the American College of Physicians
Fellow of the Royal Society of Medicine
Fellow of the Texas Neurological Society
Fellow of the American Academy of Neurology
Memory Fellow of the New York Academy of Medicine
Diplomate of the American Board of Psychiatry and Neurology

To Ethel—Sine Te Nihil

To the good people of the 21st century who still read
books. More power to you.

To fundamental facts, including the fact that $2 + 2 = 4$, and
all other truths that follow when fact is accepted as truth.
When fact is not accepted as truth, chaos follows.

TABLE OF CONTENTS

INTRODUCTION

♦ ♦ ♦

Hello there and welcome. You picked a very interesting and important book to read. You selected it because you wish to increase your mental might and look ten times smarter than you are. Good for you!

Now settle in and relax in a good chair and read. Read in solitude. One reads a book like this alone, even in the presence of others. Eliminate all distractions. Turn off your iPhone. The messages and emails and your Facebook friends can wait. If the TV in the next room is too loud, turn it down or shut the door or put on those Bluetooth noise-canceling earmuffs. Tell your friends and relations you need protected private time to study to become a memory genius. They will respect you for that, and if they don't—so what!

Doctor Bernard Patten wants to help you help yourself to a better mind and a better brain and, consequently, to help you to a better life. And he has asked me to write this book based on ideas presented in his lectures. He knows scientific research has proven mental exercise benefits the brain as much as physical exercise benefits the body. Not only does the mental exercise increase brainpower and (in some cases) brain size, but it also helps prevent dementia, including the much-feared dementia caused by Alzheimer's disease. Furthermore, the usual decline in mental power that occurs with age (known as "minimal cognitive impairment") by the proper application of techniques discussed here can be completely reversed.

Wow! Those facts are good news!

Interested?

Read on.

Not interested?

That's OK. You made a mistake. You picked up the wrong book. Put it back. It's not for you. Go watch TV.

What to Expect from Making Mental Might

Most self-help books will promise you the moon and deliver the tail end of the rocket. Not this book. In his popular course, Mental Gymnastics, Doctor Patten promised practically nothing unless you work. Brain function is an area of human activity where you have to work to get anything worthwhile, just as you have to work to get anything worthwhile out of anything anywhere at any time.

So, if you are not prepared to put on your thinking cap and do some mental work, don't expect much from this book.

Oh, I suppose it is possible that in casually reading, you might get lucky and pick up some helpful ideas and get some benefits even with minimal effort. That's possible. But if you put in time and effort, you will get better results. In fact, small efforts in the arena of brain health actually (and often) cause big returns. Yes, small efforts can = big returns, as you will soon discover should you decide to continue.

Making Mental Might (MMM) Will Not Disappoint You

At least the risk of disappointment won't be serious as we have warned you that building mental might requires work, often in the form of serious thinking and devoted actions, performance, and mental exercise.

Work!

Yes, work! Some easy work, some hard work, some work will be fun, some work which will be, well, just plain work, and some work which will be drudgery. But all of the work will, with a high degree of scientific certainty, lead you to a career featuring a marked increase in your mental abilities and performance. In fact, this book has the power to make you **LOOK** ten times smarter than you are. The objective tests of memory show that normal college students perform memory tasks ten times better (that is 1,000% better) if they use their memories trained by the techniques in this book than if they don't use the techniques and just rely on their natural memory. The same benefits may apply to you.

No bull and no kidding! Work the exercises, and you will see results. Even small efforts will reap big benefits.

About Mental Performance

Notice it was **LOOK** ten times smarter, not **BE** ten times smarter. Changing your I.Q. or your basic intelligence is possible on a small scale over long years of diligent application. But, basically, for better or worse, most of us, including me and you and Doctor Patten, and Patten's clone are stuck with what brain horsepower we got at birth. That's the bad news. The good news is with the proper training, you will look, sound, and perform worlds better than you do now. The techniques worked for me, and they worked for hundreds of my fellow students at Rice University's School of Continuing Studies, and they worked for Doctor Patten and for Doctor Patten's clone. There is no reason they will not work for you.

The secret is to apply ancient and modern techniques, great wisdom, and significant experiences to train your brain to be a more efficient, more powerful, and more dynamic thinking machine.

Hey, what!

You decided to continue reading! Good for you!

And by the way, if you picked up this book because you don't remember things as well as you did before or because you are concerned you might, just might, be experiencing the beginning of a serious mental decline, DESPAIR NOT! TAKE HEART!

You are not alone. Help is on the way. Help is here. Right here in your hands. But before we get to all that, Doctor Patten would like to add a few words.

A Personal Note from Doctor Patten

Friends, my experience helping patients and students goes back decades. First as the Fellow in Human Memory of the New York Academy of Medicine and then as the Founder and Director of the Memory Clinic at the Neurological Institute of New York and then as a practicing neurologist at the Baylor College of Medicine and last as an author of scientific papers on modality-specific memory disorders, visual methods of thinking, memory therapy for brain-damaged people, treatment of organic and functional amnesias and so forth. Last, but not least, for 17 years, my clone taught the course Mental Gymnastics at Rice University, Houston, Texas.

Why am I telling you this? Not to self-serve. Not to brag. But to clearly state the qualifications that went into writing *Making Mental Might* (MMM). The hope is your recognition of these qualifications will motivate you to actually read and carry out the forthcoming program designed to make you think faster and better, a program to make you look like a genius. It is also my express desire to take this opportunity to thank my student, Mickey, for taking careful notes during the lectures and faithfully putting those notes in manuscript to make an interesting, intelligent, practical, and useful book.

My neurological practice saw plenty of people, some with neurologic disease, but many more (usually in their fifty and sixties) who were in good health but worried because they forgot where they parked their car or where they left their reading glasses, or they drew a blank when they had to enter the PIN number on the cash machine. One left the stove on, and that caused considerable damage to her home. Another forgot her meds and had a seizure going downstairs. Burnt roasts in the oven—very common. Can't find the keys—ditto. Where is the iPhone? Did I unplug the iron? Front door locked? Garden hose still running?

Some patients told me they have on multiple occasions read a page of a book and, three minutes later, couldn't recall what they read. They have to read the page over and over, and still, they can't retain the information the way they did when they were younger or at the top of their game. One of my friends forgot where he parked his car at Bush International Airport and had to have security drive him around for over an hour until he found it. Another friend streamed *Urban Cowboy.* Twenty minutes into the movie, he realized he had watched the same movie two weeks ago. A political leader wanted to introduce me to his campaign manager but found himself in the embarrassing position of finding his manager's name had slipped his mind! Last week, I walked into the garage and couldn't for the life of me remember why I went to the garage or what I wanted to get. People have spent considerable time looking for their hat when it was on their head!

Do these things sound familiar? The foregoing examples show a poor memory is or can be a mere annoyance or a serious problem. And poor memory can be a serious life-impairing handicap, but one which, with persistence and intelligent effort, can be overcome.

The mentioned memory failures of everyday life are probably within the range of normal. If you have experienced them, do not think they forbode a dismal future. They are probably quite normal.

Remedies for the Memory Lapses of Everyday Life

Does it surprise you that there exists a remedy for each of these common problems, a simple, fast, easy technique to prevent the memory slip?

Solutions. That's what this book is about. Each step is clearly explained and sometimes repetitively explained as we go along. Repetition is the friend of memory; sometimes, it is the best friend. If, however, any point arises which is not clear to you, then write to Dadpatten@aol.com for help.

The Fun of Learning New Skills and Getting New Mental Powers

Doctor Patten designed his course at Rice University to be as entertaining as possible, but he did not omit complex scientific details about the brain, the mind, and the mechanism of human memory. Sorry, we can't go into neuroscience details here. That is how things have to be in our book, which is made especially for quick and practical advice about increasing brain horsepower. If Doctor Patten even tried to explain brain things, you would hear a lot of medical jargon that might confuse you and be off-putting. He might bore you to death, and some readers might even hang themselves.

How Do We Know Brainpower Can Be Improved?

Good question.

We know these facts from evidence that comes from the sciences connected with the biology of the human nervous system. Such sciences include solid hard sciences like biophysics, biochemistry, electrophysiology, molecular biology, neurogenetics, and optogenetics (a hybrid of optics, genetics, and virology), CAT scan, PET scan, and SPECT scan. But we also know these facts from some not-so-solid semi-scientific disciplines like neurology, psychology, sociology, and (may the gods help us!) psychiatry.

These sciences and these science wannabes provide overwhelming evidence that directed mental activity favorably changes the actual structure and function of the human brain. New brain cells are formed, new synapses are made, new networks are wired. The machine gets oiled, polished, and reconditioned.

Scans Don't Lie. They Can't.

Magnetic resonance scans of the brain show (for instance) that just 30 minutes of piano practice will alter, rearrange, and grow nerve cell connections. The new connections, the new rewiring of the brain, will last about ten days even if there is no further practice.

The results of mountains of psychological testing of normal adults, children, college students, and even the sick and the mentally deficient prove the mind can be improved and the improvements are long-lasting. Some of the more important epidemiologic studies that make this point will be covered so as to give you an immediate heads up on what you might put into practice in your own life—things, ideas, methods, treatments, approaches, tricks, clues, cues, scripts, schemata, categories, and so forth that have worked for others and that might work for you, that might give you ideas, that might give a heads-up, show you important techniques to improved clarity of your thought, give you superior powers of concentration, marvelous personal presentation, solid logical thinking, and an excellent memory.

My hope: This will be an adventure for you, an adventure that will be both productive and fun, and at the end, when the smoke has cleared, you will have made yourself look like a mental genius and a mensch. The goal is to look ten times smarter than you are. Along the way, it is highly likely you will prevent or delay dementia, which has become in contemporary America a rather cruel end to too many lives.

Understanding the biological foundations of dementia will be key to the development of targeted therapies to slow or prevent the onset of this terrible condition. But in such late-onset diseases, like dementia and other neurodegenerative conditions, delaying symptoms by even a few years can make an enormous difference to the quality of life of patients, as well as their families and caregivers. Fortunately, we now have the understanding and the means of putting that delay in place and in some cases, even preventing the actual disease from manifesting itself.

Long Haulers

COVID-19 has killed over 425,000 Americans. These are not just data points. These are real people—husbands, wives, sisters, brothers, sons, daughters, friends, and relations. A tragedy of the first dimension!

Among the survivors of COVID-19, there is a group of people, about 10% of those who have recovered from the acute illness, who, according to the *Journal of the American Medical Association* January 21, 2021, have severe problems with memory and concentration, a condition now termed brain fog. This group of sick people, called long haulers, usually has fatigue as well as brain fog. Experts don't understand brain fog and do not know what to do about it. The suggestions for memory and concentration training in this book may or may not help. There is sufficient evidence that the mental exercises to follow would probably help and would do no harm, but we simply do not know that for sure.

Take-Home Message: Your Health is Quite Literally in Your Hands. So Help Yourself.

You can do it!

What are you waiting for?

Your days (and mine) are numbered.

Our lives have definite limits.

So, before it's too late, let's get started!

WHAT LIFESTYLES CORRELATE WITH MENTAL MIGHT

CHAPTER ONE: WHAT LIFESTYLES CORRELATE WITH MENTAL MIGHT

◆ ◆ ◆

Main point of this chapter: The structure and function of the human nervous system is not fixed but may be favorably modified by directed activities.

The matter that detains us now may seem,

To many, neither dignified enough

Nor arduous, yet will not be scorned by them,

Who, looking inward, have observed the ties

That bind the perishable hours of life

Each to the other, & the curious props

By which the world of memory & thought

Exists & is sustained.

Wordsworth's *Prelude*

As previewed in the introduction, this chapter covers some of the recent scientific studies that have shown that lifestyles relate to mental might. These studies encompassed large populations of normal people who were looked after and repeatedly examined over a number of years. The studies cost the National Institutes of Health (and the American taxpayer) a great deal of money. Many physicians and scientists spent considerable time, effort, and talent ensuring the studies were done in a scientifically acceptable manner. In most cases, there was a control population so that the results in a certain lifestyle could be reasonably compared to the results in those who did not have that particular lifestyle.

Can we be frank? Your muscles are not developed or strengthened by looking at pictures of physical exercises or reading how to perform them. Only by carrying out the exercise yourself will those exercises do any good. The same is true with mental performance. Your brain and your mental powers will not benefit much by simply reading about the techniques. Only by attempting to do things yourself, augmenting your lifestyle, working the problems, and doing the memory exercises will you benefit your mind and brain.

Facts Speak Out Loud and Clear

The results of the aforementioned studies cannot be reasonably questioned. They are scientific facts. They are facts and should be accepted as such. The fact is the sweetest dream that labor knows, said Robert Frost, and he was right.

But the extensions of the results, the extrapolations from the data, the applications of the facts to you or anyone can be questioned and should be questioned.

Here's why:

It is one thing, for instance, to find that CEOs of corporations (compared to non-CEOs) have larger than average English language vocabularies, and it is quite another thing to conclude from that fact that increasing your English language vocabulary will make you a CEO.

Get it?

There is more to being a CEO than having a larger-than-average vocabulary, much more. No doubt CEOs have larger-than-average English vocabularies, but that is not the main reason that they are CEOs. Many other important items and skills are involved.

Some of you may have read that drinking wine increases your chance of living longer. Multiple studies have shown that people who drink wine actually live longer and have a lower-than-average incidence of dementia. That's a fact. People who drink wine have by and large lived longer than control groups of people who did not drink wine.

So what?

Does that mean you need to start drinking so you can add some years to your life?

Well, drinking wine may or may not help you increase your life span. And studying your English language vocabulary may or may not help you become a CEO. Chances are that those activities will help, but chances are that neither of those activities will help much. To be a CEO, you have to go to school and learn about business. A master's in business administration would help and lots of luck, insight, imagination, market acumen, hard work, creativity, and so forth.

What about wine? We just don't know for sure because people who drink wine may be living longer for some other reason than the wine per se. Their longevity might relate to the wine or it might not. Some other thing might be more directly related to living longer, and that other thing happens to correlate with wine drinking. Most wine drinkers probably have better nutrition. Perhaps they exercise more. Perhaps they take better care of their teeth and so forth. Who knows? Probably the whole package of lifestyle that goes with wine drinking is more important in increasing life span than is just drinking wine.

Correlation Does Not Prove Cause and Effect

The point is correlations like wine and life span and vocabulary and CEO suggest a connection but do not necessarily imply a causal relation. Therefore, correlation does not prove a cause-and-effect relationship; it merely proves a correlation. The situation with correlations and cause-and-effect relationships is usually more complex. The cock crows, and the sun rises. So what? The cock did not cause the sun to rise, though those of you who have lived on a farm know the cock is the trumpet to the morn. Daybreak and the cock's crow are correlated but are not related to each other as cause and effect. The cockcrow calls the hens to mate and has no effect whatsoever on the sun. In fact, if you killed the cock, the sun will rise. Hence, we have arrived at one of the very important principles of straight thinking that you should memorize right now.

Lesson: Knowing correlation doesn't prove cause and effect is your first step to becoming a mental giant.

Two events linked in time together do not prove one causes the other. If one event follows another, it does not mean the second event was caused by the first. This error in thinking has a fancy Latin name that makes it sound more scientific than it is: Post Hoc, Propter Hoc.

To Prove Cause and Effect Requires More Evidence than Just Correlation

Some examples:

A doctor gives a medicine, and the patient recovers. Did the medicine cause the patient to recover?

Stop right here. Formulate your answer.

I pause for reply.

Answer: Nope, not necessarily. The patient could have recovered naturally. Most people do recover on their own.

A doctor gives a medicine, and the patient dies. Did the medicine cause the patient's death?

Stop right here. Think! What's your opinion?

I pause for reply.

Nope. The patient could have died for any number of reasons, including the disease for which the medicine was given.

Lifestyles that Correlate with Health and Long Life

So also, with the lifestyle changes you are about to read about. Here, you will discover that playing a musical instrument correlates with a significant reduction in the risk of dementia and risk of developing Alzheimer's disease.

Will playing the piano do the same for you?

Probably it will, but in a scientific sense, we can't guarantee that result without looking at credible other data, preferably real evidence, that supports a definite causal relationship between playing a musical instrument and the decrease in dementia risk.

We do know from the study at the Albert Einstein College of Medicine that, in an adult population studied for years, playing the piano correlated with a decreased chance of dementia and that not playing an instrument increased the chance of dementia. Thus, comparison with a control group of people matched for age and sex and living in the same environment (Bronx, New York) showed playing an instrument probably does, in fact, decrease the risk of dementia. But in the case of piano playing, we have other evidence that shows the same thing and therefore supports the conclusion. We also know, for instance, from the brain scans that piano playing people increase the size of their brains when they play and when they practice. We do know that (in general) the bigger your brain and the more efficiently it functions, the greater will be your reserve power (known in neurological circles as "cognitive reserve") to ward off the clinical effects of diseases that cause dementia. Other studies show a marked improvement in mental and motor skills in those who play an instrument compared to those who don't. In other words, we look for the correlations, and then we look for other collateral evidence that the correlation does actually reflect a cause-and-effect relation.

In the case of playing a musical instrument, the overwhelming evidence from many sources supports the view that playing a musical instrument is good for your brain. That said, what about listening to music? Does that prevent dementia?

The Mozart Effect

The Mozart Effect (listening to music makes you smarter) is controversial.

Oliver Sacks, one of the best-known neurologists in the world, was Artist in Residence at Columbia University. Perhaps you have heard of him. His recent book *Musicophilia* has been a best seller. Here's what Oliver Sacks (OS) said in an interview with Neurology Now (NN) (January/February 2008):

NN: Is there any therapeutic difference between playing music, singing it, or listening to it?

OS: I don't think there's much to be said for the so-called Mozart Effect, which has to do with casual exposure to music. But I think there's a great deal to be said for active involvement with music, whether it takes the form of music therapy in a hospital or learning an instrument and following a score.

Active Mental Involvement is the Key to Building Mental Might

Notice how the great man, Oliver Sacks, emphasizes active versus passive involvement, an important point that will come up again and again. In general, playing and at the same time thinking about the piece you are playing is better than just playing the piece, which is better than just thinking about the piece, which is worlds better than just passively listening to the piece. We will return to this important idea which is that the **more actively the brain is involved in an activity, the better the brain will benefit.** Listening to music may be entertaining and fun, but actively creating music requires much more mental effort and focused attention and would therefore be expected to help your brain much more than the passive activity of just listening.

MMM Will Not Discuss Scientific Methods or Emphasize Controversy

Years ago, I made the mistake of having dinner with two neurologists. It was the most boring dinner of my life (so far), and I shall not make that mistake again. The reason these neurologists were so boring was their anal compulsive attention to details. A good scientist and a good neurologist is always questioning the received standard wisdom in order to make sure that what was and is considered truth is actually true. In some sense, these people can be as boring as some lawyers and some engineers.

In this chapter and in this book, we don't have time to question everything, for I, Mickey, am trying to write an interesting book and not bore you to death with the nitty-gritty. What you will get here is summary—usually a summary of personal opinions of what is important and what is likely true and what is a good practical betting horse to help you build mental might. If you need details about the nitty-gritty, consult other books of which there are many.

Aims for Mickey:

> 1. To write an interesting, useful, and reasonably intelligent book that is more entertaining than watching TV.
> 2. To help you add a rather large set of items to your storehouse of mental delights.

Mickey's aims for you:

> 1. To help you help yourself to mental might
> 2. To help you understand what things are good for your mental fitness
> 3. To help you know what things are not good for your mental fitness

7

4. To help you know what things are bad for mental fitness

5. To help you understand the crux of the problem

Crux of the problem?

What problem?

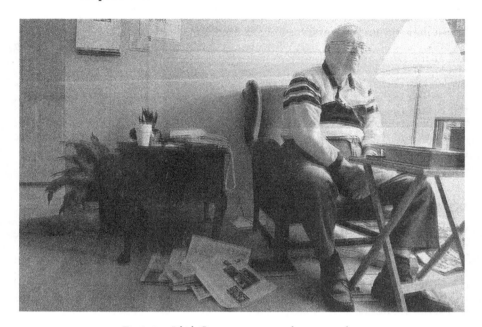

Fig1.1 - Phil Garner, nursing home resident

This is the crux of the problem. His name is Phil Granger. He is 84, a resident of a care facility, and is quoted in the New York Times, January 30, 2005: "There is everything anyone could want here. The only thing wrong with this place is that we are all old. We remember what we used to do and can't do anymore."

Phil is right, according to the National Center for Assisted Living. Half the people in his place have trouble thinking, three-quarters can't wash themselves, eight of ten can't manage their own medicines, and 90% are unfit for any kind of work, including cooking or cleaning for themselves.

Ugh! This is a bleak picture. Anything you can do to prevent this kind of disability would be all to the good. You must fight aging and the changes it brings as much as you can for as long as you can. Agree?

Who Wrote the Paragraph That Follows and When?

"It is our duty to resist old age, to compensate for its defects by watchful care, to fight against it as we would fight against a disease. Practice moderate exercise, take enough but not too much food and drink. Nor, indeed, are we to give our attention solely to the body; much greater care is due to the mind and soul, for they like lamps grow dim with time, unless we keep them supplied with oil. Intellectual activity gives buoyancy to the mind."

The above advice is over 2000 years old and was written in a very famous essay called "On Aging." The author, Marcus Tullius Cicero, knows whereof he speaks and much of the advice, nay all of it, still applies today.

Moderate exercise. You bet.

Enough but not too much food and drink. Right ho, Jeeves.

But it isn't my job to tell you to obtain regular exercise, put out those cigarettes, socialize with others, maintain good nutrition, get a good night's sleep, maintain a happy, upbeat, optimistic outlook on life, and so forth. You know what's good for your general health, and you know what isn't good. If in doubt, consult *Health is Wealth: Small Changes Reap Big Benefits*, a book that covers basic advice about environment, exercise, and diet.

So, for the most part, let's skip the health, nutrition, and medical stuff and concentrate on Cicero's next item: building brainpower.

Much greater care is due to the mind and soul. About the soul, I know nothing, but we shall have several chapters on how to keep the lamp lights of the mind working bright, including a super-duper chapter on memory augmentation and a chapter on mental math. In the middle of the chapters and at the end of the chapters, there will be suggestions and exercises for you to consider (these are called mental gymnastics) and to help yourself to mental might. Meanwhile, let's talk about evidence that the brain can change, and let's talk about evidence that we can change our brains.

Sidebar by Doctor Patten about Scans—Evidence That the Brain Can Change

Many years ago, never mind how many, when I was in neurological practice, a young artist came to see me because he was losing his mind. He had painted several paintings that had sold for a lot of money and, though he was young, he did have a national and international reputation for his work.

His problem was that over the course of a year, he had noticed a fall-off in his creative abilities, and he had noticed that his memory was failing. On more than a few occasions, he would start to say something and then forget what he was talking about. Despite a valiant effort, he just couldn't get back to the subject. Whole evenings would slip out of consciousness, never to be recalled again.

Except for impairment of ability to remember and poor ability to subtract numbers mentally, his neurological examination was OK.

The brain scan (this was the era of CAT scan) showed tremendous loss of brain tissue with dilated ventricles (the fluid-filled cavities in the center of the brain), narrow gyri, and enlarged sulci (the gyri are brain tissue ridges and the sulci the valleys between ridges).

Dilated ventricles usually mean loss of brain tissue, narrow gyri ditto, enlarged sulci ditto. Looking at the scan, I estimated that my patient had lost over 40% of his brain tissue. That was not good. Consequently, the prognosis was not good. In fact, the prognosis seemed grim.

His personal history was significant because he had been drinking a quart of rye whiskey a day. (Yes, that is what he said, and there is no reason to think he was bragging. If anything, at least according to his wife, he might have been underestimating the dose of booze.)

"If you continue to drink like that," says I. "You will soon be dead."

Notice I did not say, "You must stop drinking." That kind of medical advice is paternalistic and takes part of the patient's personal power away. This man is an adult, and he has to decide what he wants to do with his life. My job, as I saw it at the time, was to give advice in the form of a realistic warning about death. "Death is a bad thing," I told him. "It spoils your weekend."

And then, to emphasize the seriousness of the situation, I showed and explained the CAT scan to him. He was impressed by the visual image of his rotted brain, much more impressed by the picture than he was by my warning. After all, the man is an artist, a great artist.

"Will my brain grow back?" he asked.

"Certainly not. Brain tissue, once lost, is lost forever. The best you may hope for is to arrest the brain loss at the present level. Your brain will never recover, for it never can recover."

The Dogma of the Inability of the Brain to Recover is Now Passé

Long ago, never mind how long, during medical school, internship, and residency, my professors told me emphatically that once brain tissue is lost, it can never be recovered. So, what I was doing in advising this patient was merely repeating the neurological dogma that had been drummed into my head during my medical training. At the time, it was considered no more possible to regenerate brain tissue than it was possible to fly to the moon. We now know, of course, that humans can do both.

What Happened Next?

Three months later, the artist returned for a follow-up examination. He felt that he had recovered completely. His wife gave it for her opinion that he was better than ever. My examination confirmed that thinking, memory, and even the subtractions were now not only normal but superior. What had happened?

He stopped the booze, of course. Remove the cause of a disease, and you usually get an improvement, and his improvement was dramatic. But what happened to the brain?

The artist wanted a repeat CAT scan to answer that question. But, of course, I told him that a repeat scan would be a waste of time and money because there would be no change. Besides, I was pretty sure his insurance wouldn't pay for a repeat scan. Why should they when it was generally known that the brain cannot regenerate?

Sure enough, the insurance company wouldn't pay for another scan, but the patient did pay the $850 (scans were cheaper in those days). He wanted to see the picture of his brain again, and he was willing to pay for the picture, an attitude totally consistent with his vocation as a visual artist.

Seeing is Believing

Seeing is believing: If you see something, you believe it. If you don't see it, you don't know. Shakespeare called this "ocular proof." Seeing is believing. But if you don't see it, does that mean it isn't there, and you shouldn't believe it?

Aye, there's the rub. It could be there, and you missed it. Or the tools you are using could have been wrong for that particular observation. For instance, if I say there are no bacteria on this paper, and I am using a telescope to look for the bacteria, I will be using the wrong tool and reaching the wrong conclusion. You can't see bacteria with a telescope. To see bacteria, you need a microscope, not a telescope. Actually, there are billions of bacteria on this book and on your pillow at night. You can't see them. But they are there.

The Artist's CAT Scan

Holy Cow! What to my wondering eyes should appear?

A **NORMAL** scan.

The brain scan was now normal, as normal as the patient. For me, this was an earthquake, as you can imagine. You can't appreciate this kind of revelation. That is unless you have been brainwashed (like me) by eight years of typical neurological training.

MENTAL MAKING MIGHT

The scan proved the point: The brain, just like so many other body organs, just like so many other body tissues (liver, skin, bone, etc.), has the potential to recover. And under the right circumstances, it will recover. And in this case, it did recover. It recovered functionally, as evidenced by the artist's normal mental status examination and his return to creativity, and the brain recovered structurally, as evidenced by the repeat CAT scan that was now normal.

Since that time, scans have proved the point time and time again; hence, we are sure of the fact that diseased nervous tissue, given the right circumstances, can recover, re-grow, look normal, and be normal.

Yep, that is the answer for diseased brain tissue. But what about normal brain tissue? Can we, by directed mental activity, grow brain tissue to suit a particular need? The answer is yes, yes, yes.

Mickey already mentioned the changes in piano players after only one practice session. Magnetic scans of violin players show that the area that controls the strings is bigger than the area that bows because the hand that strings has more to do. Another study that proves the point best is the London Taxi Driver Study.

The London Taxi Driver Study proves that the part of the brain concerned with the geography of London (after diligent application and study) increases in size four-fold (400%) according to a ground-breaking study by Maguire, E et al., published in 2000 in the Proceedings of the National Academy of Science, 47(8) 4398-4403.

London is an old town probably named after an ancient Celtic god of light (Lug or Lugh). Julius Caesar in De Bello Gallico says Lugh was the most revered deity in Gaul. The name Lug town said differently and corrupted by time and usage became what is now called London. Lugdunum (fort of Lugh) was the capital of Roman Gaul and is now modern Lyon. London is just one of many cities (too numerous to mention) named after Lugh.

Lug town was laid out before the Romans arrived. It was once one of the dark places of the earth. Hence, London does not have a grid street pattern like more recently established cities. What you have in Lug town became a London where a bunch of old trails and cow paths subsequently turned into major roads. Consequently, the geography of London is not rational but chaotic (like human anatomy), and to learn the geography of London (or human anatomy), one must study and memorize the lay of the land. There is no other way.

People who want to get a license to drive a Taxi in London must first pass a test to prove that they know the shortest distance between any two points in that fair city. To learn enough to pass the test usually requires about two years of diligent application, sometimes longer. Multiple books are available to help people learn the lay of the land and to pass the test.

What if we took a group of people who wanted to drive a taxi and scanned them before they started to study and then scanned them after they passed the London geography test to see if the brain changed? What if we took a group of London bus drivers and did the same brain scans? The bus drivers have a set route and do not have to memorize anywhere near as much as the Taxi drivers. Question:

Would bus driver brains grow tissue like taxi driver brains or not?

Neurologists know that the part of the brain that controls visual-spatial orientation would be most likely the region that would have to do the work of memorizing London, so particular attention would be focused on that area.

And bingo! The predicted area (posterior hippocampal of the right temporal lobe) is the area that increased in size an average of four-fold (400%). The longer the individual studied the geography of London, the larger became that area of the brain. Bus drivers had no significant change in brain size in any region. There was a suggestion that the anterior hippocampal region in the taxi group had decreased in size, a possible cost of the training. The brain is like that. Work some part a lot and some other part may suffer. There was no clinical deficit found in those drivers who had a slightly smaller anterior hippocampal.

Another takeaway message from this study is that the brain response is task-specific. The typing center did not expand because typing was not involved. The language center did not expand because it was not being trained. This modality-specific response of brain plasticity is normal and natural and reflects the way the brainworks.

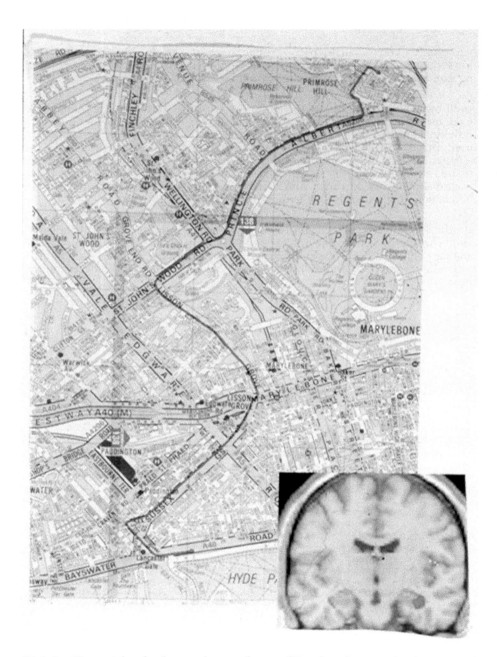

Fig1.2 - Here with a background map of part of London showing the shortest path to the Primrose Hill district is the part of the brain in the right temporal lobe that expanded in the taxi drivers. The area in question shows up as a gray blob.

Lifestyles That Prevent Dementia

Okay, let's talk about some of the controlled studies that have shown what life-styles correlate with better brain function. We will start with the study done at Albert Einstein College of Medicine.

The Verghese Study

The Verghese Study (Verghese was the head author) done at the Einstein College of Medicine worked with the elderly from the Bronx, New York. There were 469 subjects, 91% white, 64% women, who were enrolled in 1980 and 1983, and followed up every 12 to 18 months for over seven years.

The idea was to see what lifestyles correlated with a decrease in dementia risk and what lifestyles did not. At the end, it was found that only one physical exercise correlated with decreased risk of dementia, and that was ballroom (social) dancing. No benefit was observed in the following physical activities: tennis, golf, swimming, bicycling, group exercises, team games, walking, climbing stairs, housework, babysitting, or playing with grandchildren.

Positive findings among the thinking (what they call cognitive) tasks were reading books or newspapers, playing board games or cards, playing a musical instrument, and social (ballroom) dancing. Notice ballroom dancing is both a physical activity and also a thinking activity. Those of you who ballroom dance know that is true.

No effect on dementia risk was observed for creative writing, group discussion, or crossword puzzles. The more thinking involved in the activity, the more the cognitive score on the thinking test, and the more dementia was prevented regardless of age, sex, education, or baseline cognitive status.

Post-Study Reanalysis

To ensure that lesser levels of cognitive activity were not the consequence of pre-clinical cognitive decline, analysis was done after exclusion of those who became demented during the first seven years of the study. The association of cognitive activity and reduced risk persisted.

The study was published in the New England Journal of Medicine. Dr. Joseph Coyle, in an editorial in the same journal, concluded that the study showed: Effortful mental activity "not only strengthens existing synaptic connections and generates new ones, but it may also stimulate neurogenesis, especially in the hippocampus."

By way of other comments, Doctor Coyle also mentioned the importance of not watching TV.

We will talk more about TV and its adverse effect on the brain later. Meanwhile, keep in mind that during TV watching, all the great powers of the human brain are quiescent. TV watching is fundamentally a passive activity. It is probable that the metabolic level of the brain is less while you are watching TV than it is while you are sleeping.

Lesson: TV Is Junk Food for the Mind

Junk food for the body is empty calories of no nutritional value. Junk food for the mind is content of no intellectual value. So, do yourself a favor and don't reach for that remote. Get a life. Life is what happens when you are not watching TV. That's another consideration: The opportunity cost of watching TV. Why watch it when you could be doing something better with your life? When you do something, you exclude something else that you could have done. That exclusion is the opportunity cost of the first activity because it deprives you of doing the second. Part of the cost of watching TV is that you don't do something else in its place, something that might be or probably would be more useful.

Opportunity Costs: Lost Opportunities Are Opportunities lost

As discussed: The problem with TV is the time spent watching it could have been better spent thinking or reading or learning or playing a musical instrument or playing chess or bingo, social dancing or doing any one of a number of activities that have been scientifically shown to improve brain function. Any one or any combination of those activities, just mentioned, has been shown by neuroscientists in prospective, controlled, blinded, long-term scientific studies to augment brainpower and reduce the chance of dementia.

Watching TV, on the other hand, has been shown (I am not making this up) to increase your chance of developing heart disease, diabetes, cancer (cancer of the colon in particular), obesity, and dementia. TV has been shown in numerous studies to seriously degrade attention span and memory capacity. Significant evidence indicates that watching TV causes autism in some cases and that stopping TV stops the autism in those cases. If it sounds like watching TV is really bad, it is because watching TV is really bad.

Doctors Are Against TV

And the austere, usually laconic, and rarely committed *New England Journal of Medicine* came out in an editorial against TV as detrimental to the brain. If doctors don't know what's good for the brain and what isn't good for the brain, who does?

How Much TV Do Kids Watch?

Nielsen Company says in a study released October 26, 2009, that children ages two to five watch more than 32 hours of television each week (*Wall Street Journal*, October 27, 2009, page A4). Kids six to eleven spend a little less time in front of the TV screen—more than 28 hours. But that is partly because they have to go to school. TV isn't called the electronic babysitter for nothing. Think of all those young brains that are not getting the exercise that they need for proper development. Think about all those young muscles that are not getting the exercise they need for proper development. Think of all that wasted life. The kids are better off playing with blocks or dolls or toy trucks or playing stickball with friends than they are watching TV.

If you are not convinced kid TV is junk, go watch your kids in the living room in front of the television, within its electromagnetic field. They are watching cartoon characters beat each other over the head with bananas. Linger a while, and you will want to smash the set. Letting them sit before the tube is as bad as feeding them a diet of Hostess Twinkies.

Twinkies? That will remind the lawyers reading this book about the Twinkie defense used by Dan White to explain why he killed Harvey Milk and George Moscone. In the famous 1979 San Francisco trial for murder, the jury concluded that White had diminished capacity to premeditate murder in part due to depression and in part due to a diet of Coca-Cola and Twinkies. White was convicted of voluntary manslaughter and sentenced to seven years in prison. High-sugar diets are probably not a good idea for children or murderers or anyone, for that matter, and may be as bad for your general health as watching TV.

But what, you may ask, about educational TV?

Educational TV is Not All That Educational

How about educational programs on PBS and TV programs of that ilk?

Next time you watch such programs, pay attention to three things: The presentation, the information density, and the content. The presentation will be entertainment. You may find that the information density is slight and the content does little more than flatter your ego by showing you stuff you already know.

One producer from Disney (Mr. Lesiter) explained this directly: "The public will not tolerate anyone showing them stuff they are not already familiar with. The public wants affirmation that they already know all they need to know. Try to teach them something new, and your chance of staying in business is close to zero."

Seeing Is Believing

A word about negative data. As mentioned, if you see something, then you know. If you don't see something, you don't know. It could have been there, and you missed it. Some of my fellow students resented the fact that there didn't seem to be any benefit from playing with grandchildren. That doesn't mean much. Positive findings are much more important than negative ones. And it certainly doesn't mean the grandchildren didn't benefit from the play, and it doesn't mean they did benefit either. When we just don't know something, we just don't know.

Lesson: Stick with the positives.

It is possible that some study in the future will show a benefit of playing with grandchildren, but all we know now is that particular item did not show a benefit in dementia prevention in this particular study from the Einstein College of Medicine.

Why Is This Study of Dementia Prevention Not Widely Known?

Your guess is as good as mine. The study is scientific, and it did reach some definite conclusions. If you had a pill that prevented dementia, it would be all over the papers, and people would be paying to get it. Instead, you just need to do some social dancing, or read, or play an instrument, or play board games or cards or bingo. In other words: Get involved. Use it or lose it. In fact: Use it and improve it.

The Brain Benefits from Thinking Just as Muscles Benefit from Exercise Because Thinking Is the Exercise of the Brain

Notice all of the activities that correlated with dementia prevention involve thinking. Notice also that the amount of brainwork needed to get benefits is really quite small—minimal indeed. How much thinking do you need to play two-card bingo? And yet, two-card bingo once a week might reduce your dementia risk considerably. It is estimated that playing one-card bingo once a week for three hours might reduce your dementia risk about 20%. Two-card bingo would do even more.

Reading Is Good

It doesn't matter what you read to get the benefits from reading. A book will do, and so will a magazine or newspaper. The benefit from reading occurs even with minimal amounts of reading. By the same token, it doesn't seem to matter what board games you play or what card games. It is the playing that counts and the brain effort involved in thinking about the next move in chess or checkers or whether or not you should hold or fold those cards in poker.

Musical instruments ditto: Any one will do. But from what we know from collateral evidence, the more complicated the instrument, the greater the brain benefits. It, therefore, seems safe to say that a keyboard instrument, the master of all instruments, probably gives more brain juice than other lesser instruments. Many people think keyboards are music's most versatile instruments. We can back that statement with some facts:

Keyboards (piano, organ, harpsichord, harp) have a great range of volume from soft to very loud. Sure, your neighbor can play her bugle loud or soft, but she can play only one note at a time. Your friend with the violin can play two notes, three max at a time, and the pitch range is sometimes less than that of a piano.

Keyboards can sound more than one note at a time. Piano uses pedal, sometimes even two feet, one on each pedal at different times or at the same time. That requires coordination. The right and left hand have to balance the voices to bring out the melodies of the complex polyphonic textures of the music. That requires great control and sensitive and attentive ears. Memorization of piano music is a lot harder due to more complex structures and hence better for the brain. Notation of piano music requires reading in both treble and bass clefs which look different because different lettered notes are assigned to spaces and lines in both. That difference is challenging from the start. Hence, more brainwork and more brain benefits.

Keyboards are toned. That is, they produce different musical notes. A drum is usually unpitched, as is a triangle, as is a cymbal.

Keyboards have the widest pitch range of any musical instrument, from very high notes to very low. In fact, the 88 keys on the usual piano just about cover the entire range of the human voice: Soprano, alto, tenor, bass.

Keyboards can be played solo or with others. Ensemble is a plus because it is a form of socialization, which is good for us.

So, given the choice of instrument, if the goal is to get the maximum brain benefit from playing a musical instrument, then you might come down for a keyboard instrument like the piano, organ, celesta, harp (like a keyboard, only positioned vertically and plucked) and so forth. But if the bugle turns you on, that's OK. The bugle is a complicated instrument and hard to master. But it is not as hard as piano. The same idea of the benefit of complexity probably applies also to reading.

Reading: The Same Again

From what we know from other collateral evidence, it seems safe to assume that the more complicated the reading material, the more complex the game, the more mentally demanding the musical instrument, the more the brain will benefit.

This idea will turn up in other studies. A little mental exercise is good and goes a long way in preventing dementia and in building mental might, and the more complicated or demanding the brain exercise, the more benefits are to be expected. The ACTIVE study is another case in point.

The ACTIVE Study

- Advanced cognitive training for independent and vital elderly
- Prospective six-year study, four groups
- Three groups got two-hour sessions for five weeks
- And four remedial sessions at 11 and 35 months
- 2,832 people, mean age 76, 26% black
- Sessions consisted of three categories of instruction: memory, clear thinking, hand-eye coordination. Those were the modalities that were trained, and the hope was that the training would improve brain function in all areas.

The bullets pretty much summarize the ACTIVE study, which would be too boring to go through in detail.

ACTIVE is the acronym for the nine words in the first bullet—advanced cognitive training for independent and vital elderly. The results showed that brain training is modality-specific. If you train people to memorize, by the gods, that's what they get good at. If you train them to think clearly, by the gods, that's what they get good at. If you train them to have hand-eye coordination, you guessed it.

Bottom Line:

- Brain training is modality-specific:
  - Trained in memory? That's what you get
  - Trained in critical thinking? Ditto
  - Trained in hand-eye coordination? Ditto

Amazingly: Despite minimal effort, measurable improvements remained after five years or longer. For unknown reasons, critical thinking improved activities of daily living long after the lessons in critical thinking stopped. The benefits of critical thinking are enormous, and that is why you might consider reading Doctor Patten's book *Truth, Knowledge, or Just Plain Bull: How to Tell the Difference*. Or his other logic book: *The Logic of Alice: Clear Thinking in Wonderland*.

In fact, the group that received instruction in reasoning skills, when tested five years later, did 40% better on the tests of reasoning skills compared to the control group not so instructed. The reasoning-instructed group also experienced a marked benefit in ability to do activities of daily living, including taking care of their own personal hygiene, keeping all parts of the external body clean and healthy. Personal hygiene is crucial for maintaining both physical and mental health. Why instruction in critical thinking was associated with these extra benefits is not known, but it did.

The memory group, compared to controls, did 75% better on memory and the visual group did 300% better on visual tasks. Again, minimal effort resulted in useful and significant measurable improvements long after training stopped.

Which Is Better? Use the Weak Hand After a Stroke, or Use the Strong Hand?

Put on your thinking cap and answer the question. Now that you understand that the brain benefits by doing and thinking, decide what kind of rehabilitation would work best on a patient who had a stroke. Should the patient use the good hand that is not weak? Or should they use the bad hand that is weak? Pause now for 15 seconds and tell yourself the answer and support your answer with a reason.

Constraint Therapy Is Effective in Stroke Rehabilitation

There are in the United States 700,000 strokes per year. Of those people who have had a stroke, 570,000 survive with some impairment. They need lots of care, and in fact, 58 billion dollars are spent each year on stroke care—about half for rehab. The EXCITE study proves (again) the point that making the brain work makes the brain work better:

EXCITE assessed 106 stroke survivors with CIT (Constraint Inhibition Therapy), which prevented the patients from using the unimpaired arm and hand by making them wear a mitt for much of their waking hours. One hundred sixteen control patients got no CIT, just the usual rehab treatments.

Measurements made: Wolf Motor Function tests of time, strength, quality of movements, as well as measurement of how well and how often 30 activities of daily living are performed and how long it takes to do those activities.

The results speak for themselves: CIT patients did better than control patients. Results persisted for at least a year. CIT prevents and often reverses the learned nonuse of the affected limb.

Next question: Which hand is the weak hand? The patient is on the left. Doctor Wolf (one of the developers of CIT) is on the right.

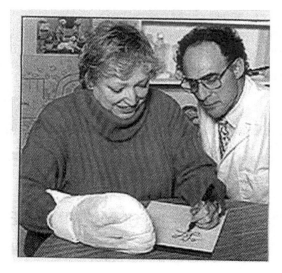

Conclusion: Use it or lose it, and use it to improve it.

Answer to the above question: The mitt is on the good hand. She is trying to write with the weak hand. Because she is writing with the impaired hand, the brain will try to and often does rewire itself to better direct motor function in the hand that has been weakened by the stroke.

Fig1.3 - Doctor Wolf (right) and patient (left)

Amblyopia

Amblyopia, informally called "lazy eye," is reduced vision in an eye due to abnormal visual development as a child. When the brain receives poor information from one eye, it stops communicating with that eye and relies on information from the other "stronger" eye. Treatment consists of correcting vision in the bad eye by correcting refractive errors (nearsightedness, farsightedness), strabismus, or cataract. The next step is to work on training the brain to use the weaker eye again to help it get stronger. This may be done with a patch over the stronger eye. The patch forces the brain to use the other weaker eye and thus improves vision in that eye. Kids who struggle with the patch get eye drops in the good eye (usually atropine) to blur vision in that stronger eye. The principle here in this standard therapy for amblyopia is the same as that in CIT: improve poor brain function by making the damaged part of the brain do work. Reference: Journal of the American Medical Association January 26, 2021, volume 325 Number 4 page 408.

Other Studies

There are about 10,000 other studies that show that the brains of animals and mankind regenerate. There are studies of Long-Term Potentiation (LPT) and Short-term Potentiation (STP), synapse formation, neurotransmitter release, and so forth. There are studies that show the more toys, the better the brains. The more play, the better the brain. The more activity, the better the brain. It is not necessary for you to know anything about these things for you to build mental might any more than it is necessary for you to know the detailed working of the internal combustion engine for you to drive a car. The general idea will do. And having convinced you the brain can be favorably modified by directed mental activity, here are some cautiously made recommendations.

No program is right for everyone. You have to pick and choose what is right for you. Mental exercise should be fun. Physical exercise should be fun also. Studies have shown that forced physical exercise (as opposed to voluntary physical exercise) is not effective in building physical fitness. By the same token, it may well be possible that forcing mental exercise will create a kind of resentment that would be detrimental to what you are trying to accomplish. When you make up a mental fitness program for yourself, make sure you like it, and it likes you. By the time you finish this book, you should have a good idea of what you wish to accomplish and how much and what you are willing to do to accomplish what you wish. Know what you want to do and then do it. This planning is a kind of future memory that is handled by the anterior frontal lobes of the brain. You imagine what you wish to plan to do in the future, and then you remember that plan and work it. People with injured anterior frontal lobes can't do that task. They can't plan ahead. But normal people can.

What Specific Tasks Are Recommended?

Reading: As noted before, it doesn't seem to matter what you read, a book, the newspaper, a magazine. They all use a tremendous amount of brainpower. To read, you must see the words, then convert the visual image into some kind of lexical meaning and so forth. The process is quite involved, and the brain scans show that during reading, the brain lights up in many places all at once. That is the desired effect. In fact, there doesn't seem to be any other activity that lights up the brain as much, except reading a new score of music, which I guess is also just another type of reading where instead of words, the brain is reading symbols that represent pitches and notes.

It probably doesn't matter how much you read. Twenty minutes a day should be quite enough exercise to maintain mental fitness for reading. Reading too much and not doing anything else is probably not a good idea either. So read, but don't become a reading drudge.

Playing board games: The social aspect is probably just as important as the game itself. Therefore, play with others. A game that requires thinking is best. Games that just rely on chance alone are not good because the brain doesn't get a chance (pun intended) to do its thing. Scrabble is great to work out the left hemisphere, which is primarily responsible for language. Blockus, 3D and 2D versions, is great to work out the right hemisphere because it requires lots of organization of sizes and shapes. Chess, checkers, cards—OK. How much game playing is needed? Who knows? Once or twice a week is probably good and maybe just as beneficial to the brain as once a day.

Playing a musical instrument: Highly recommended. And don't say it is too late for you to start. People have started playing the piano in their eighties and nineties. Doctor Patten tells me he went back to the piano at age 67. Having a good teacher is important, and you should make sure the teacher likes you and you like the teacher. Most people learn best in a calm, happy atmosphere and not in one where there is strict musical discipline. How would you like to have had Ty Cobb as your batting instructor? Or Julia Childs as your cooking teacher? These teachers are way up there, and their standards are high. With teachers like that, as a student, you are in a no-win situation. Perfect is the enemy of the good, and sometimes good enough is good enough. Playing a musical instrument well will take years of study and hard work. But remember, it is the mental effort that benefits the brain, so the work will pay off not only in much musical joy but also in building mental might.

Learning and singing songs will benefit the brain because the voice is a musical instrument. Songs have an advantage because usually you can learn lyrics more easily than a poem or script because of the cues in the melody and the repetitions.

Dancing: Ballroom has a good track record for building mental might. In a ballroom you need coordination, rhythm, recall of the dance's style, spirit, and steps, and at the same time, you are socializing with a partner and a group. Start easy with Foxtrot and then work up to Waltz. With Foxtrot and Waltz you will be able to do 90% of the dances played on cruise ships or at your local adult venues. Once or twice a week for an hour or so should be sufficient. Starting lessons can be painful (especially to your adult ego), but if you stick to it, the results are worthwhile. Some people go for tap dancing and jazz. The benefits are enormous in terms of coordination and grace. Most adult tap groups do shows for retirement homes, senior centers, nursing homes, daycare centers, Japanese tourists, and so forth. Performing in front of a group can be a mental stress at first, just like every other new brain task, but with persistence, the rewards are enormous.

Our local tap group (the Silver Stars of Pasadena, Texas) ranged in age from 63 to 95, with an average age of 78. The group has a repertoire of over 40 dances. Each dance has about 12 different steps. Each step is divided into multiple little steps and maneuvers. You get the idea: tap is a fine physical workout and a fine brainwork out. Hooray for tap dancing!

In addition to memorizing all the choreography notes, the group has memorized what costume goes with what dance, where the cane goes and where the hat goes, when, and how, and so forth. The mental horsepower needed for effective tapping is tremendous, as tap dancing is an art form so deep no one will ever completely master it. Tap dancing is also a musical form where the rhythmic percussive notes are struck by the taps on the floor. Therefore, every real tap dancer is also a percussion musician. The benefits of playing a musical instrument, therefore, apply, at least in part, to tap dancing.

By the way, dancing and playing a musical instrument have lots in common. They both involve physical exercise and

- Rhythm is involved
- Memory is involved
- Coordination is involved
- Many brain areas are involved at the same time
- Social skills are involved

- Listening and following the music, melody, and lyrics may be involved
- Mental Math: A neglected area that should be studied more. When you do mental math, you will actually feel your brain straining, so you know math is good for the brain. A chapter on mental math is included in this book. Besides the brain workout, mental math has practical applications. When the computers are out at your local gas station, and the woman at the desk can't make change, you can do it for her fast, easily, and accurately. Often using a calculator gives the wrong answer, as the following example illustrates.

When my best friend died, Helen, his widow, asked me to go with her to make the funeral arrangements. While the funeral director added up the cost on his calculator, I did the additions in my head. Chapter 6 will show how you can do this. The funeral director was off by $1,735 because he punched in the same number twice. Was he cheating? Or was this an honest mistake? We'll never know. Cheating or mistake, still it pays to be on your toes.

OK—full disclosure: You can also use the mental math tricks to show off. They are especially effective in impressing grandchildren. Show-off mental math is also featured in chapter six. But my work at the funeral home was to help Helen and was not showing off. It was checking the calculated results to make sure they were correct. When I corrected the director, he looked at me as if I had grown two heads, one red and one blue. Helen assured him that "he can do that, and you are probably off." Sure enough, the redo showed the mental math was correct, and the director by hook or by crook had punched the same number twice.

Recitation: As people get older, their vocabulary usually increases, but their verbal fluency declines. We can't see you right now, but if you are over 65, we will bet that you are smiling because you know what we mean. If your speech has become hesitant and if you experience blocks or other fluency problems, despair not. Reciting poetry aloud will often solve the problem. Oral recitation activates massive amounts of brain tissue in both cerebral hemispheres and in the cerebellum and spinal cord, a fact proven by the scans done during that activity. To recite, you have to activate the speech area, the speech planning area, monitor what you say, impress emotion and prosody on what you say, and so forth. Just for grins, let's list a few brain areas, shown by the MRI scans, that you will use when you recite aloud:

- Broca's area—the motor speech area in the front part of the left side of the brain
- Wernicke's area—the reception speech area in the back part of the left side of the brain
- Motor cortex—both areas on the right side and left side of the brain in the central region of the cortex
- Premotor cortex—both areas on the right side and left side of the brain in front of the motor cortex
- Parietal lobe—both areas on the right side and left side of the brain in back of the motor cortex
- Monitoring and encoding centers for emotion in right hemisphere and limbic system

- Basal Ganglia—the large collections of neurons at the base and inside of the brain that play a major role in controlling muscle function
- Cerebellum—the massive part of the brain in the back region which helps control, organize, and memorize motor sequences
- Recitation in front of an audience, or a mirror, or a video camera will also use multiple body parts, including:
- Brain
- Lips
- Tongue
- Pharynx
- Larynx
- Respiratory system and associated muscles
- Hands and body

Expected Benefits from Periodic Recitation Aloud:

- Greater oral presentation skills—includes more fluent speech, larger vocabulary, greater intellectual range, and a greater emotional range.
- A decreased chance of getting Alzheimer's disease or other forms of dementia
- A remarkably improved memory for verbal and visual items
- A greater awareness of the multiple realities of life on this planet and their complexities, especially if you recite poetry and prose that has literary merit.

Mental Gymnastic

Memorize and recite verbatim the immortal poem by John Donne, *No Man is an Island*. Review it and repeat it until you get it right. Keep a record of how long it took to get it into your memory. It will take much longer than you think. Do small bits at a time and keep track of when you start practice and when you end practice so that in the end, you will know the total time spent on this memory project. This time will be your baseline time. Chances are, you will notice after you have learned the memory tricks in this book that the time needed to memorize anything will have decreased significantly. Memorize in less time with fewer tears: That's the ticket.

During your practice of the *No Man* poem, simulate playback conditions as much as possible. As for me, I usually close my funereal orations with this poem. Therefore, for me, the playback of this poem is a funeral where I have been asked to say something about the dearly departed. Dearly Departed—Sounds like they went on vacation or something. As you get older, the funeral scene gets more frequent. Be prepared. The effect is magnificent, with lots of watery eyes in the audience.

When you think you have the poem memorized by heart, perform it in front of a mirror or, better still, in front of a video camera. Record and review your performance. Use the analysis to improve your style, tone, pace, body language, posture, and verbal fluency.

No cheating! Everything should be in your head and nothing on paper. Remember, the result is not as important as the mental effort to get to the result. Mental effort is what builds brainpower. The result reflects it merely.

Summary of Chapter One:

Overwhelming evidence that is relevant and adequate proves that directed mental effort can favorably modify the structure and function of the human brain. This idea is called the principle of neuroplasticity, an important term which recently has been surfacing in newspapers, magazines, and on National Public Radio. Why not memorize the definition now so when the word shows up again, you know what idea is in reference, and you can look super smart during the next dinner conversation?

Definition: A Neuroplastic Is a Nervous Tissue That Can Modify Itself to Suit The Needs It Is Called upon to Fill

In most cases, the neuroplasticity is modality-specific such that the brain is modified to produce a specific effect. Therefore, it is not enough to decide you want a better brain. You have to decide what you want a better brain for; that is what you want your brain to do better for you. For instance, you just can't wake up in the morning and decide you want a better memory. That is a wonderful wish, but it is too general and non-specific to be of much practical use to you or to your brain.

You have to decide you want a better memory for a reason, usually a specific purpose. Perhaps you want to remember better to recite poetry, or play *Rhapsody in Blue* from memory on the piano, or remember the name of everyone you meet, or all the special features of the automobiles you are trying to sell or all the trading symbols on the New York Stock Exchange so you can easily read the tape and so forth. Or maybe you wish to learn French or Latin or Hebrew or nuclear physics. What's your bag?

MENTAL MAKING MIGHT

The Brain Is a Focused Instrument of Learning

Once you decide what you want your brain to do for you, then you work out a program to train your brain to do it. The reason you need to focus is that the brain itself is a focused instrument of learning. Studying auto mechanics is unlikely to help you learn touch-typing. But thinking and working on touch typing will do the trick. Working on Chinese will not help you much when you want to speak French. But taking a course in French will be of benefit. Studying chapter ten in the physics textbook will not help much if tomorrow's test is on chapter nine. Get it? Get specific, and you may get somewhere. Remain abstract and nonspecific, and the chance of significant progress goes way down.

The next chapter will give you some ideas about building a better memory for all sorts of tasks. Most people complain of lack of memory. But none (you will note) complain of lack of judgment. Mark Twain said people complain about the weather, but no one does anything about it. Bruno Fürst, one of the greatest mnemonists of all time, said many people complain about their memory, but few do anything about it.

About training judgment, little is known. About training memory, a great deal is known, as you will see in the next chapter.

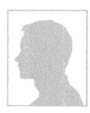

CHAPTER TWO

MEMORIES ARE MADE OF THIS

CHAPTER TWO: MEMORIES ARE MADE OF THIS

◆ ◆ ◆

Main point of this chapter: Human memory is a complex brain function that is modality-, time-, brain state-, emotion-, and lesion localization- dependent. An understanding of the nature of human memory and how it functions will help you develop techniques and strategies that improve memory performance and mental might.

Before we get to the real memory stuff, let's pause for a brief discussion of what is not real about memory augmentation techniques, especially the memory augmentation techniques that are touted by charlatans.

Introduction to the Desert of the Real

Get straight on a few things:

First: Stick to the desert of the real. When it comes to memory, forgetting is the default mode. It is normal to forget almost everything and anything.

So, if you can't recall much about what you have read so far in this book, don't worry. Chances are your memory is normal. If you can't recall what you ate for breakfast yesterday, don't fret. Chances are your memory is normal. If you forgot to pay the electric bill, chances are your memory is normal. But you had better pay it before they turn off the lights.

The Human Brain Is Made to Forget

The reason that forgetting is the default mode of the human brain is to prevent our conscious lives from being cluttered with unimportant stuff. We need to remember the important things and forget what isn't important. Otherwise, our memories would be intolerably cluttered. The Irish have a proverb that relates to this idea. But I forget what it is. I am trying to remember the proverb, but no dice. Perhaps if I make a mental picture of my Irish grandmother telling the proverb, it will come to mind. Nope—that didn't work. Forgetting things like that is annoying, but that happens to me rather often, and I would bet that it happens to you. Forgetting is normal. Remembering takes effort and repetition and sometimes plain bloody work.

The best approach is not to worry much about what you can't recall. Chances are, the item is in your memory bank somewhere. I know the Irish proverb is there somewhere. The usual problem is a problem of recalling the item to consciousness. Think about something else, and your unconscious mind will work on the problem. After some time, the answer may pop into your head, or the answer may be with you in bed when you wake up. The reason for this is our memory, like all other functions of consciousness, is not entirely inactive during sleep; it works on and on, in a more restrictive mode, replaying (in part) the electrical equivalent of sensory experiences in order to register them more deeply in the mind or to sort out the important from the unimportant.

Sleep helps consolidate procedural memory (memory for doing tasks like making coffee or tying shoes, or playing Beethoven's *Moonlight Sonata*). Recent studies confirm that a good night's sleep is essential for you to learn to perform any motor task. The exact mechanisms by which sleep helps memory need to be worked out in detail. Most sleep researchers believe sleep benefits memory by enabling the brain to replay information encountered earlier. The evidence comes (again) from imaging research where physicians studied brain activity during memory acquisition and during a subsequent sleep phase. Neural pathways that were activated during the learning period were reactivated during sleep. This dream activity is memory consolidation at work. The reactivation strengthens the neural pathways that hold the new information. Furthermore, sleep decreases stress hormones known to damage the hippocampus, where many memories are processed. Shakespeare was right: Sleep knits up the raveled sleave of care, sore labor's bath, balm of hurt minds.

Tip of the Tongue

Later, we will discuss specific techniques and tricks to recall information you know is in your head or that you feel is on the tip of your tongue. The suggested techniques were discussed by Aristotle himself in his famous book entitled On Memory. The great thing about these tricks is they work! When and if you have finished this book, it is likely your friends will ask how the devil you got such a good memory, giving you an excellent opportunity to improve Doctor Patten's economic status by your wholeheartedly endorsing *Making Mental Might*.

Memory Training Is Work

Face up to the fact that there is no easy street to a good memory.

Training your memory is going to be work. To develop a good memory, some people will have to work hard; some will have to work not so hard. But all will have to work.

Rest assured, however, that great abilities are not required to become a memory genius. All you need are a few facts (soon to be supplied), some imagination (suggestions to follow), and practice, practice, practice. Penetration, accuracy, attention, and focus on the details will fit you for the task if you can give the task the application that is necessary.

Positive Mental Attitude Is a Positive

Studies have repeatedly shown that if you think that you can memorize something (a music piece, a poem, a formula to calculate the behavior of the hydrogen atom, the Kepler orbital equations—anything and everything), the probability you will memorize that piece of music or poem or concept in astrophysics, and so forth, goes way up. Conversely, if you think you can't memorize a poem or the formula or something, the chance of your mastering those things is far less, probably close to zero. This little poem summarizes this idea:

If you think you can, you can

If you think you can't, you're right again

For whatever you think you can or can't

That's what you can or can't

If you haven't already, you may wish to discover the story of *The Little Engine That Could.* It is a classic tale of kindness and determination that has inspired millions of children around the world. "I think I can, I think I can…" And because she thought she could, she did pull the train full of wonderful things over the mountain to deliver to the children on the other side.

Failures Now Do Not Mean Failures Always

Let's say you have two or three times failed to recollect a particular passage of *Evangeline.* Do not assume and do not imagine you will forget it on the next occasion you try to say it. A person who says to himself: "I know perfectly well I shall break down in the usual place; it's no use, I simply can't remember it" is doomed to forget, for this form of auto-suggestion is likely to be fatal. Conclusion: Don't say anything bad about yourself or your abilities because you might believe it. In general, don't say anything bad about yourself to other people because they might believe it.

Lesson: To imagine you can't do a thing is to very often render yourself incapable of doing it.

Moreover, it is of no service to a person (or to anyone else) to will himself to remember something he has assured himself he cannot remember. Thus, when the imagination is in conflict with the will, the imagination will usually win. We are not saying the will doesn't exist or that it is totally disabled. We are saying that under these self-imposed restrictions, the will to remember will function feebly or arbitrarily or not at all. There is a long and complicated factual explanation for this failing, but let us illustrate the principle in action:

Any normal person can, without much difficulty, walk along a twelve-inch wide plank placed on the ground. No particular balancing powers are required for such a feat. But if the same plank were projected over the edge of a cliff, not one person in twenty could walk it. Why? In the last case, the person fearing he may fall imagines he will do so—tells himself that he will and then believes what his imagination has told him. Some of this imagining may be unconscious, but it is there and playing a role influencing performance. From that moment, the actual power to walk the plank will significantly degrade so much so that he may indeed obey the compulsion of the imagination and actually fall.

Believe in Yourself

Bottom line: It is evident that in training the memory, one must at the same time cultivate the confidence in one's own powers. Without self-confidence, very little can be accomplished in any sphere of endeavor. You can do anything within reason. Your music memory is much better than you think. Your verbal memory is much better than you think. Your visual memory is much, much better than you think. Your motor memory is superb. Doctor Benjamin Spock reassured new parents with the unforgettable introduction in his famous book on childcare: "TRUST YOURSELF." That is exactly what we want to convey about your mental might and memory adventures. TRUST YOURSELF! You can do it!

Human Memory Has No Limits

Neurologists know there is no practical limit to the powers of human memory in general and visual and motor memory in particular. Many of our great pianists have a repertoire of two or three hundred pieces, included among which are four or five concertos, say, a dozen sonatas, several works of the dimensions of Schumann's *Faschingsschwank aus Wien*, two or three of Liszt's *Hungarian Rhapsodies*, and perhaps 60 or 70 compositions, each of which takes eight or ten minutes to perform. These humans acquire this enormous repertoire without any particular strain, and though, of course, some of them are specially gifted, there is no reason why the average musician who takes his work seriously should not at least memorize fifty works. No kidding. The human brain is that good when properly instructed and motivated.

Question: Who do you think needs to do the instructing and motivating?

Answer: You! No one else will do.

Personal Sidebar by Doctor Patten

Seventy-five years ago, I set out to memorize poems. One a week or once every two weeks was my goal. Each night while taking my nightly bath, I spent 30 minutes going over the poem of the week. Now I can recite verbatim over 500 poems. Don't get me started. It sounds almost impossible, but after a time, committing to memory became second nature. The more you memorize, the easier it will become to memorize. Have faith in your own ability. Trust your memory, and it will trust you. Rewards will follow. Success is a great reward, and your personal rewards will feed your personal success.

American Memory Competitions

In the memory competitions held in New York City (March 2008), contestants memorized 99 faces and the associated names in 15 minutes. They memorized thirty 25-digit numbers in 15 minutes and the order of a pack of 52 cards in just five minutes. These people are not freaks, geeks, or geniuses. They have, however, devoted attention to training their brains, their memories, and their attention spans, and so could you. Whether or not you should is entirely up to you. Life is full of choices. You have to decide what you want and what you want to do. Are you going to embrace this opportunity for growth? Why or why not?

Walter Hilse, a conductor friend, has pretty much memorized multiple operas and symphonies. He has the score before him, that's true, but it is there chiefly to give confidence rather than reference. Walter occasionally eyes the score, not so much to read it as to assure himself that his memory is not about to betray him. Only those of you who have examined a full orchestral score can form an adequate notion of the high degree of mental training required to memorize it and fifty more like it.

The Gift of Memory is Nothing Special

This gift of memorizing—especially when it is as highly developed as it is in our great conductors, pianists, singers, orators, actors, and memory athletes may seem a rare and special thing. Rest assured: It is not! Memory is one of the lowest functions of the human brain. Even idiots have it. Even earthworms have it! Your cat and your dog have it. Our ancient ancestors needed it to find the berries and to recall where the hunting grounds were. Without memory and its continued improvement, our species would not have survived, and you, dear reader, would not be here.

But, You May Say, What If I Really Do Have a Poor Memory?

If you have trouble memorizing a Chopin waltz, don't assume you have a poor memory. An untrained memory—yes! If you can't memorize that Robert Frost poem about apple picking, don't assume you have a poor memory. An untrained memory—yes! If you don't recall the chemical name of MPTP, the neurotoxin that causes Parkinson's Disease (1-Methyl-4-phenyl-1,2,4,5-tetrahydropyridine), don't assume you have a poor memory. An untrained memory—yes!

Your ability to memorize is not likely to be below average, and the capacity of the average memory is astonishingly high. But, alas, real achievement in memory depends on training, training that can be hard work. Yes, work is involved, but not that much considering the results. The basic trick that memory experts use is to have an organized and associating framework on which to peg the information to be memorized. Structure and pattern recognition—that's the ticket. And, of course, repetition and review. The more you know, the more you can know by attaching new information onto the old.

Example: Mister Green's address is 365 52 Street, Manhattan.

Mentally organizing the information into more easily remembered patterns or chunks, we get Green things grow year-round (365 days) and a year has 52 weeks. Thus, Green's address is 365 52 Street. Now try to forget Green's address. You can't.

Considered Organization of Material Is Key

Even the best memory expert and most expert musician cannot memorize a page of random notes. No sir! They, like you, need an organizing framework, a logical development of faculties, and the right appreciation of memory techniques, including pattern recognition, graphs, pictures, hooks, pegs, clues, cues, scripts, schemata, stories—all of which will quickly bring about astonishing results as you will soon see as you work through this project.

Mental Gymnastic

Recite in random order the 52 cards of a deck. Do not omit a card, and don't count the same card twice. This is hard—in fact, almost impossible to do in a **random** manner. But now do the same thing by organizing your recital. Name the four suits, clubs, hearts, spades, diamonds. Name all the cards, Ace to 10 in each suit. Then name the picture cards—four Jacks, four Queens, and four Kings. Presto! By organizing the task, you can easily recite all the cards in a deck without hesitation or duplication. If you did this exercise, you proved to yourself how important organization and pattern recognition is to looking like a memory genius. An impossible task became possible.

As you work on memorizing easy memory, things will get easier, and memorizing hard memory things will get easier. Don't believe? Read on. And, more importantly, try it.

What Does Not Work

Ginkgo biloba doesn't work, so the $90.2 million spent on it yearly in The United States benefits only the companies that make it and those people who sell it. Quote the Raven: "Ginkgo biloba is good for my potency, and I forgot what else." (The Billy Christal joke here is Ginkgo biloba is advertised to and is supposed to augment memory.

Supplements and Vitamins = Useless

In general, tons of vitamins, salts, special herbs, and so forth are of no avail. Forget the bullshit. Stick to the real. Some memory books written by physicians who should know better still recommend daily vitamin E even though scientific studies have proven vitamin E not only useless but even harmful because it causes heart problems, including congestive heart failure. Vitamin E has also caused dangerous bleeding in people taking large doses. So, stay away from vitamin E.

Furthermore, any product that you put on your head or rub into your scalp to increase memory will not work. Consider this advertisement from Shaper Image:

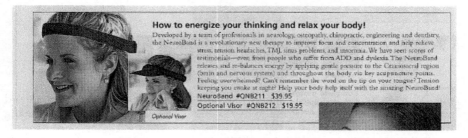

Fig2.1

Mental Gymnastic to Heighten Attentiveness and Concentration

Careful observation and concentration are the foundations of a good memory. Unpack and take apart this advertisement in detail and prove that it cannot possibly be true. After you have studied the advertisement, answer the following questions:

1. How likely is it that neurologists would have anything to do with chiropractic, much less collaborate with chiropractors to develop a neuroband?
2. How in the world can neuroband apply pressure to both the cranial and sacral regions at the same time to the same person?
3. What is the real purpose of neuroband?

Answers:

1. Unlikely
2. It can't as the two regions, cranial and sacral, are far apart.
3. To get your money.

MENTAL MAKING MIGHT

Introduction to the Science of Learning

Long ago in Paris during the spring of a year, a young German (or was he Austrian?)—no matter—was standing at one of those bookstalls by the Seine, the river that runs through that fair city.

There and then, he picked up a book, the name of which is not recorded in his autobiography, and he read something. What he read is also lost to history. But at that moment, that man had a sudden flash of inspiration—an idea that changed the course of human history, an insight that has significantly changed many lives for the better and that we hope will soon change your life for the better.

A Brief History of The Dawn of the Scientific Study of Human Memory

The idea was to study human memory scientifically. Yes! Scientifically!

And to a scientist of that era (especially a German or Austrian scientist), the word "scientifically" meant quantitatively. By quantitatively, that man meant reducing memory to numbers by essentially measuring what was memorized and measuring what was forgotten, and (more importantly) measuring when, why, and how it was forgotten. "Measurement began our might," said the Irish poet William Butler Yeats. And he was right. All scientists believe if you can't measure something, you can't study it all that well. Numbers and direct measurements—very important in giving us insight into the nature of nature, the nature of reality. Business people know if you can't measure something, you can't manage it. The government understands this principle, and that it why it often issues figures about employment, unemployment, inflation, pandemic deaths, and so forth.

Ebbinghaus, the Father of Modern Scientific Memory Research

The man at the Paris bookstall was Hermann Ebbinghaus (1850–1909), a doctor of Philosophy and a genius. Hermann promptly returned home from Paris, kissed his wife, and then locked himself in his upstairs study to work on the complexities of human memory.

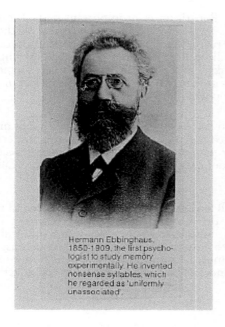

Hermann Ebbinghaus, 1850-1909, the first psychologist to study memory experimentally. He invented nonsense syllables, which he regarded as 'uniformly unassociated'.

Hermann Ebbinghaus, the first psychologist to study memory experimentally. He invented nonsense syllables, which he regarded as uniformly unassociated. Most textbooks will tell you he got his idea of studying memory quantitatively from reading Gustav Fechner's book *Elements of Psychophysics*, and that was the book he found at the Paris bookstall. But if that were true, why did Hermann not mention that in his autobiography?

Fig2.2 - Herman Ebbinghaus

Hermann Ebbinghaus' Experiments

Using himself as the one and only subject for his experiments, Hermann Ebbinghaus devised 2,300 three-letter nonsense syllables for measuring memory. In a typical experiment, he would pick the nonsense syllables at random from a hat, review a list of 16 of these until he could recall them perfectly in two faultless executions aloud, and then retest himself at various time intervals recording the results. All in all, he had 420 lists, and each took about 45 minutes to memorize. He estimated he did at least 14,000 repetitions. While the time spent memorizing the lists and the number of repetitions were closely correlated, Hermann found the number of repetitions done was more important than the time spent. There are important physiologic reasons why this is true, reasons we now know to be true, reasons that do not concern us here. In fact, the Nobel prize in Medicine was awarded for the discovery of the brain mechanisms that underlie repetition as the major mechanism of learning. Just remember this: Neurons that fire together, wire together. And then, it follows as the night the day, neurons that are wired together will fire together. Key ideas like these are often more easily memorized as verse:

Neurons that fire together

Wire together

Neurons that wire together

Fire together

The lesson is clear: Repetition counts. Repetition is an important part of learning and memory. Without repetition, very little learning takes place. Without repetition, very little learning can take place. We repeat: Repetition is important. I repeat: Without repetition, there will be little learning. One-step learning is possible but usually for only simple tasks. Large projects and important memory tasks require repetition. Was there ever anyone who could memorize *Casey at the Bat*, all 52 lines, without repeating the poem many times?

Repetition causes neuronal networks to fire together and wire together, and once they do, they tend to be more easily fired together, the very process that underlies human memory. When you start your memory work in earnest, you will recognize how repetition starts to make recall easier and easier until, at last, recall is automatic.

Repetition is so important that you will find that things are often repeated in this book. No harm in that, and actually, the repeats will help you remember. But hear this! Stupid parrotlike repetition, especially when you are not mindful of what you are repeating, does away with concentration. Our repetitions must be patterned and organized. Repetitions must be mindful and focused. Rote memory = bad. Repeat out loud: Rote memory is bad. All repetition, to be effective, must be mindful.

Repetition Has a Dark Side

As we learned, when you repeat something over and over, the nerve cells in the brain form new connections. This is how you learn things and how you form new habits. The more you repeat something, the stronger the connections between the nerve cell networks. But there is a problem. You may have noticed that once you have developed a habit, it is really difficult to change it. That is because the connections in the brain that form the habit have been formed by lots of repetitions over time. To unlearn a habit or to replace it with a new one, you have to repeat the new habit many, many times so that the brain changes the old connections and forms new ones. In piano practice, for instance, if we repeat the passage many times incorrectly, the brain will actually learn the incorrect form of the music, and there will be a devil of a time correcting the mistakes and getting the piece played right. The key point here is that in repetition of anything with a view to remembering, make sure that you are repeating as carefully as possible, avoiding any and all errors. This applies to memorizing music, songs, poems, history, math, or anything. The important part of repetition is to repeat correctly and not repeat incorrectly. Each time you do a correct repetition, you are writing a protected spot in your brain. Each time you do an incorrect repetition, you are also writing a protected spot in your brain, a spot that will be difficult to erase or change without lots of work. Practicing errors will not give you the results you want or need. Therefore: Always practice right! And never practice wrong!

OK, Hermann Locked Himself in His Room and Repeated Nonsense Words—So What?

So what?

No way, so what. You should be thinking: Wow!

Think about it! Locking yourself in your study for three periods each day 10–11 AM, 11–12 AM, and 6–8 PM for over four years and memorizing masses of meaningless lists. That's dedication, dedication to science. And mind you, all this must have been tedious and boring. Tenaciousness is considered by some as a particularly Teutonic trait. If that were true, then Hermann's work would be a great example. He carried on, despite the fact that his work must have been boring.

Must have been boring?

YeeeAhhh!

What are we talking about? It was boring. Hermann says so in his famous book published at Leipzig in 1885, Über das Gedächtnis (Memory, A Contribution to Experimental Psychology).

Hermann, in confidential moments, admits his brain loses its "freshness" after 20 minutes and becomes bored. When each test required longer periods of concentration, say—¾ of an hour, he admits, "and toward the end of this time exhaustion, headache, and other symptoms were often felt which have complicated the conditions of the test."

One wonders how many headaches were generated to learn that lesson.

What lesson?

Lesson: The human brain fatigues quickly. The human brain quickly loses its focus, becomes bored, and begins to shut down. If you are tired or bored or sick, forget about memory work until you ready and eager.

At-TEN-shun!

Failing to focus is one of the biggest things that interfere with memory. You can't remember something to which you didn't pay attention. Think about that. It could be the reason you are not doing so well in piano lessons or in science class or in everything else that you are not doing well. You are mentally absent instead of mindfully present. What's the treatment for that?

Answer: Pay attention! Also, take frequent breaks to refresh your brain. A break every 15 minutes is good. During the break, focus away from what you are doing on to something different so as to refresh your brain. How about now? Let's focus away from this memory stuff and do problem four in the problem chapter. It's a math problem about horse racing taken from Lewis Carroll, the author of *Alice's Adventures in Wonderland*.

Pause now to consider the horse-racing odds and how to always win no matter what horse comes in first. When you have worked the problem or tried and failed to work it, come back here to resume the discussion of human memory mechanisms.

Get It or You Will Forget It

You have to get it. Or you'll forget it. But this idea begs the question. The more important question is—How do we get it? That's the key question: How do we train ourselves to pay enough attention in the first place to get the items we want to remember into our memories?

Lesson: Boredom prevents and often kills memory.

The best bet is **AVOID BOREDOM:** Do a small amount of mental work at a time, take frequent breaks, and vary the subject matter. Work on things that are fun and that interest you—about those techniques, more later. Meanwhile, let's talk about what our hero Hermann accomplished despite the boredom, and despite the headaches he endured.

Despite the headaches, the dull, dreary, mind-numbing humdrum, Hermann persisted. He exercised willpower, something we all can use to our advantage in our mental exercises.

After he got an individual list memorized (as was mentioned), he retested himself at timed intervals, recorded what he recalled, and recorded what he did not recall. Along the way, he proved human memory is a complex process that is time-, modality-, emotion-, and state-dependent. Some, not much, of the complexity will be covered later in this book. But it might be useful for you at this time to memorize the definition. Memorize it either as a statement:

Memory is a complex brain function that is time-, modality-, emotion-, brain-state-, and brain-lesion-localization-dependent.

Or memorize the definition by its divisions:

Memory is a complex brain function that is dependent on:

1. **Time**
2. **Modality**
3. **Emotion**
4. **Brain state**
5. **Brain lesion location**

Each of these items is important and will be explained, except for the brain lesion thing. That is the realm of neurology. Neurologists know there are special sections of the brain, which, when injured, prevent verbal memory. Other sections, when injured, prevent visual memory. And, yes, there are sections for particular types of memory, such as memory for a fire alarm or a ringing phone. Those patients understand speech and can talk quite well, but they are blind to the meaning of the non-verbal sounds like a bird call or mountain lion roar. There are people who have sections of their brain injured who can speak and understand words but can't repeat anything you say to them (known to neurologists as a disconnection syndrome conduction aphasia wherein the speech detection system is disconnected from the speech production system due to a lesion in a deep white matter tract in the left hemisphere known as the arcuate fasciculus). There are patients who can write their name or anything you dictate but can't read what they just wrote. That syndrome is known in the business as dyslexia without agraphia and is due to a lesion in the posterior corpus callosum and the right visual cortex. Fascinating right? But not important for you at this time.

What is important is knowing how time, modality, emotion, and brain state affect memory. Knowing how those items work and what role they play in memory will help you get through any memory task.

The Famous Forgetting Curve

Despite the complexity, our man Hermann proved memory, under certain experimental conditions, can be measured almost exactly. His most important discovery, and the one for which he is very well known in psychological circles, was the "forgetting curve" that relates the amount of forgetting to the passage of time.

Yes, time! Time is the real enemy of mankind, and time is the real enemy of memory because human memory degrades with the passage of time. The forgetting curve proved that fact now and forever. As time goes by, you remember less and less. Is there any doubt about the adverse effect of the passage of time on memory?

Human Forgetting Is Both Active and Passive

In fact, recent neuroscience research proves that forgetting is not entirely just a passive process. The brain actually uses physiological mechanisms to erase memories, and with the passage of time, this erasure will be permanent. Review of the memory before the complete erasure will freshen the memory and promote recall. Lack of review with the passage of time may actually erase the memory entirely. There are many memorized piano pieces uploaded onto YouTube ten years ago that are fully and completely forgotten. It would take about the same amount of time and effort to get those pieces back in the memory. On the other hand, pieces uploaded last year or two years ago can be (and have been) relearned in record time without much difficulty. Therefore, recently memorized material is more easily recalled than remotely memorized material. You already knew that. Right? This is called the recency effect. A short review before you are actually tested will work wonders, especially on multiple-choice or short-answer tests.

Lesson: Review time is never wasted. Review what you want to remember and forget the rest.

Back to Hermann and the forgetting curve:

The forgetting curve remains one of the eternal verities about human memory performance. There are other eternal verities about Human Memory, which we will cover, but that one, the forgetting curve, is among the most important. Never ever forget the forgetting curve. Another way of saying the same thing: Always remember the forgetting curve.

Not incidentally, there is also a learning curve. It is exponential, just like the forgetting curve, with the sharpest increase in learning occurring on the first day. After that, the learning curve levels out much like the forgetting curve.

Time-Dependent Processes in Human Memory:

There are two important time-dependent phenomena in human memory that Hermann studied quantitatively:

A. Forgetting, and

B. Encoding

Let's look at these items one at a time. Forgetting first.

A. Forgetting Is the Default Mode of Human Memory

In a certain sense, the news about the forgetting curve ain't good: The default mode in human memory, as mentioned, is to forget and to forget quickly.

In the list of 16 nonsense words (like WUX, CAZ, ZOL, BAZ, etc.), for instance, which Hermann had memorized perfectly, only eight could be correctly recalled one hour later, and only five could be recalled after two days. Thus, overly learned material that had been recalled perfectly twice had slipped out of the memory at the rate of about one percent per minute for the first hour. After two days, the rate of loss tends to settle down until a relatively constant level of retained information is reached two weeks later. Hence, if you can recall only a fraction of what you have read in the introduction to this book or a fraction of what happened to you two hours ago, don't fret or worry; your memory performance is quite normal. If you have played a piano piece perfectly twice from memory, say *Für Elise* by Beethoven, don't be surprised if you forgot half of it the next day. And don't be hard on yourself if, without review, two weeks later, you forgot 70% of it. That's the norm: 30% correct recall after two weeks and 70% forgotten. Expect the same thing if you recited from memory Lincoln's *Gettysburg Address* perfectly twice. You will forget almost half of it the next day, and one week later, you will recall less than 30 or 40%. However, despair not: a brief review will work wonders in bringing back the previously learned material if you have learned it well and were able to reproduce it perfectly at least two times. With each review session, the time to relearn the material will shorten. If you don't believe me, try learning the *Gettysburg Address* and retest yourself at intervals.

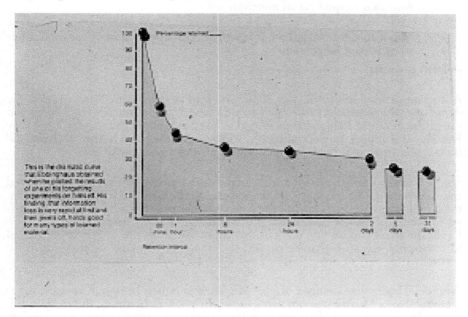

Fig2.3 - The forgetting curve for unassociated perfectly learned three-letter items. Note the dramatic drop in retained material after just one hour. Within 24 hours, over 60% is lost forever.

But what's the deal? How come we forget so easily? How come we have to work to remember?

Here's the answer:

We Need to Forget Almost Everything

There are important reasons that our brains are biased to forget: Most of the stuff we come into contact with in our everyday lives just ain't that useful or important or that memorable. Just think of what a nightmare life would be if you remembered every little detail of every little thing that happened every little moment.

Whoa! Now that I have been thinking about forgetting, I now remember the Irish proverb. That is a good illustration of how our minds work. One item tends to help recall others. Once two items are associated in the consciousness, each tends to recall the other. In this case, all that thinking about forgetting and remembering helped me recall the Irish proverb about remembering:

> **To remember everything is a form of madness.**
—**Irish proverb**

> **And that helped recall another:**

> **May you never forget what is worth remembering nor ever remember what is best forgotten.**
—**Irish proverb**

A Russian psychologist, A.R. Luria, discussed (in an interesting book entitled *The Mind of a Mnemonist: A Little Book about a Vast Memory*) the case of S. who had the problem of not being able to forget. S. has a real name that is very long, very Russian, and almost unpronounceable, so S. is usually known to the psychological literature simply as S. because (guess what) his name starts with S.

Yes, S. had trouble forgetting, and in many cases, he couldn't forget. He suffered the disadvantage of having a mind perpetually bombarded by past memories, most of which were irrelevant to the present situations that S. wanted to or needed to work on. What S. needed and wanted in a most desperate way was to forget the trivia and only remember the important stuff, the stuff that he wanted to remember, the stuff that he needed to remember to make a difference in his everyday life.

We, too. That's what we need. Right? We want to remember what we want to remember, like a Mozart piece or *Für Elise* or the spouse's birthday, the electric bill, and so forth, and we don't want to remember what we don't want to remember. We want to remember the French word for cat if we want to buy a cat in France or say the word correctly in French class tomorrow.

Goal #1: Forget Trivia; Remember the Important Stuff

That begs the question. What is important? The answer is what is important is what is personally important to you. What interests you, and what you want to remember. No one can tell you what is important. You have to decide for yourself. Your brain usually doesn't know what is important. You have to tell it. The brain assumes something you do often or think about often is probably important, and that is why repetition and habit fix memories.

Remember What is Important

It's nice to remember the important stuff like your spouse's birthday or when the mortgage needs to be paid or when the garbage gets picked up, to bring the math homework back to school, where you parked the car at the airport, that the door is locked, stove off, and so forth. A good memory can come in handy in many ways.

The trick is to remember the things that are important and forget what is not important. The techniques discussed in the pages coming up will allow you to do both (remember and forget) and give you control over your memory that you (perhaps) never thought possible.

Not Discussed—Psychological Amnesias

What will not be discussed is the form of active forgetting psychiatrists see in people suffering from neurosis. In that form of illness, unwanted material is actively and unconsciously suppressed from the consciousness because the material tends to cause an unpleasant mental state called anxiety. The official psychiatric term for this kind of active exclusion of memories from the consciousness is repression. Repression is an exaggerated form of the normal tendency—but not an invariable tendency—for human nature to forget what is painful. We do so for sake of peace of mind. Instinctively, we struggle for happiness, and in that struggle, we dismiss from our minds much that is hurtful. Repressed memories do tend to surface in dreams, during psychotherapy, and under the influence of drugs, particularly alcohol. Repressed memories usually have no direct application to general memory tasks and therefore do not enter further into the scope of this book.

Repression is not always bad. Soldiers who refuse to recall battle experiences or to discuss them often have better mental health and fewer post-traumatic stress disorders. All of us will die sooner or later. If we went around thinking all the time about our ultimate doom, life would be quite unpleasant. Instead, most of us just forget the obvious bad news and carry on.

"What's too painful to remember, we simply choose to forget," sings Barbara Streisand. And she's right.

Ugh! Thinking about Barbara reminded me of a professor of psychiatry at Columbia who looked like Barbara. And that memory made me recall that repression might have a direct application in memorizing certain things. So let's take it a step farther:

Repression May Cause Loss of Memory

In the realm of music, for instance, failures of memory are due to the same causes as they are in the circumstances of everyday life. Most pianists, even of little experience, know what it is to interpret and perform a piece of music with the score, not before the eyes, and break down time after time at precisely the same place. There are various reasons for this failure (which will be discussed), but one reason is not that the music has suddenly become more difficult, but because their memory in that particular passage has failed them due to active repression. In the mind of the player, this particular passage of music may have associations with something that has been repressed and forgotten. The pianist is unconscious of the associations; nevertheless, because they exist, the pianist is prone to repress the music around which these associations cluster.

Sidebar by Doctor Patten

With me, I have great difficulty playing or memorizing even simple pieces composed by the Russian composer Dmitri Shostakovich. I believe this difficulty is due to the associations that come forth when I see his name or read his notes. These negative associations derive from the rather negative impressions I have of Shostakovich personally and the negative impression of his circumstances during the time that I took care of him as his physician. What's the solution? I guess several years of intensive (and expensive) psychotherapy might rid me of my repressions and enable me to play his pieces. Or, I might handle the problem by just playing the pieces of other composers, of which there are many. That last solution works for me. How you solve situations like this is up to you. Denial of emotionally unpleasant things often works.

Another Problem: Some Parts of an Item May in and of Themselves Distract Us

For some reason, known only to God, at a particular part of the e minor section of the *Minuet in* G from the Anna Magdalena Notebook, my mind thinks of Sarah Palin, the Republican candidate for vice president of the United States. Something about the notes in measure three brings forth the Palin idea and the feeling that she was poorly qualified to be president, and that tends to make me lose focus and foul up at that point in the piece.

Actually, why those notes summon the idea of Palin is a not a mystery. My wife interrupted my playing exactly at that note cluster to tell me about McCain's ill-advised choice of Palin as a running mate. So, we could make a case that there was a temporal association of Palin with the notes of that section and that the two items (Palin and the e minor part in question) once associated in the consciousness each tend to recall the other. The evidence that this analysis makes sense is the fact that if someone tells me about Palin, I immediately recall the e minor part of the piece. In other words, the association works both ways: Palin recalls the e minor section, and the e minor recalls Palin. Later, I may explain how I get around this difficulty. What works for me might work for you.

Virginia Woolf describes a shock she received as a child while on vacation in St. Ives, the impact of which lasted her whole life long: "We were waiting at dinner one night when somehow I overheard my father or my mother say that Mr. Valpy had killed himself. The next thing I remember is being in the garden at night and walking on the path by the apple tree. It seemed to me that the apple tree was connected with the horror of Mr. Valpy's suicide." This is an excellent example of the associative properties of the brain. The apple tree has nothing to do with Valpy's suicide except when Virginia's mind made it so. When Virginia thinks of apple tree, suicide pops into her mind. Palin has nothing to do with the minuet save that association makes it so.

B. Encoding

Human memory encodes in time-dependent stages. Most neuroscientists talk about a working memory that lasts for a minute and a half. (Some memory books mistakenly say this stage of memory lasts only 10 seconds. That is wrong!)

Next in sequence, there is a short-term memory lasting about two hours, and after that, there is a long-term memory capable of lasting a lifetime. The physical basis for the working memory is electrical activity in the brain, probably close to the frontal lobes; the physical basis of short-term memory is chemical changes at synapses with increased release of transmitters that facilitate synaptic transmission and a decreased release of inhibitory transmitters, which also facilitates transmission at the synapse. The activities of short-term memory occur for the most part in midline structures of the brain. We know this fact because lesions in those midline structures abolish short-term memory.

With long-term memory, the actual memory trace is delocalized and stored diffusely and is based on the actual structural alteration of the brain with the growth of new synapses, the growth of more connections between nerve cells, and the production of new nerve cells and linked networks of responding cells. Different modalities of memory like taste, touch, light, sound, smell are stored in their own brain areas as well as stored in networks that often connect with one another. Motor memories (also known as procedural memory) are stored over the long-term diffusely and are also concentrated in the cerebellum and basal ganglia. Motor memories are the firmest and most long-lasting of human memories. Some examples of motor memories include: Riding a bike, tying shoes, driving a car. Try to forget how to tie your shoelaces—you can't. Try to tell someone how you tie your shoelaces. That is difficult in the extreme because motor memories are mainly non-verbal.

A detailed knowledge of the agencies that control these (quite complicated) stages of memory encoding is not needed for you to use the information constructively in performing memory tasks, any more than a detailed knowledge of the (quite complicated) workings of the internal combustion engine is needed for you to successfully drive a car. But, in the hope that a not-so-detailed general knowledge of some memory mechanisms might help you memorize better, faster, and easier, here are the basic ideas related to the time-dependent encoding of human memories:

Time-Dependent Stages In Human Memory—Four In Number

Receptor Stage

All sensory modalities have receptors that convert energy in the environment into electrical impulses, which are then sent to the brain for organization and interpretation. The brain knows nothing about the environment, save what it receives in the way of electrical impulses from sensory nerves. Take the visual modality, for instance: Light (a form of energy) hits the chemical in the eye, which changes the chemicals configuration and excites a retinal receptor, which starts a chain of electrical impulses that eventually arrive at the brain. The retinal receptor does not turn off immediately. It continues to discharge for a fraction of a second, depending on the intensity of light and the situation surrounding reception. Because of this continuation of discharge after the stimulus is removed, we are able to maintain continuity of vision even when we blink, and we are able to see moving pictures as a single continuous image even though multiple frames of the image are actually being projected.

Thus, there is a very primitive stage of human memory based on receptor function and based in receptors. You can recall that this stage exists by remembering what happens when you prick yourself with a pin: The pain continues after the pin is removed, and in fact, you can exactly locate the place where you were stuck even though the stimulus (the pin itself) is no longer in your skin. The pain receptors are still discharging, and that is why you can exactly locate where you were stuck. In a certain sense, the continued discharge of the receptor makes you remember what happened and makes you remember where it happened.

The R Stage, the Receptor Stage, Is the Start of All Memories

Most memory books don't even mention this stage of memory, but as for me, I do, and I call this stage of memory the receptor stage and abbreviate this stage as R, where R stands for receptor, any receptor of any sensory modality: Touch, vision, hearing, smell, taste, and kinesthetic. These receptors are important, so make sure your receptors are in the best shape possible. Get your vision checked and corrected to the best you can do. Get your hearing checked and improved to the best you can do. With vision and hearing up to snuff, you will miss less of what is going on and remember more.

Pause now. Consider whether you have made sure your receptor systems are in the best shape possible. Hearing is especially important in the older age group. So get tested and corrected.

What happens next? What happens after the R stage? Remember, the encoding of memory is time-dependent and occurs in a set fixed sequence.

Stage I Memory or The Working Memory

Once information passes into the brain from the receptors, it is processed in the working memory. The working memory is what we use to think. All conversations take place in the working memory. All conscious thinking takes place in the working memory. In the verbal working memory, the normal human can hold only seven items forward and five backward.

If someone asks you to repeat the number 474 7670, you should be able to do so, and in the process, you will be using your working memory. If someone asks you to repeat the number backward, if you are like most people, you will have trouble and will only be able to repeat 5 of the seven digits backward. If you don't believe this is true, try this on your friends or have your friends try it on you. The storage limit of short-term memory is seven items forward and five backward. This is one of the important facts about human memory, a natural fact and a natural limit to the short-term memories of most of us. There are other facts about this memory item that you might keep in mind. This stage is fragile and is easily erased by distraction or interruption, and this stage (as mentioned) is very short-lived, lasting only about a minute. This phase of memory is extremely accurate and never makes a mistake, and never creates a false memory within the limited span of seven items forward. Other stages of memory make mistakes and can create false memories. Not this one!

The usual telephone system is built on this fact of working memory, and that is why currently we have telephone numbers of seven digits. For some reason, the seven digits are more easily recalled if they are grouped into clusters of three and four digits.

Example of Short-Term Memory Failures

Unfortunately, the working memory has a short-term of existing, as mentioned, usually a little longer than a minute. That is why when you look up a number in the telephone book and prepare to dial it, you will fail to remember that number if—

1. The period between lookup and dial without mental review of the number is significantly over a minute or
2. Your attention is, just for an instant, focused onto something else.

You will not fail to dial correctly if you say out loud or otherwise consciously rehearse and review the number until the number is dialed. Short-term memories are supposed to be fleeting. That's their nature. They turn over at a fast rate and are easily erased by distraction. That is why you can only keep a limited amount of information in your mind at one time.

Mental Gymnastic

Test your working memory by reciting this number aloud once. Then go someplace and write it down. 6392067.

By the way, if you don't do the gymnastic, you will cheat yourself of a learning experience.

Most people will be able to easily recite and write down this number forward. How did you do? Now without much ado, write the number backward. This is harder, and most people will fail to write the whole number backward. Usually, most people can do only five digits backward.

Now, look at the number in three groups: 639-20-67. This trick allows the memory to better handle the number, and you will notice it is easier to visualize the number and recite it backward. Say mentally the first group is 639 (and encode these numbers easily because they are part of a familiar pattern (369) but with the 6 first, then the 3, and then the 9. Next, see the 20 and the 67. To go backward, think of 67 and reverse the digits to get 76. Think of 20 and reverse to get 02. And last, picture in your mind's eye if you can the 639 and reverse to 936. Conclusion: By imagining patterns and breaking the memory task into smaller bite-size pieces (chunking), we can partially overcome the limitations imposed by stage one memory.

Let's try another experiment. These experiments are useful, and you are doing them on your own to explore the nature of memory and to see where your memory is good, and to see where it is not so good. Look at this number and recite it aloud. But look at it in the sophisticated way of chunking or analysis of patterns or developing a little narrative story to help you get it right.

818604726

Now go somewhere and write the number backward. How did you do? When I did this task first, I grouped the digits into 818 60 47 26. To recall it backward, I took the 26 and said 62, then took the 47 and said 74, and then for some reason, the 06 popped into consciousness, followed by 818, which is the same forward or back. OK, here's the point. This is a nine-digit number, and I have just recited it backward. If a psychologist were testing me, she would write down that I did nine digits backward, a performance much better than then the expected 5, in fact, a performance level 80% above normal. The lesson here is that applying some simple grouping made me look 80% smarter than I am.

Performance of Any Memory Task Requires Working Memory. Working Memory Is Also Known as Stage One (Stage I).

For instance, all playing of music from memory uses the working memory to read notes and play them and to play the piece by reading out of other stages of memory into the working memory. Because the working memory is based on brain electrical activity, the stage will be interrupted by a convulsion or by electric shock or by distraction. In patients with severe dementia, this stage of memory is often preserved so that a patient may carry on a reasonably coherent and fairly intelligent conversation and, yet, if distracted, even for just a moment, the demented person will be unable to recall what they were talking about, who they were talking to, or even where they were talking. The lesson here is that distraction is the enemy of stage one memory because it is the enemy of focused attention. Continued focused attention is the friend of stage one memory and is necessary to memorize any complex material and is necessary to read out any complex memory from storage.

Comment by Doctor Patten

Years ago, my wife and I decided we wanted to raise genius children. We both read a book entitled *How to Raise a Genius Child.* My copy was given to a student at Rice University who didn't return the book, so I can't tell you who the author was or the publisher. But I can tell you the main point: Train your children to pay attention to everything. And I mean **everything!** Train them, so they pay attention to everything and remember almost everything almost automatically without apparent effort. Eventually, get the kids to the point where minute and detailed observation is spontaneous and natural, just as natural to them as play or eating, or sleeping.

Training the Memory of Children

At the dinner table, explain about your new patient from Chicago who had Myasthenia Gravis and a Thymoma in the anterior mediastinum, and then stop talking and ask your kid what the diagnosis was, where the patient was from, what was in the mediastinum. After insistent questioning about all sorts of details, the kids become automatically attentive and observant. Soon you will find it difficult to think of a question that the kids can't answer. This like potty training. After a while, the kids are potty trained and don't have to expend much effort to take care of the calls of nature. After a while, their trained brains will latch on to ideas, information, and facts without much effort.

In addition to dinner table quizzes, there were quizzes after watching a movie or visiting a museum. What was the number the detective dialed in the movie? How tall is the David, and who was the sculptor? They will know it! The side effect will be that you yourself will become more observant. You will be paying more attention to what you say and see so you can make out questions that might stump the kids. It's a win-win. You get smarter, and so do your children.

Your kids may become valedictorians of their high school and Phi Beta Kappa in college and earn doctorates. They may not be geniuses, but they sure will look like they are.

Lesson: Memory has no greater enemy than lack of concentrated attention. Train yourself to concentrate your attention intensely.

Mental Gymnastic

The present emphasis on political crisis, trade wars, and sensational news is an enemy of concentration. TV keeps switching items, so concentration and attention degrade. Make up your mind to fight back. Try the following exercise with a view to improving your concentration:

Stretch out in a comfortable chair or couch in a quiet room. Relax all muscles. Have no stress or strain on any part of your body. Close your eyes and visualize something. Try to visualize something even if you can't actually visualize. Make it something simple like a Coke bottle or the American flag or a light bulb. Concentrate your thoughts on this item to the exclusion of everything else. Do not let your thoughts stray away.

Suppose you choose the Coke bottle. Keep your mind on it and nothing else.

Prediction: At first, it will be extremely difficult for you to keep focused on this one item for more than a few seconds. The national average is four to five seconds before a new thought or distraction pops up. Yep, the modern attention span is that bad. By gradual and regular drill, try to hold your attention on that one item, the item you yourself selected, for ten seconds. It is difficult but important training. Then when you can do ten seconds, start to work on a more difficult task by doing the experiment not in a quiet room but with the radio or the TV playing. Impressions on eye and ear will make it more difficult for you to hold your thoughts. The goal is to develop your mindfulness so that you can concentrate on anything without distraction for as long as you want wherever you are, no matter what the environmental distractions may be.

Take an Example from Fakirs

Indian fakirs and yogis have this faculty so firmly under conscious control that they can focus away from pain and on to the idea of the absence of pain. They are able to pierce their tongues, cheeks, and the muscles of their upper arms with long needles while they smile and carry on a normal conversation.

Rest assured, you will never reach that degree of concentration. But you can try. Try entering and swimming in cold water by concentrating your attention away from the cold by singing a song like *Swing Low Sweet Chariot*. Not only will you not feel the cold, but also you will like the experience of being in control of the situation by sheer mental effort and willpower. One of the major things you need to learn in life is how to suffer. Once you know how to suffer, everything else comes easy.

Reminder: If you don't suffer through the exercises, you are the one who loses out. You are the one who is cheating yourself.

Stage One Memory Is Preserved at Cocktail Parties

This stage, stage one, of memory is also preserved at cocktail parties, but other stages may fail due to the adverse effect of alcohol. Hence, someone may appear quite intact on the basis of small talk, and that someone may carry on a reasonably coherent and fairly intelligent conversation, and yet when they wake up the next morning, they will not recall anything about the party, much less what was said to them or by them.

Note: Because the working memory is really the first stage of human memory, we refer to it as stage one, but other people may call it the "working memory" or the "ultra-short-term memory."

Attention! Stay awake! A key point is coming. Are you still with me?

Stage One Memory Is the Beginning of All Memories (after Receptors Have Fired).

If you don't go through stage one, you don't get to stage two or to stage three. Therefore, to remember anything long-term, you must conform to the requirements imposed on you by the biological imperatives and limitations attached to stage one:

The To-Be-Remembered Item Must Be Consciously Thought About

The short-term duration of stage one and its limited storage capacity means it is unlikely that you will be able to put into long-term memory items larger than the storage capacity of stage one, which is, as you recall, about seven items. This means it is unlikely that you will be able to memorize any piece of anything except in small chunks, measure by measure, as Shakespeare points out. So, for instance, when you set about to memorize music, a poem, a shopping list, or anything of that ilk: Divide the task into small units and memorize them. Later on, connect the smaller units into a whole with a chain narrative or some other clue or cue. Some people can make a picture of what they need to shop for and then call up the picture in the store and read the items from the image. You have the capacity to do this, but the ability has been highly suppressed. More about this subject later. Little children have no trouble making mental images, and they think it is fun. "Reality is nice," says my granddaughter Callie. "But pretend is nicer."

Stage One Examples

Sometimes that small chunk, say in memorizing a music piece for recital, will be one measure with its complex structure. Sometimes that chunk will be a sequence chunked by a category clue such as scale structure or cadence or a repetition. The seven-item limit applies to fingering. It would be hard to memorize the fingering for more than seven notes at a time. In general, keep the fingering to seven notes or less at a time.

By the same token, stage one will limit the memorization of poems, lists, numbers, faces, names, dates, and so forth. It is possible to make it appear that you have augmented stage one memory by chunking the information and using category clues or using the tricks that were mentioned and by using other tricks discussed later—tricks that take advantage of chunking, associations, category clues, and mnemonics.

Lesson: Start now to be aware of category clues and chunking and how to use them as memory tools. When confronted by a memory task, stop and think about ways to make it easier for you to remember what's what.

Meanwhile, just keep in mind that to memorize anything, you must at first effectively deal with stage one. To memorize anything in stage one, you must pay attention to that thing long enough for you to become consciously aware of the thing itself, and the number of items that you are aware of, the number of items to be placed in the long-term memory must be about seven, no more. Otherwise, the probability of success is small. Indeed, the secret of learning anything by heart, in view of the severe limitations of stage one memory, is to concentrate attention on one (small bite-sized) thing at a time. One line of Shakespeare at a time, as the bard suggests, measure by measure. Or, as the Romans knew: Divide and conquer. To get a big item into your memory, you divide the task into small bite-sized pieces. The small pieces are easily digestible, whereas big pieces will choke you. An amorphous gaseous cloud of information must be compressed into a bite-sized, easily assimilated pellet. Just the way you compressed the task of reciting all 52 cards in a deck into categories (four suits and numbers 1–10) that made the recall easy and accurate.

Students who try to learn a dozen things at a time, changing what they are concentrating on, and varying the phrasing or to-be-remembered-items from day to day, or even minute to minute, and so forth, will get utterly bewildered. Is it surprising that some people can remember anything at all?

The Cause of Most Memory Failures

Most memory failures are either due to inattention or too many items in the stage one memory (stage one memory overload).

About Natural Attention

Natural attention is also known as spontaneous attention. Complete concentration is typified by a child when playing a game she loves; so absorbed is she that, for the time being, nothing else exists for her. That animals have natural attention we can guess merely by watching a sporting dog on the scent of a rabbit or a cat hunched and ready to strike at a mouse. Natural attention arises when the object (or idea or whatnot) upon which the mind is centered is associated with interest or enjoyment or both. If something is emotionally important to us, we will naturally pay attention. Think now about what is important to you and why you have a natural tendency to remember those things.

Older people concentrate naturally for periods of time, varying with the attraction of the thing attended to. Most studies show the older group pays particular attention to health information and ideas about living longer as that seems to be their major area of interest. Attention and concentration vary from individual to individual. Some have a lot. Some have a little. Some have none.

Intense Interest

Not only the lover, but the artist, scientist, and businessman, may experience moments (sometimes over many years) when emotion so intensifies interest that a person, idea, or ambition may become an obsession, occupying the mental field exclusively. That is real attention, the kind of attention that has been productive of some of the greatest achievements of the human mind. Marie Curie comes to mind. Pasteur. Milton. Thomas Jefferson, who was a devoted student of literature. Newton. There are many others. Think of a few and wonder what really turned them on and kept them interested.

For Most Memory Tasks, Natural Attention Doesn't Work

To practice your French lesson with this kind of natural attention may not prove possible. But with willed attention (that is forcing your attention) on to the material at hand, you should be O.K. And, if you get interested enough, the material itself will help focus your attention because it has movement, interest, enjoyment, emotion, color, sometimes passion,—something of interest (otherwise why bother with it?) and most important of all: a reward for having memorized the item. What many students experience is that initially, they are learning because they have to, but after some time, an interest in the subject itself develops and propels the learning forward and without much difficulty.

Mental Gymnastic

Let's work out on attention and recall by an intense and focused examination of how to spot a concealed handgun. Read and examine in detail the exposition in the chart and then answer the questions:

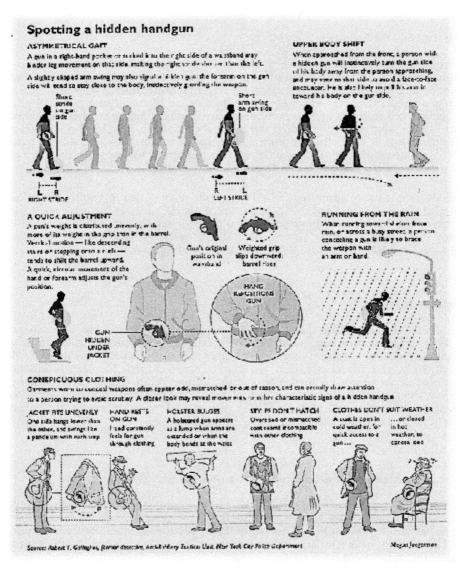

Fig2.4

Questions:

List three items under the title Conspicuous Clothing that might suggest a person is carrying a gun. Write your answers so that you can check them later.

Who is the source of the primary data that was used to make this page of information?

What institutional affiliation did the source have?

What is the purpose of the text and the images?

Check the display techniques used and put an X next to the display techniques that are not used on the page:

a.   Motion curves
b.   Call-outs
c.   Multiple viewpoints
d.   Silhouettes
e.   Flatland footprints
f.   Various scenes
g.   Words and images working together
h.   X-ray vision
i.   Sequence
j.   3-D images
k.   Color and black and white contrasts
l.   Real pictures of real people carrying guns
m.   Display of revolvers and automatic and semiautomatic pistols
n.   Holster bulge at shoulder when lifting
o.   Hidden handgun at ankle

According to the display, what physical property of a gun usually requires the quick adjustment of the gun's position when descending stairs or stepping off a curb?

Name the components of upper body shift.

What happens to stride and arm movements on the gun side?

Discussion of This Mental Gymnastic

Well, did you do the work?

If not, who do you think will not benefit from the exercise? Who do you think you are fooling?

You did the work. Good for you!

Did you write your answers? Reviewing what you know is very important. Testing yourself is a key item in making sure that you actually know the material, as there is a tremendous difference between actually knowing something and thinking you know something. And the thing that really hurts is thinking you know something that is actually wrong or not true.

Did you follow the rules? Pay attention? Concentrate? Make associations? Chunk information into categories? Review? Sometimes talking to yourself about what's what helps cement the memory.

Do you want to swing on a star? Be better off than you are? Or would you rather be a fish?

OK. How did you do? Did you really notice much at all?

Most people do not have a trained mind. Consequently, they do not get much information from what they read or what they look at. With most people, the material goes in the eyes and out the window; little or nothing of substance remains. When asked to review what they learned, most people will be able to give a general idea of what's what, and some of that will be silly, simplified, or wrong. Our judgments of what we have learned well, what we don't know, what we do and do not need to practice are not as accurate as they could be.

On the other hand, those who have trained minds will get to a stage where they will automatically get the information without much effort, just as they automatically drive a car without much effort. These favored few are not geeks or geniuses. They are normal people with trained minds. Their mental might is due to training and discipline, just as much as a skilled dancer's choreographed performance is due to training and discipline. Just as much as President Obama's oratory is due to training and discipline. Just as much as Van Cliburn's performance of Chopin is due to training and discipline.

About Realizations

For each mental gymnastic in this book, I might suggest a possible rendition or "realization" for the purpose of study. These suggested realizations are not to be construed as the definitive way to do the gym work. They are merely there to provide appropriate examples to learn from. Remember, the answers are not important. It is the work, the mental work, that YOU do to get close to the answer that builds mental might.

About Spotting Handguns

Your discussion of conspicuous clothing should have mentioned the idea that any clothing that seems inappropriate to the place, person, or climate would raise suspicions. Did you list: Misfits, hand on gun, bulges, non-matching clothing styles?

The primary source of the information is Robert T. Gallagher, former detective in the New York City Police Department. He has been credited with more arrests for concealed weapons than any other policeman in history. Always check the source of information so that you can appraise the truth value of what you have been given. If you said that the source of the information was the artist Maegan Jaegerman, you are wrong. The question asked for the source of the primary data, not who did the pictures and lay out.

The purpose of the text and images was to teach you things that might suggest that a person is carrying a concealed handgun. Such information may or may not be useful to you, but it is required material for those who are studying to become policemen. The detection of a concealed weapon goes a long way in preventing fatal assaults on the police by criminals.

On display techniques, you should have had an easier time because the question itself might clue the memory. Multiple-choice tests and true-false tests are usually not much of a strain on the brain, but they are easier to grade.

Hidden handgun at ankle is not displayed. The guns shown are all revolvers. There are no automatic and no semiautomatic pistols. There are no real pictures of real people and no 3D images.

If you said the weight of the gun requires the adjustments, you are wrong. The article said that the problem is that the gun's weight is not distributed evenly, and so the gun tends to rotate the barrel up.

Upper body shift? Review the page. Ditto stride and arm movements.

Stage Two Memory or Short-Term Memory

The next stage after stage one is (you guessed it) stage two. Others call this stage of memory "short-term memory" because it is based on the neuronal mechanisms that underlie short-term potentiation. To avoid confusion, let's stick with our name and our terms and call it stage two memory because it follows stage one.

Stage II Memory

Stage two is mainly chemically based and is needed to get information into the long-term memory. Stage two is the stage of memory commonly interrupted by drugs, and the drug that most commonly interrupts stage two is ethyl alcohol. In some people, just one drink will do it, and in others, six or seven will not. Much depends on sex (women are more easily affected), previous drinking experience, and the liver's ability to metabolize alcohol.

The Sequence in Information Processing: R → Stage One → Stage Two → Stage Three

All the time-dependent processes must work in sequence for you to encode complex material in the long-term storage. First R (the receptor stage), then stage one (the working memory of consciousness), then stage two (short-term memory), and then stage three (long-term memory).

Think now how you can remember the stages of human memory processing.

Answer: chunk into easily assimilated patterns. In this case, the pattern is R123.

Stop! Name the Stages of Memory

Notice how easy it is to recall the stages of human memory because they are the same as the sequence of numbers that we all have all Overlearned by heart: one, two, three. All you have to do to look smart is remember to put the R in front of the one, two, three, and remember what that R stands for. R, of course, stands for—? Ye gods, did you forget? I hope not. Receptors!

Now you have a framework for you to discourse on the stages of memory for at least three minutes. Start at the beginning with the R and tell what you know. Then pass to stage one and give some examples and the facts and limits of this stage. You might mention the cocktail party effects, which seem to catch the interest of most people because they have seen it in action or experienced it. Next, do stage three and the little that has been mentioned about that stage—delocalized and stored diffusely and pretty hard to destroy. See? You are learning some things, and you are becoming sensitive to factual information. At this point, you probably know more about human memory than 99.99% of people on this planet.

Stage Three or Long-Term Memory

Stage three is also known as long-term memory because it lasts a long time. It is the stage in which we would like our important permanent memories to reside. Regardless of the different names, the experts agree that long-term memory is physically based on long-term potentiation in the brain, which is based (at least in part) on unusually folded brain proteins and on actual structural changes in the brain. Long-term potentiation and short-term potentiation are brain mechanisms based on brain biology, the details of which, though well understood, need not bother us here. If you really want to know about them, consult Eric Kandel's book *The Principles of Neuroscience.*

What Causes Memory Failures?

Most, if not all, memory failures are stage one failures—that is, failures to encode in the first place due to poor attention or stage one overload. "You can't recall what you didn't pay attention to in the first place," said Harry Lorayne, American Mnemonist. Cocktail party failures are stage two failures as stage one is usually intact at parties, and stage two is adversely affected by alcohol.

Readout Failures

Even if you did pay attention in the first place, the bad news is you can still fail to recall what you actually encoded into your brain. Readout failures of information correctly transferred from stage one to two and three are due to ineffectively transferring information back from stage three to stage two, then to stage one, the working memory. Most read-out failures are due to the brain being in a different chemical state from the state in which the original memory was encoded or a failure to adequately encode the memory in the first place. Or too much time has passed, and the active and complete removal of the memory by natural biological processes has already occurred.

Retrieval

Testing ourselves (retrieval) is not only a demonstration of past learning; it is also a way of re-encoding. Every time you recall information, you re-encode it in your memory banks. You retrieve it and use it, and the information is actually changed and re-encoded because you have retrieved it and used it. In this manner, although retrieval often gets thought of as a way of demonstrating previous learning, it turns out it is also an important way to improve memory over time. Retesting yourself on material to be tested on by your professor is the surest way of getting good grades and is much more effective than simply rereading the material or looking it over or saying it.

Clues and cues will often help recover from a readout failure, and sometimes just time will result in a correct readout, and sometimes just a good night's sleep will recover the memory. Getting the brain in the same chemical state and getting your body in the same place that the memory was encoded will also help. Always think place and not time. Where was I when I last had my reading glasses? Not when did I have my reading glasses last? Human memory of place is much more powerful than human memory of time. You can prove this point to yourself. Think of a place where you stayed on vacation. Recall as many details about that place as you care to. Now try to place that place in time. What was the year you visited Egypt? You recall lots about what you heard and saw, but if you are like most normal people, you will have more difficulties recalling the year, month, and other aspects of time spent in that place.

Failure of Stage One to Stage Two

When you forget where you parked your car at the airport, it is because you didn't force the information into stage two. So next time, just sit there for a fraction of a minute and tell yourself **here is where you parked.** Usually, address yourself as your last name and not as I. But if you wish to say to yourself: **here is where I parked the car**—that's fine. And it is OK if you also address yourself by your first or last name or both. Suit yourself. Addressing yourself by your last name may have a special attention-getting quality that addressing yourself as "I" does not. Try it and see.

Example: "Listen up, Patten—you parked on the roof of D in the blue area with the front of the car facing north toward the control tower. That's roof, D, blue."

Note the surroundings and prominent landmarks that will help clue the memory when you return from your trip. This will take about a minute. Once you make a mental note of where you parked, try to forget where you parked. You can't!

When you walk into a room and don't know why you are there, that also is a stage one to stage two transfer failure. Next time deliberately tell yourself, "I am now going into the kitchen to get the scissors." If you did do that, that is, if you actually consciously told yourself why you were going into the kitchen, then you may think of anything else you wish. When you get to the next room and ask why you are there, you will know. Don't believe me? Try it!

Review and Repeat Aloud: Most Memory Failures Start With a Failure to Pay Attention in the First Place

Thus, most memory failures are due to failure to pay sufficient attention in the first place. You would be surprised how much information that passes into the working memory goes immediately out the window. How many times have you seen a traffic light? Yet, are you sure which light is on top? How about when the lights are displayed horizontally? Which light is on the extreme left, red or green? I bet you don't know or are not sure.

Which way does Washington face on the dollar bill? If you are like most people, you have seen his face on the dollar bill thousands of times. And yet, and yet, you might not be sure which way he is facing. What about Hamilton on the ten? Is he facing left or right? Which of these bills, 5, 10, 20, 50, has *We the People* written on it in gigantic red letters on the right and a gigantic red torch on the left? A smaller, denser red version of the torch appears on the right just before the serial number. How many letters are omitted from the touchpad of your portable phone? You have looked at that pad many times, but you did not observe that 7 has pqrs and 9 has wxyz. From a dial phone? From your home phone?

On the modern quarter dollar, what is the order of print size of the words "LIBERTY," "THE UNITED STATES OF AMERICA," and "IN GOD WE TRUST?"

These things are not important to most people, and no one is trying to beat up on you. Most people have seen these things repeatedly, and most people don't care about them. The point is that these common things have been seen but not observed. You saw them, but you did not consciously pay attention to them enough, and consequently, you didn't memorize what was what. On the other hand, if you suffered from red-green color blindness, you needed to know the light on the extreme right in a horizontal display is red. When that light is lit, you stop even though you don't see it as red.

Whoa! Did you believe that last statement? See how easy it is to accept as fact something not true. Check it out. The light on the extreme right of horizontal display is not red. It is green!

Most people don't care about the print size on the quarter, nor should they, except recently, "Liberty" has been degraded to much smaller print than on previous U.S. coins. Now the United States of America has the biggest print. What this means, I'm not sure, but it doesn't seem good. Is it an idea that means liberty is less important than the idea of the United States of America? I hope not!

You See a Lot by Looking

Yogi Berra famously remarked that you see a lot by looking. That's true.

Unless you make a conscious effort to study and observe the details of your current memory task, you are doomed to failure. You should have learned that fact from the handgun gymnastic. You look with your eyes. You observe with your mind.

Unless you make a mental note of where you parked your car, you are probably doomed to have trouble finding it when you get back from that long vacation to Rarotonga. Unless you make a conscious mental note of where to start the Mozart piece at that high B, you might not know where to start. Unless you make a mental note that you locked the front door, you are doomed to go back and check. Ditto, is the stove off? Windows closed? Lights out? Cat fed?

Failure of Stage Three to Stage One Is a Common Cause of Breakdown

This will be covered later with multiple ideas on how to avoid the problem and how to facilitate accurate readout of a stored memory from long-term into the consciousness and the working memory of stage one. At this point, it is sufficient for you to know that once the memory is in the long-term storage space (which we are calling stage three), it must, to be used, be called out and put into stage one, which is (as you remember) the working memory and the modality of consciousness.

Modern Memory Studies and Research

Since Hermann's original studies, over ten thousand memory studies have been done, and over a hundred books have been written on the subject. We will now cover each and every one of these in great detail:

Only kidding, of course.

Even a pseudo-scholar like myself wouldn't do that. Besides, I am trying to write an interesting, helpful book, not bore you to death. The details of memory mechanisms are the bailiwick of scientists, not of us.

So here is a summary of memory truths to help you understand your memory and, with that understanding, use your memory skills better. Pay attention to these principles. They will give you a head-up (and a leg-up) on performance of any mental task. As you read them, actively imagine how you might apply them to your next memory task. Recall the brain works best when it is doing and thinking. Another hint: Reread each of the principles each night just before you hit the hay. Reread them until (you guessed it) you can recite them from memory. Learn them as well as you learned the cycle of fifths or the major scales, the alphabet, the numbers from one to infinity, the times tables, and the prayers you said as a child, and so forth. Without this foundation to build upon, no satisfactory progress can be made with this or any other rational system.

Summary of Chapter Two

The default mode of human memory is to forget.

To overcome the default mode requires mental work.

Most memory failures are due to mental laziness, failure to pay attention, and boredom.

Most memory successes are due to active engagement of the brain while actually doing work on the memory task. Thinking and doing = good.

Stage one memory lasts about one minute, has a storage capacity of seven items forward, and is easily interrupted by distraction and easily improved by chunking, clueing, repetition aloud or under breath, and associations, especially visual associations. When not overloaded and when there is no distraction, stage one never fails.

Stage two and stage three memory can fail and can produce false memories.

Time spent in review and repetition is never wasted.

Repeated self-testing is the key to exact learning.

The more thought, the more effort, the more ingenuity you put into memory, the more you get out.

We are, in general, poor judges of what we know and what we don't know. Hence, when exact memory is needed, it is a good idea to test ourselves.

Now, Friends, We Move on to Chapter Three. Have Fun!

Chapter three will tell about principles of learning. None of these principles by themselves are particularly important. But all of them, taken together, are the key to information storage in the human brain. You have heard, no doubt, that genius consists of trifles, but genius is itself no trifle. Spectacular memory consists of trifles, but in and of itself is no trifle. The more thought, the more effort, the more ingenuity you put into memory, the more you will get out.

Good luck and happy practicing!

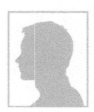

CHAPTER THREE
PRINCIPLES OF LEARNING

CHAPTER THREE: PRINCIPLES OF LEARNING

◆ ◆ ◆

Summary of this chapter: This chapter gives ideas for you to consider. Some of these ideas might apply to your learning tasks and work for you, and some might not. One size doesn't fit all. It is up to you to see if a particular idea likes you and you like it. Read over the chapter quickly. Apply what seems practical in your situation and disregard the rest. You are the master of your fate. You are the captain of your soul. You decide what's good and what's not. Here are, offered for your consideration, suggestions merely.

Review Time

Item one: Time spent in review is never wasted. Multiple studies show that the students who do best are, by and large, the students who study. (Did you have any doubt about that?) Furthermore, the more you study, the more you learn. You get what you pay for: Spend the time, and you will get the results. But don't overdo it. You don't want to develop a reputation for being a hopeless drudge or a grub for grades.

Most of the scientific studies indicate the most **efficient** study is to spend the same amount of time reviewing as you did during the initial exposure. A one-hour lecture would then get one hour of review time. About this, more later.

Ignacy Paderewski (1860–1941) famously remarked that if he missed a day's practice, he would notice the ill effect of that omission on his playing; if he missed two day's practice, his wife would notice something wrong; and if three days passed without his touching the piano, the public would notice it.

Paderewski had more than the usual problems with technique. But what worked for him (daily practice) might work for you. He claimed the reason he lost ability by missing just one day of practice was his fingers got stiff. They may have stiffened alright, but not that much. The brain is especially equipped to rid itself of complex material that is not renewed on a daily basis. So, the effect that Paderewski noticed was more likely due to a degradation of brain engrams (memory traces), which directed the motor control systems assigned to move the fingers. The degradation would slow fingers and make them appear stiff. The problem, dear Brutus, is not in the fingers but in the brain and in the nature of the forgetting curve.

Practice What You Need to Practice

Item two: Also, don't forget you have to study the right material. Human memory is modality-specific. If the French test is going to be on chapter seven and you study chapter eight, you might not do as well as you deserve. In fact, Professor Hermann discovered that maximum efficient learning occurs when review time equals the exposure time to the same material. So, in general, for a one-hour lecture you attend, you should spend at least one hour in review of that lecture. For the 57 minutes or 90 minutes or 120 minutes or the 17 hours it took you to read this book so far, you should spend the same amount of time reviewing what you read.

Maximal Efficiency for Time Invested Depends on Review Time

Item three: Yes, maximum effective learning occurs when review time equals learning time. Review time = exposure time gives the best return for time spent in learning.

What does that mean? If you are interested in maximizing the **efficiency** of what you learn, that is, learn the most in the smallest amount of invested time, the best bet is to review the material for the same time as the initial exposure. In the mental gymnastics course at Rice University, we have one 90-minute lecture a week. As this is the case, students should, for maximum efficiency, spend 18 minutes each weekday reviewing what was said in class. Recall that $18 \times 10 = 180 / 2 = 90$, the reason that it is suggested that the student take 90 minutes of review, 5 times $18= 90$, but the easy way of 18 times 5 is to multiply by 10 and divide by 2. We use 5 because usually there is no study on the weekend. The weekend is a sacred time. Most students wouldn't study on the weekend, so why should you? Rice students don't study on the weekend, most of them anyway. All work and no play makes Jack a dull boy—Jill too.

But—More Time Usually Means More Material Mastered

Item four: Because maximum efficient learning occurs when study time equals exposure time, it does not mean that more time will not result in more learning. The exposure rule is concerned only with getting the biggest reward for the smallest amount of time invested. The exposure rule is about efficiency of learning. The exposure rule is not about maximal mastery of material or total learning. It is not about proficiency. Proficiency is a horse of a different color. Proficiency will take much more time and many, many repetitions and reviews and self-tests.

Reminder: Review should be mindful. As soon as you are fatigued or bored, take a break to refresh your body and brain.

Hence, if you had a one-hour piano lesson a week, maximum efficient learning (the highest rate of reward for invested time) would occur at one hour of review, and the best and most efficient way to review would be to space the reviews at 12 minutes a day Monday through Friday. No kidding—that's what the scientific studies indicate. Piano teachers who have just read that fact are probably screaming.

The latest research findings in the domain of memory development reveal mere repetition in study is not enough. Focus on the subject is important. Also, there is a distribution factor to consider. Memory professors Ebbinghauss, Dueer, Menmann, and Fürst have provided the following data:

In the majority of experiments, as a general rule, material that required 68 repetitions in one day could be mastered with only 38 repetitions if these repetitions were spread over three days. This proves, by the way, that the student who waits to the last day to "cram" would have actually saved half her time if she learned the subject gradually over a period of several days. Why this distribution rule is true is not entirely clear. Current opinion favors the idea that sleep between repetitions makes the learning task more efficient and easier. Regardless of the mechanism or mechanisms, it is an established fact that dividing the review time and dividing the repetitions over several intervals of time augments the memory and makes encoding easier and more solid.

Lesson: Complete mastery of the material takes time, as every real student and every real teacher knows.

Sickness Slows Learning and Makes Memory Defective

Item five: Sickness and fatigue interfere with memory and learning by making our brains less alert and less effective. The reason for this is that the encoded memory traces are stored in a particular brain part called the neuron. Neurons are cells, and when they are sick, they don't work right. Sometimes, neurons will respond to a short nap or a cup of java, but if you are really sick, forget any serious mental gymnastics, music memory, poetry memory, advanced calculus, trying to figure out that American Express bill, Trump politics, or other mental tasks. Concentrate on getting better. Decreased brain function caused by sickness is a natural and expected thing, a consequence of our having a brain made of cells and meat and not silicon or germanium or zinc oxide.

Associations Facilitate Recall

Item six: Recall of memories is facilitated by association. In fact, once two items are associated in the consciousness, each one tends to recall the other. This is the basic principle of all memory, which, believe it or not, was discovered long ago by our ancient ancestors. It is the major way that long-term, previously encoded memories are brought to the consciousness. That is, it is the major way that stage three memories are brought into stage one. Let's listen to the master about this:

"Ideas developed simultaneously or in immediate succession in the same mind mutually reproduce each other, and do this with greater ease in the direction of the original succession and with a certainty proportional to the frequency with which they were together."

–Aristotle (384–322 BC)

Wow! What the ancients did not know could fill volumes. But in this case, Aristotle gets it right. But Aristotle did not make that discovery. He just talks about it. The real discovery was made in prehistory, somewhere and somehow, in a time out of mind—in a time older than the time of chronometers, when an unknown human learned that making mental images and associations of items and places facilitates recall and that two items, once linked in the consciousness, forever tend to help each recall the other, especially if the items are originally encoded in a visual and vivid way. Friends, this is the basic human mental mechanism behind memory and is the "discovery" that is at the basis of ancient and modern memory arts. The discovery, we can speculate, facilitated finding the berry patch after an absence or the hunting grounds when territory is revisited. Thus, associations are necessary to memory. And more than one neurologist and psychologist has noted that the brain is a coincidence machine.

Lesson: The brain remembers items that are coincidental in the consciousness.

Two items, once associated in the consciousness, forever tend to recall each other. And the two items don't have to be related to each other logically or in any way. The brain doesn't care about anything but the fact that the two items appeared in the conscious mind at the same time. Two neuronal networks responded together, and that is what will link them. That is what ties them together. When one item activates its neuronal network, some or all of the other item's neurons activate, and presto! Item two comes to conscious attention.

When I say A, what do you think of?

Most people think B because, in their youth, A and B were associated together in that order. What do you think of if I say C?

As associations make memory links, the question then devolves to what associations work best?

Associations That Get Our Attention Work Best to Preserve Memory

Associations are best when they are vivid, visual, violent, emotionally related to us (our self-interest) and in motion. And as Aristotle notes above, the more frequent the associations are made, the more certain will be recall of one idea by the other. Repetition cements memory and facilitates recall.

About how to make better associations to augment memory, more later when we cover the Ancient Art of Memory, a system of memory tricks our ancient Greek, and Roman ancestors used to memorize immense amounts of material such as the entire Iliad and the Odyssey, which many of them could recite verbatim. This ancient art of memory was also used by musicians from the 12th century to the 16th century to memorize music. In fact, the music was often modified to facilitate the direct application of memory arts to the piece, not vice versa. The Ancients considered memory an art because it was a created, individual, immediate, personal, technical, and imaginative craft requiring adroitness and cunning for successful performance.

Active Attention and Mental Engagement Is Needed to Memorize Most Things

Item 7. Active engagement is better than passive. We talked about the reasons this is true. And it was explained why in view of the enormous benefits of active mental activity, people still prefer passive watching. One answer is mental passivity is a lot less work, and the easy path is tempting even if we repeatedly are disappointed in ourselves and in the results. If you just zipped through the concealed gun demo, you didn't learn much, and that's a fact. If you concentrated, reviewed, repeated items to yourself, made associations with the pictures, in other words, put in some effort and work, then you are now an expert on spotting a concealed handgun.

Harry Lorayne, the great American mnemonist, categorically states you can remember any new piece of information if it is firmly associated with what you already know. He says one of the fundamentals of a trained memory is what he calls "original awareness." Anything of which you are originally aware is difficult to forget. When you make an association, you are automatically forcing an original awareness. Anything you wish to remember must first be observed. Once the observation is made, associations will usually take care of the rest.

Practice What You Need

If you want to learn how to touch type, for instance, you should not take a course in which you merely watch others type. That is unlikely to get you anywhere. Nor can you become an efficient typist if you just read about typing. Remember, the human brain learns best when it is actively involved in doing something that it is thinking about. Doing and thinking together—that's the ticket. The magic is in the mix of those two things.

So, if you want to learn how to type, you have to get in there and think about typing while you are actually physically typing. You can't learn to read by watching someone read. And by the way, don't forget the modality thing: Human learning, Human memory is modality-specific. Your piano playing will not be significantly improved by fixing your bike tire. Your piano playing is much more likely to benefit from (you guessed it) playing the piano.

Do you want to become an expert taster of wines? Well, that's what you have to work on. How about working for a company testing perfumes? Yes, there are such people, and you can bet they have a highly trained sense of smell. Frank Sinatra, even after he was famous and rich, practiced singing at least four hours a day. Muzio Clementi (1752–1832), who had an enormous reputation as a musician, practiced at least eight hours a day, and if he missed time one day, he made it up the next day. Why? For him, that was his thing. He devoted time and energy to it because he loved it and wanted to be good at it.

Imagined Practice Is Effective

While active playing of a real piano is the best way of encoding music memory, multiple studies have also shown that mental review is almost as good. While waiting in line at the supermarket, you can, with profit, go over your piano piece, the poem you are working on, or that formula in calculus, and so forth. Working things in your mind is effective in creating memories that can be used when needed. It is a conscious act and almost as effective as doing the real thing.

Mental review can be visual with mental construction of imagined notes of your music, or it can be auditory with humming or tapping. Or mental review can be both visual and auditory. The same technique is effective in memorizing your tap-dancing routines. Effective mental rehearsal is almost as effective as the real thing. You don't have to work out the proof of the general theorem of calculus, you can do it in your head, and that review will be almost as effective as doing it on paper. Get the idea? Mental review works, and mental review probably works because it activates the same brain areas (or similar brain areas) as practicing the real thing. The advantage of mental work, as opposed to the actual physical and mental work, is you can do it without the equipment usually needed. My tap shoes are not on, but I am reviewing my latest tap show dances while waiting for the parade to begin, the bus to arrive, or the doctor to see me.

For Most People, Visual Associations Work Best

Objective tests favor visual methods of recall as they are proven to be more effective for most people. Doctor Patten's studies showed visual memory is at least 1,000 times better than verbal memory. This is why photos and photo albums are so effective in bringing back memories of past events. That is why a picture is worth a thousand words.

Like it or not, humans are mainly visual animals. You are human, and therefore you are mainly a visual animal. Over 80% of the total sensory input to your human brain comes via the visual system. So, try to make associations that have some visual connection. Recall the forgetting curve and the importance of review just prior to playback. Thus, instead of sitting dumbly on the bench awaiting your turn to go into the performance examination, the lecture you are to give from memory, the interview for that big job that requires a detailed knowledge of high-energy physics, and so forth, you might profit by going over your task, the poem, the formulas, whatever, particularly the most difficult parts, in your head and do it in pictures. Believe it or not, the big thinkers think in pictures.

Einstein Used Visual Methods of Thought

Albert Einstein says in his autobiography that visual methods of thinking were the basis for his discoveries. If you read his book on relativity, you will find that most of the ideas are illustrated with images, moving trains, flashes of light, bright golden cages accelerated in space, and so forth. About how to do this best, more later. The benefit to memory and recall about review just before recall events is called the "recency effect." What you review just before the test is still in your mind, and that helps. Try to keep in mind: Images and recent review facilitate correct recall.

The Brain Gets Bored Fast

Item eight: Variety is better than a single task. Our brains get tired and bored fast.

They are specially constructed to pay attention to anything new and different. That is why you will do lots better by varying the task at hand than trying to do the same thing over and over. It is better to read a non-fiction book for 15 minutes and then switch to a novel for 15 minutes and then switch back to nonfiction, alternating back and forth as you go. Each time you switch, your mind will be eager to get back to the other book before the usual ennui sets in, or you begin to nod off. The net result is that you can often read two books in the same time it would have taken you to read either book alone.

Try this: Study two music pieces or two poems in the same sitting. Review one for ten minutes and then switch to the other. Keep switching back and forth. You should find that you learn both pieces or both poems more efficiently. But get this: Because the brain likes novelty, you will actually do better alternating work on your music piece with work on the poem. Two dissimilar things are more easily encoded than two similar things. In fact, if two things are too similar, the memory of the first will interfere with the memory of the second, and the memory of the second will interfere with memory of the first. The effect of the first on the second task is called proactive inhibition in psychology circles, and the adverse effect of the second task on memorizing the first is known as retroactive inhibition. This phenomenon has been demonstrated repeatedly in laboratory studies, so we know for sure it is real.

Notice I said switch at ten minutes. This seems to be an important point. Your brain tends to fatigue at 20 minutes, so you are better off stopping the project while your brain is still fresh and interested in that item. The brain will then be eager to return to the interrupted task. Don't believe me? Try it and see for yourself.

Personal Example

When I do my piano work, I usually pause after ten minutes and go read a magazine or a novel. This refreshes my brain and makes me eager to do both tasks. I know this may not sound right to those of you who were trained up to sticking your nose to the grindstone and doggedly keeping your nose on the grindstone until the task is done. But try this system just to see if you like it and to see if it likes you. If it works for you, great. If it doesn't work for you, at least you learned what doesn't work for you.

The Brain Has a Mind of Its Own

The brain has a mind of its own but techniques can trick the brain into remembering more material faster. Reminder: Each person's brain is different, so the above advice applies in general, but not in particular. Some brains get bored in far less time than the 20 minutes stated by our friend Hermann Ebbinghaus and other brains never get bored no matter how much time passes. What's true for your brain?

Retroactive and Proactive Inhibition for Lists

Another thing to keep in mind about the above advice is a memory phenomenon called proactive and retroactive inhibition that applies most commonly when two similar lists are memorized one after the other. The first list will tend to interfere with the recall of the second list (proactive inhibition), and the second list will tend to interfere with the recall of the first (retroactive inhibition).

The Treatment of Proactive and Retroactive Inhibition

This phenomenon is not present when the lists are encoded using associative techniques like the ones about to be discussed. It is doubtful that in the course of memorizing two pieces of music, one after another or two poems and alternating the tasks, that either of these memory processes (proactive and retroactive inhibition) will operate. If they do or seem to, then just concentrate on one piece at a time. With me, I have not noticed any proactive or retroactive inhibitions except in memorizing tap dance routines where the two routines are similar to each other. The more similar the two tasks you are working on and switching back and forth to, the more likely that there will be trouble. If you have trouble, just stop and work on one memory task at a time.

The Distributive Rule: Don't Cram

Item nine: As discussed, distribution of effort over time is important. If you are trying to learn how to touch type or tap dance or learn a foreign language, you are much better off and will achieve better results working one hour a week for 40 weeks than, say, working eight hours a day for five days. The evidence for the benefits of distribution of tasks is overwhelming.

A study that proved the point was done by the British postal service. One group of workers were given one-hour typing lessons once a week for 40 weeks. The other got 40 hours in one week. Of course, the group whose task was distributed did much better on the objective tests of typing.

Distribution of the task in time is the ticket. This is simply true and will remain true on this planet for the next 4.5 billion years when our sun will become a super red giant and burn Earth to a crisp. Scientists hope by the time that happens, humans will have emigrated to another solar system to pollute another planet. Science magazine recently reported there are over 300 million planets with liquid water just in our galaxy. Our species will have plenty of new homes to choose from.

Stop!

Think and discover for yourself why and how you recognized the above repetition about humans leaving Earth. What was it about this repetition that got your attention and made you aware that you had encountered that idea before?

Lesson: Little bits over a long time are much better than a lot of material all at once. In other words: Don't cram!

With the distributive rule in mind, determine which approach is likely to result in the most progress if you have two hours to devote to memorizing the famous poem *In Flanders Fields* by Lieutenant Colonel John McCrae, MD, and one hour to do housework:

Restatement of problem:

You have three hours, two to memorize a poem and one to clean. How should you proceed? Which answer is best?

Answer A. Do the two hours of the poem first, then do the hour of housework.

Answer B. Do the hour of housework, then do the two hours of the poem.

Answer C. Do one hour of the poem, then an hour of housework, then an hour of the poem.

(Notice: Those morons who did not circle answer C or otherwise know C is the answer must go directly to jail and not pass Go.) Those who did get the correct answer should reward themselves by doing something nice.

Mental Gymnastic

Now that you have read the facts twice, summarize them. List as many facts about the postal system study you recall. Tell why we know for sure that distribution of a task is an effective way of mastering a memory task. Write out your answer or recite it into a recorder or video. Then, check your answer with the information provided. Note what you got right and what you missed. Try to figure out why you remembered what you did and why you forgot what you forgot. The usual reader gets only the main point and misses the details. Grade yourself to see how many key points and details you actually mentioned in your answer:

1. The study was in England.
2. Postal workers were trained to touch type.
3. Because the postal system was switching to zone codes.
4. Zone codes in England have both letters and numbers.
5. Touch typing has standard tests.
6. Postal workers were divided.
7. One group got 40 hours of typing instruction in one week.
8. One group got one hour a week for 40 weeks.
9. The results proved intensive typing instruction was far less effective.
10. Therefore, don't cram!

Well, how did you do? If you got less than three of the above points, you need to concentrate more on concentrating more. Mental laziness is the reason most people know very little definite information about most things. Most people are airheads. "Dull heads among windy spaces," according to T.S. Eliot.

Details are important because they are the evidence supporting your points and your conclusions. Citing evidence makes you look smart, and evidence protects you and others from believing things that are not true.

Don't beat up on yourself if you missed most of the points. You're reading this book to improve. You want to be better at observation and attention to details. Even the great master Aristotle had some problems with proper and detailed observation. He famously said the common housefly had four legs. That error was copied and repeated for centuries. Not until the 1880s was he corrected by people who decided to take a look and prove: **Flies have six legs.** Aristotle categorically stated that heavy objects fall faster than light objects. That is hogwash. All objects fall (in a vacuum) at the same accelerating rate.

BERNARD MICHAEL PATTEN, M.D.

The Devil is in Details

Consider this story told to Bruno Fürst by a furniture manufacturer who was taking Fürst's course in memory:

There were two candidates sent down, after the usual questions about training, experience, and references, to find out about a load of lumber being delivered. Both candidates then reported back what they saw.

Candidate #1: "The lumber is being delivered."

Candidate #2: "The shipment which is being unloaded is walnut from the Blank Company in Cambridge, for which you placed an order. It is exceptionally fine wood. About two-thirds of the shipment is unloaded, and it will take about one hour more to complete the task. The yard foreman is supervising the unloading. He gave orders to store the wood in Warehouse 3."

Candidate #1 was considered unsuited for the job and sent away. The report of candidate #2 was more detailed, almost comprehensive. It showed the candidate was a close observer and was resourceful in asking pertinent questions about points that did not come under his own observation. Candidate #2 was actually thinking about what was what. He got the job.

Ask Questions

Asking questions is good. Ask them of yourself to clarify your thinking and to prove to yourself you are mastering the stuff you are trying to master. Ask questions of others to clarify their thinking. If someone is telling you something and you don't quite get it, ask them to repeat or explain more or explain themselves better. If you didn't hear what they said, ask them to repeat louder. If you really can't hear well, get a hearing aid.

Remember, there is usually no general rule that applies to all situations. So thinking is involved before mechanically applying any rule or protocol. In general, people will be flattered that you are interested enough in what they say to ask them questions.

Trisha Greenhalgh (Oxford University), warned by a teacher that the University of Cambridge did not admit women of "her sort," applied nonetheless. Tim Hunt (Nobel Prize in Medicine) interviewed her and asked seven questions. When he told her she got every answer wrong, she asked him to explain, and together they reviewed the problems one by one until she fully understood her errors. She got her place at Cambridge because "research is not about knowing the right answers before you start. It's about how you ask the questions and how systematically you go about finding the answers."

Greenhalgh is famous for her work in challenging conventional wisdom. Her 2014 paper on the mistake of prescribing statins to a 74-year-old woman is one of the most widely read and quoted papers ever published in the British Medical

Journal. The statins caused muscle pains (a common side effect of statins) that prevented the woman from exercising and interfered with her hobbies. The prescribing physician was following a standard protocol without much thought about how the patient lives. Such scenarios are "a good example of the evidence-based tail wagging the clinical dog." Trisha refutes any mechanical form of reasoning, be it guidelines or specific research design. Her statement, "I oppose categorically the most overused and under-analyzed statement in the academic vocabulary: that 'more research is needed.' What we need is more thinking." Bravo! Cookbook medicine = Bad medicine. Doing anything mechanically without thinking about what might happen is not a good idea. Think first, then act. If President Trump had followed this rule, the United States would not be in its present pickle.

Note from Doctor Patten

Applicants who wanted to do medical research with me were required to read *Arrowsmith* and take a test on the details of that book. A candidate who did not know the details of the book in extenso would not make a good medical researcher and would not be hired. Any candidate who did not know the answer to the following two questions was automatically disqualified:

How did Arrowsmith's wife get the infection?

Answer: She smoked a contaminated cigarette.

Why was Arrowsmith's experiment a scientific failure?

Answer: He treated the control group with his serum and therefore couldn't prove the serum actually worked.

Repetition is needed. One-step learning for complex tasks almost never works. Be sure to pay attention to brain state during repetition. Stay in focus and don't be bored or tired. But quality of the repetitions is important and sometimes key.

Item ten: Repetition and review are the major ways to learn. This book repeats things because repetition is basic to all memory. In a sense, this is the same as principle #1 above, but in a sense, it is not. The best repetitions must be similar to the test conditions under which you expect to use your knowledge. If you are interviewing for a job, you must rehearse your responses to the usual questions in front of a mirror or in front of a good friend or, better still, a cam recorder and a person. The cam recorder is there so you can review your performance. If you don't know what about your performance is bad, how will you correct it?

Practice makes perfect, and the perfect practice is that which mimics as close as possible the conditions under which recall is needed. This immortal truism is known in the psychology business as state-dependent memory.

State-dependent learning: All memory is dependent on the state of the brain at the time encoding is attempted.

Item 11: Suppose, for instance, a patient came to clinic and told you that they were a parish priest and had recently received a big donation of money (in this case, the big amount, according to the priest, was $3,000). The priest then invited his fellow priest out to celebrate this wonderful gift. Along the way, both got very drunk. The next day neither the priest nor the friend could remember anything about the night's activities, much less where the money was. Think about this: What advice would you give to the priest to enable him to recall where he hid the money? Think about this in terms of the state-dependent memory principle mentioned.

Get it? Don't get it? DON'T CARE?

If you DON'T CARE, then give up right now. You are not going to make it. You are reading the wrong book. Go watch TV.

If you get it, that's great. If you don't get it, that is greater because you are about to learn something. The mental work to get an answer is much more important than the answer itself because the work to get the answer is what stimulates the human brain and promotes mental might.

Results count, but not that much. It is the effort to get to the result that builds brainpower. Once an answer is known or a result obtained, the brain benefits are not worth talking about. Kids who are trying to master a video game, for instance, have brain scans that light up all over the place, reflecting the enormous brain activity involved in learning that task. Once they get it cold (that is, know how to work the game automatically), the activation scans show little activity.

What Advice Would Work for the Priest and Help Him Recall Where He Hid the Money?

OK. Pause now and state your advice aloud. Then check your advice against what was actually given in neurology clinic.

Pause for Thinking

The priest was advised to get drunk again while in the company of his fellow priest, who would remain sober. Start drinking at the same rate, the same whiskey at the same time of day in the same room wearing the same clothes that you wore on the day the money was lost. Try to get into the same celebratory mood you had on the day the loss occurred. Duplicate as much as possible the brain state that occurred when the money was misplaced. What happened to the money should then flash into consciousness.

Result: It worked.

The priest had hidden the money in the light fixture of his room because he didn't want his housekeeper to get a hold of it. (Was he copying the excellent movie *Lost Weekend*?)

The priest's brain hid the money while under the influence of alcohol. Getting the brain under the influence again helped facilitate recall. Multiple other examples could be given about state-dependent learning. This is a very important item to add to your knowledge of human memory, so pay attention.

State-Dependent Learning Is Real and Really Important

Astronauts who have, while on Earth in one-G gravity, performed the same task over 100,000 times often can't even recall how to start the task when they are in free fall simulating zero-G in space.

How come?

Answer: The brain of the astronauts is not in the same physical state or chemical state in space that it was on Earth. Therefore, recall will be impaired.

Astronauts who Overlearned a specific task in space (that is, in free fall simulating Zero-G) can't recall it so well when they get back to earth. But when they go back in space, they know it.

How come?

Brain recall is state-dependent, and the more closely the recall situation resembles the situation during learning, the better the chance of recall.

Divers who learn a task while they are underwater have trouble recalling the task while they are on land. But when back underwater, they can recall the task without apparent effort. Ditto the reverse: What's learned on land, they have trouble remembering during the dive.

Tell why this is true.

Think about an actor who prepared at home to play Othello. Now he is on stage blinded by footlights, headlights, spotlights, shadow lights, and intimidated by the presence of an audience and the other actors. That actor's brain will need to adjust to the new surroundings and a different situation. Since the law of state-dependent learning has been violated, the highly sensitive subconscious mind will not function normally. It may become confused and break down.

Margaret, a seasoned tap dancer, suffered loss of her memory for one tap routine that she knew so well. The apparent loss of memory occurred when she put on her new tap shoes to do *Tea for Two* on a different wood floor in front of a vast new audience. Very interesting that even a slight alteration may adversely affect recall. The confusion cleared, and her memory returned when she put on her old shoes. Eventually, she relearned the tap dance in the new shoes, and all was well. You will notice that minor deviations in brain state will cause problems if the overly learned task is complex. You played *Fur Elise* perfectly today but don't be surprised if there are problems tomorrow. Some things tomorrow will be different than they were today, and that may affect recall and performance.

My experience with *The Promenade in Pictures at an Exhibition* by Modeste Moussorgsky is a case in point. After months of work, I was able to play this piece without apparent effort, almost automatically, and did play it hundreds of times without difficulty. One day, I had serious acid indigestion. Surprise! No matter how much I tried, I couldn't get things right. The next day, when I felt normal, there was no problem. The indigestion put my brain in a different state from the state during which I usually play this piece, and that different state did not have the memory down pat.

An Example of State-Dependent Learning from a Classic Novel

Willkie Collins wrote a wonderful novel where the plot structure revolves around state-dependent memory. The main character spends most of his time looking for the thief who stole a precious gem. When the main character came under the influence of opium a second time, he discovered, much to his chagrin, that he himself had stolen the gem while he had been under the influence of the opium the first time. Naturally, under the influence of the opium, he also remembered, at the time he stole it, that he gave the gem to someone in the hallway, but he couldn't recall who that person was. The plot structure of *Moonstone* makes sense in terms of what we know about state-dependent learning. There are many other examples of state-dependent learning, many from situations and problems of performance in music, art, sports, surgery, theater, airplane piloting, and so forth. See if you can discover state-dependent effects in your own life. Control these effects as best you can to improve your performance.

Think about this: A drunk driver is a poor driver. Why? Is his brain in a different state? Would that affect his performance? You bet. How about a sleep-deprived intern at a teaching hospital? Studies show the more sleep they need, the worse their medical judgment.

What Does State-Dependent Learning Mean in Relation to Music Memory And Performance?

State-dependent learning means that for maximally effective recall, the brain must be in the same physical state or a state that is similar or reasonably similar to the state it was in during the actual learning process. Otherwise, there may be problems. Also, it is a good idea to store your memorized music piece in both your conscious and subconscious mind. Traditionally, memorizing music is done by playing through a piece repeatedly until it becomes automatic. Musicians who practice this method rarely attempt to put the music also into their conscious mind or awake mind. Thus, the music exists in the artistic and expressive part of the motor brain and is subconscious. During a performance, when the pressure on the musician is great, it might be difficult to stay subconscious, where the music was memorized. If the brain shifts to the other state—the conscious state—where the music is not located, the performer will think he/she has gone "blank." He/she will think that they have gone blank because (what else?) they have gone blank.

State-Dependent Learning Is Real and Really Important

The other take-home message about state-dependent learning is that practice conditions should match performance conditions as much as possible, and multiple encoding of the same items should be done under different conditions.

Multiple Encoding in Many Different States Helps Prevent Performance Blank Out

The brain in performance should be in the same state as it was during the learning state. To correctly simulate the performance state requires lots of work with lots of attention and focus. Most performance will benefit from simulated performance before a group to try to duplicate the setting of recital. Wearing the same clothes that you intend to wear for the recital and having the same chemical brain state would also help. For instance, if you learned your piano piece, your poem, or speech and practiced it most mornings at 10 AM after you drank two cups of coffee at 8, then your best performance would be under the same exact conditions 10 AM and two hours post two cups of coffee. If the recital will use a real piano, practice on a real piano and not on a keyboard, and so forth. Pay as much attention to your performance during rehearsal as you would during performance. At your rehearsal and at your performance, no one should be listening more attentively to the music you are playing than yourself; no one should be listening to your recital of McCrae's poem more attentively than yourself. No one should be monitoring your golfing performance more than yourself. It's hard to understand why this is necessary for superlative performance, but if you would just try some memory task using that approach, you will notice a great benefit. Focused attention and duplication of playback conditions do count; sometimes, they count a lot.

Anxiety and stage fright alter brain chemistry and electrical activity of the brain, often placing the brain in a state different from the brain's state during practice. Thus, during anxiety, playback conditions differ from learning conditions. Consequently, there may be trouble.

Some of the recital, poem reproduction, job interview, and other memory difficulties stem from anxiety changing the brain's chemical state such that the brain's condition during performance no longer matches the brain's condition during learning. Hence, inexperienced pianists are often surprised that during recital, they flub the piece they did so well so many times at home. Amateur poets are surprised when their recitation flops. The tyro politician forgets plank three on his platform. The treatment for these things varies.

How to Cope with Fear (Also Known as Performance Anxiety)

Experience helps calm recital and public speaking fears. Good teachers teach how to avoid performance anxiety. Overlearning of the task also helps. The reason good Catholics can recite the prayer *Hail, Mary full of Grace* is they have literally recited it over 100,000 times. In fact, they can and do recite it automatically while not thinking of it. In fact, they can recite it while the mind is mindlessly a million miles away thinking of something else. They can recite it when they are sick or when they are well. They can recite it when they are driving a car or taking a bath. They have practiced it so much under so many different circumstances that they can recite it without actually thinking.

Some years ago, I took a course called *Elements of Moral Philosophy.* It was the most boring course imaginable. Two years after the course was over, I met, at a cocktail party, the professor who taught the course.

"You know, Professor X," I said to him. "Your course was so boring, I firmly believe that five minutes after you started your lecture, you were the only one paying attention to what you were saying. The rest of the class was thinking of something else."

Says he: "Oh no, Patten. You're wrong! I wasn't there either. After teaching that course so many years, I have trained myself to give the lecture while thinking of other things, usually what I was going to do after class was over, like take my wife to dinner, or take the car in for service. Things like that."

No wonder this professor was so boring. He was himself bored with his lecture. His lecture occupied a space in his mind similar to the space occupied by the *Hail Mary* in the minds of some Catholics.

Really Important Things Should Be Encoded under Multiple Brain Conditions to Ensure Effective Readout During Playback

Learning under multiple conditions of brain function will also help. Repeat the task when tired, when wired from too much coffee, when unhappy, and when elated. Repeat whenever you can before whatever audience you can drum up. Repeat at different times of the day and night. Try to encode the information sequences at several levels of brain states and conditions. That way, you will have stored McCrae's poem in many different brain states in many different brain areas, and you will have increased your chance of correct readout from the long-term memory no matter what the environmental conditions or situation.

MENTAL MAKING MIGHT

Pause to Take a Lesson from Public Speakers

Experienced public speakers will actually visit the venue of their speech time ahead and check out the lighting, acoustics, podium position, slide projector, and so forth. They will also deliver their entire talk with slides to make sure their brain is familiar with the performance setting and all the technical stuff is working. This review technique is called "rehearsal." Rehearsal is a form of scripting in which we go through the expected events and use that frame to augment our memories.

Scripts

We get scripts in many ways, and many scripts are acquired almost automatically by experience and repetition. A script for eating out at a restaurant, for instance, would include entering the restaurant, taking a seat, reading the menu, ordering, eating, and then asking for the check. Going to the bathroom or examining the quality of wood in the chair would not be part of the eating-out script. Job training often consists of scripts to help the new hire learn how to do the job. If you know in advance the plot and characters in the movie you are about to see, you will better recall the movie than you would have if you did not know such things. Shakespeare, in the prologue to *Romeo and Juliet*, tells exactly what to expect from the play. This device (explaining the plot in advance) makes the play much more memorable. Lawyers use opening arguments to preview their case for the jury to help the jury follow events that follow in the trial and to help the jury remember their side of the story. Children were divided into two equal groups. One group was told what to expect from the visit to the zoo about to occur, and the other group was not so informed. The group that received the preview script recalled much more and much more vivid detail of the visit than the group that did not receive the script.

Experienced public speakers will not only know their talk by heart; they will have memorized the proper tone, facial expression, body language, pace, style, and tempo of the talk. They will have a clear vision of the aim and purpose of the talk, the mood and the reason for the content, and the character of the audience. They will know the material so well and will have rehearsed it so much that the whole performance will appear natural, relaxed, spontaneous, and even extemporaneous. They will know in advance as much as possible who will introduce them, when, and how.

Let's Pause for a Story about Memory Failure and Success in Public Speaking

At a Veterans Day ceremony, a nine-year-old student was supposed to recite the famous poem *In Flanders Fields* by Lieutenant Colonel John McCrae, MD.

The Master of Ceremonies introduced the lad, who came to the podium, looked over the eager faces in the audience: then he paused for 20 seconds, made a face that expressed horror, and said in a panic, "I forgot my poem."

It was a sad scene. This boy had probably recited that poem hundreds of times at home. What he may have needed was the first line of the poem, which he could have easily read from the program as the title of the poem begins the first line. After that first line, automatic memory would have possibly carried him through. But we will never know. They didn't give him a second chance. They pulled him off.

Another boy, about the same age (nine or ten), who had just finished reciting Lincoln's *Gettysburg Address,* stepped forward, volunteered to fill in, and flawlessly recited McCrae's poem.

Wow! What a demonstration. It turned out that the other boy, the one who did both recitations, had, over a seven-month period, practiced both Lincoln's Address and In Flanders Fields literally thousands of times. That boy's great-uncle (who at the time was a state senator) trained the boy to recite both the address and the poem. The Senator had reasoned that the kid doing Flanders might clutch, in which case the Senator's nephew could step right in. And that is exactly what happened.

Question: Why in the world am I telling you this story?

Question: What in the world does recital of an Address or a Poem have to do with memorizing?

Stop for two minutes. Put your feet up on the desk or go get a drink of water or cup of tea or pace the floor. Think up answers to the questions. Then compare your answers to what is written below.

You were told the story because we like stories, and we think stories teach great lessons, especially when the stories are true. The lessons apply to memory because that's what recitals are—a reproduction from memory. Poetry recitals and public speaking and music performances are similar; each is based on considerable memory. The features they share are:

1. They involve musical instruments. In one case, the human voice, which is a string instrument that is activated by human breath. In the other case, the musical instrument is the piano (or such like) which is a string instrument activated by hammers hitting the strings.

2. Both recitation and recital are in public places in front of an audience, and both require memory and not only direct, intelligent expression of meaning but also expression of emotion. People who read their poem or their speech are far less effective than they could have been.

3. We learn what is correct by knowing what is not correct. In the case of the boy who failed, we learn that better preparation might have helped. And it is an acknowledged fact that better preparation would save lots of music recitals as well. We think the boy who failed might have been cued or clued by the first lines of the poem. Knowing the first notes of your music will set you on the right track. It is an acknowledged fact that if you don't know where to start, you will have trouble starting. And if you

can't start, you sure as hell can't finish. We also understand that the brain of the boy who failed was in a different chemical state from the state in which his brain had encoded the poem. Review the sections on state-dependent learning if you feel vague on how this applies to music recital or poetry, or public speaking. Thus, the boy who failed probably failed for many reasons, among which was stage fright and inadequate preparation.

4. We learn what is correct by copying the success of what is correct and the methods used to get to that success. In the case of the boy who flawlessly recited the address and the poem, we learned that there was an enormous amount of preparation involved, much more than anyone would have imagined. According to the senator uncle, the practice sessions were always done in front of a mirror so that the boy himself could see his performance. The uncle would correct body posture, hand gestures, facial expressions, tone, tempo, pace, syntax, diction, and so forth. In other words, the preparation for recitation was on a high, almost professional level. We also saw how an experienced public speaker like the Senator could predict with remarkable accuracy the likely failure of a young and very inexperienced speaker who would be set before an assembled multitude the likes of which that boy had never seen before or imagined. There were 1,000+ people in the audience that day.

Senatorial Overkill?

Furthermore, in order to train the nephew to control stage fright, the senator arranged for the nephew to do the recitation before several different audiences, including the Chamber of Commerce and the Elk's Club. The senator asked the school principal at the nephew's elementary school, New York City public school 109, to arrange for the recitation to take place before a general assembly of students and teachers. That happened also. In addition, on the day before Veterans Day, the senator and the nephew visited the venue where the recitation was to take place. The venue was a large public park, and the men had already put up a platform that would overlook the assembled crowd. The nephew did a recital from that platform. And, get this (this should really impress you), the senator inquired as to where the ceremony might take place in the event of rain. The senator and the nephew then went to the Queens theater, the rain venue, two blocks away, and recited the two items from the stage of the dark and empty theater.

On Veterans Day, the rain started just as the *Gettysburg Address* was to go on. The announcement was made about the change in venue, and a half-hour later, the program started again, this time inside the theater where the nephew had rehearsed the day before.

Was this overkill? In a certain sense, it was. But in another sense, it wasn't. The Senator was training the nephew to become an accomplished public speaker. The recitation preparation was a preparation, not just for this event on Veterans Day, but also for a lifetime of political activity that the Senator had envisioned for his nephew. The Senator knew the value of over preparation and the value of practicing as close as possible to performance conditions.

Remember: Practice should simulate playback conditions as closely as possible. If a phrase is meant to be soft, why practice it loudly? To play softly is not easy because it requires strict control of motor habits. Why should a melody be practiced as a succession of even notes if the composer intended it to sing with varied tones above a soft accompaniment? If a passage has four notes to the beat, why rehearse in triplets? Apart from these considerations, expression is a great help to the memory. Actors with the best memory for words are those who concentrate on their meaning, associating expression through voice and gesture. They also master the emotions expressed and the personality of their character. You should do the same.

Sometimes, Even Experienced Performers Need Tricks

If tricks are needed, experienced performers will use them. In 1926, George and Ira Gershwin mounted a show called *Oh, Kay!*, with Kay played by a frail and not-altogether-confident Gertrude Lawrence. Although *Oh, Kay!* was fluff, it produced one of Gershwin's greatest songs, *Someone to Watch Over Me*. Lawrence was too nervous to effectively deliver *Someone to Watch Over Me* before the large audience. George Gershwin saved the song from being dropped from the show by instructing Lawrence to sing it to a sad-looking doll instead of to the audience. Forget the audience and sing to the doll. The original presentation of the song brought boos. The new presentation with the doll as ploy brought standing ovations. The trick was that by singing directly to the doll, Lawrence was able to screen out the audience and concentrate her full attention, heart, and soul on the performance. By concentrating on singing for the doll, Lawrence was able to achieve beauty, something that had been lacking when she sang directly to the audience.

Friends, those of you who suffer stage fright, despair not. There's hope. Three decades later, Gertrude Lawrence played the female lead in Rogers and Hammerstein's *The King and I*.

Denial as a Mental Mechanism to Get You Through

Some pianists handle the stage fright problem in the same way that Lawrence did. They concentrate completely on the piece and thereby mentally isolate themselves from everything else in this wide world, including the audience. What works for them might work for you.

Other Tricks

The Norwegian composer, pianist, and conductor Edvard Grieg controlled his anxieties by carrying with him three mascots: a red troll, a pig with a four-leaf clover in its mouth, and Grieg's lucky frog. Grieg's favorite was the frog, which he carried in his coat pocket when he conducted or performed. Before stepping onto the stage, he would put his hand in his pocket and rub his lucky frog. And he always had the troll and the pig on his bedside table. According to Nina, his wife, he always said, "Good night" to them.

Leopold Bloom, in James Joyce's novel *Ulysses,* won't leave his house without touching the potato in his pocket and saying to himself, "Potato I have." For the Irish, the potato is a luck charm the way a rabbit foot is for others, or a miniature Shinto shrine is for Japanese students about to take an exam. The best thing you can say to an Irishman is, "Good luck to you." The worse thing you can say to an Irishman is "Bad luck to you." Good luck. Bad luck. Who knows? The point is if they believe the potato will get them through, it probably will help.

Pause for a Brief Sidebar about Lesson Jitters:

Lessons jitters are similar to and different from stage jitters. How many times have you been able to play a piece straight through from memory at home or sing a song well at home and yet failed rather quickly during your lesson with the teacher or at that dinner party? How many times have you recited a poem at home perfectly and yet failed when in class? How many times have you discussed an important political issue with your family but bungled it badly in front of a larger audience? If that problem doesn't sound familiar to you, you haven't taken enough lessons or memorized enough, or done enough public speaking.

My explanation for this commonly experienced phenomenon is threefold.

First, there might be the state-dependent effect because, after all, practice alone and play before the teacher or performance in a different place are two different things. In the same way, speaking before friends and family and public speaking are two different things. And two different things will have two different brain states.

Second, perhaps, there is the element of fear and anxiety in the lesson situation. Many people also experience fear and anxiety when speaking before an audience. Certainly, fear and anxiety play a role early on, but as time goes by, most students love their teacher and have little fear. And most experienced public speakers have no fear or anxiety whatsoever.

Third, in this setting, under the scrutiny of the teacher or under the observation of the audience, there are interruptions of the motor sequence. The usual scenario in a music lesson is that the student starts to play and the teacher notices a wrong finger, a misplaced note, wrong rhythm, or some mistake, or the teacher tries to steady the pulse of the music by playing in a higher register or playing on another piano or even humming or singing. In other words—the student is interrupted with the aim of improving the situation. But the motor sequence is broken in the process, and the addition of new and different sounds makes the performance flummoxed.

Interruption—I hate it because it throws me off, and to avoid interruption, I tell my teacher not to interrupt. "Let me get through it, and then you correct what's wrong."

But the thing that has most often fouled up my playing in recitals and in lesson is the break in the circuit caused not by my teacher but by my own thinking too much about my wonderful performance and how well I have been doing so far into it.

I have seen some very accomplished and experienced public speakers get unglued by a rude question from the audience or other such interruption. I have seen speakers lose their sang-froid when their joke falls flat. The subsequent confusion is pitiable.

Avoid interruptions by telling the audience at the beginning of your talk that you will welcome comments, suggestions, and questions at the end.

When your joke falls flat, think nothing of it; just step over the fallen joke and move on. It's no big deal. Some comedians will make a joke of the joke that fell flat by saying something like, "Jesus, my wife told me that no one would laugh at that one."

"A man entered a bar with a piece of concrete under his left arm and said: Joe, make it one for me and one for the road." No laughs? The trained stand-up comic just hunches shoulders and tells another: "Two men walked into a bar. The third saw it and ducked." No laughs? He hunches and tells another: "A man at the bar started screaming 'Lawyers are assholes.' A drunk in the back stumbled to the bar, tapped the guy on the shoulder, and said, 'I have serious objections to what you just said.' 'Why, Sir? Are you a lawyer?' 'No, I'm an asshole.'"

Interruptions Destroy Sequence and Damage Memory. Avoid Them like the plague.

Tell the Gong-Qi master you wish to do the moves through to the end no matter what. "After I finish, there will be time for corrections."

The real damage of interrupting student practice for recitations is that the student has not been permitted the freedom to try to get through to the end. The student has not been permitted even the semblance of a partial success. Failure to succeed is a serious problem and is often the root cause of future failures, which, not surprisingly, will often occur at the exact place where the teacher interrupted the playback. In general, failure breeds failure. The reverse is also true: success breeds success.

Practice Playing from Memory Should Simulate Playing from Memory Conditions in Every Way, Including NO INTERRUPTIONS

When the student is asked to play their piece in the studio, they should not be interrupted. They should play through as best they can. Then, and only then, should the teacher go over the mistakes one by one.

1. This policy will build confidence because the student will have proven to himself/herself that they can get through the piece because, after all, they did. They may not have been note-perfect or rhythm perfect or fingering perfect or perfect in any way, but they did get through. Anyway, few human things are perfect. General George S. Patton said, "A good plan today is better than a perfect plan tomorrow."

2. This policy of letting the student play through will give the student excellent practice in how to cover mistakes and continue on. Covering mistakes can make a gigantic difference in how the audience perceives the performance. Multiple techniques can cover. Become an expert at covering mistakes because you will make lots of them. In general, it is much better to cover mistakes or disregard them than to stop or shake your head "no" or to apologize for the errors.

Repeat: NO excuses! NO apologies! NO stopping! Continue on as if everything is OK. Better yet, smile and continue on. If you are smiling and look happy, the audience will think that everything is OK. Most of the audience will be half asleep anyway, so don't worry about your mistakes, and most of them won't know you made a mistake, and if they did know, most of them wouldn't care.

General Rule: Do Not Start Again

Starting again is an admission of error and is sometimes interpreted by the audience as a discourtesy. It is often better to continue on than pause and start again.

Furthermore, starting again doesn't guarantee success, and indeed starting again may result in the same failure at the same place, a blackout, which is usually due to too much reliance on kinesthetic memory (to be discussed later) and not enough on intellectual memory (to be discussed later).

Rather than start again, preplan a place ahead of the trouble spot so that you can jump over the trouble spot and land on the prefigured place of rescue. In poetry recitation, skip ahead to the next line or the next paragraph or even the next idea that you really know. If you don't hesitate, if you don't seem to have missed something, the audience usually will not know something is wrong. If you do stop and try again, or hesitate, or hit your head and say I forgot my poem—something stupid like that, then they will know for sure that something is amiss. Try to keep with the spirit, tone, and feelings of the poem so that your fumble remains concealed.

In your rehearsals, have multiple spots in the musical piece, poem, or speech you can skip ahead to. But don't tell your teachers I said you can skip ahead: Here now, for the record (and only for the record), I advise you really should not skip anything. But, you know, this is an imperfect world, and desperate situations call for desperate measures. If you do blank-out, skip ahead to the part you know, your lifesaver. These spots are called lifesavers as their employ does seem to save the performance from looking bad. Was it not Franz Liszt who said, "Never mind the wrong notes—Play!"

Memory Is Modality and Task-specific

Item 12: Memory and learning are task-specific. If you wish to learn touch typing, it is unlikely a course in auto mechanics will help you. Though, anything you learn will tend to help prepare your brain for other new learning. Thus, a course in auto mechanics will tend to help you learn touch typing. It will help, but not that much. Touch typing results will be world's better if and only if you study touch typing. By the same token, studying French won't do much for your algebra grade. Old Chinese motto: Want bean? Plant bean. Want corn? Plant corn.

Focus your attention on the things that count, and focus your attention away from the things that won't count much. The problem is most people don't have the foggiest idea of what they want for themselves and therefore are adrift. You and you alone need to decide on what you wish to work and what you need to do to make that wish come true.

Question: With the task-specific memory principle in mind, what task should you concentrate on if you wish to become a flutist?

The Brain Sorts Items on the Basis of Similarities and Differences and Amount

Item 13: Analysis of similarities and differences enables you to make the associations that facilitate recall. Aristotle pointed out that the best way to compare things is by analysis of the similarities and differences. This is the basis of the High School English essay "compare and contrast." It is also the basis of our present scientific classification of plants and animals. The similarities are represented in the genus, and the differences are in the species. But what happens if things are exactly the same? How do we compare, then?

Again, our friend Aristotle has the answer: We compare things that are the same by measuring amount. For instance, Aristotle tells us that one talent (an ancient unit of money) is the same as another. That makes sense because we know one dollar is the same as another. So, to compare one pile of money with another, we count. By the way, Aristotle, master of those who know, gives it for his opinion that it is better to have more money than less. Most of us would agree. But talking about money reminds one about spending. (Notice how the brain associates money with spending.) The idea of spending reminds us that we are spending time on similarities and differences and amounts because those are the analytic tools that give us a handle on the associations that will facilitate specific recall of memorized passages in memorized material, especially pieces of music, dance routines, car invoices, grandchildren's birthdays, and other material things like that that have similarities and differences.

Mental Gymnastic—Similarities and Differences and Pattern Recognition

Problem: Using Aristotle's method of comparing and contrasting by doing an analysis of similarities and differences, work your right brain on pattern extraction by completing the following sequences.

1. 1 3 5 7 __
2. AB CE CD EG EF G_
3. blowhard hardhat hatcheck _____mate
4. toner tone ton __
5. stone tone ton __
6. astray stray tray ___
7. snit in snot on prod or mode __
8. bib bib ton, not 399 993 pin ___
9. din don fan fen pep pip cod ___
10. 289735 897352 973528 735289 _____
11. stops _____ top to
12. polygram 12345678 pray 1674 ploy _____
13. gum gun bar bat sun sup lip ___
14. hole pit seed kick punt boat edge shore strengthen hurt _____ clever
15. bird crane stretch sprint run snag lozenge mint new note _____ beak
16. 7913 992 488 569 72155 614_
17. Q O M K I _
18. A E I O _
19. JK KJ LM IH NO G_
20. retire rite strafe fart inept pen peruse _____

Norms: Age 20–39: 8–12 correct = average; 13–16 correct = above average; 17–18 correct = superior; 19–20 correct = gifted

Age 40–59 6–10 correct = average; 11–15 correct = above average; 16–18 correct = superior; 19–20 correct = gifted

Age 60–79 4–6 correct = average; 7–10 correct = above average; 11–17 correct = superior; 18–20 correct = gifted

Stop! Did you do the mental gymnastic?

If not, please go do it.

If you did do the gymnastic, good for you.

Here's how I worked the problems. Answers other than the ones I gave might be OK. Your realization and approach may differ from mine. In fact, I am sure it will. It has to. You are you, and I am me. If you didn't get the same result as I did, don't worry. The answer is not important. It is the mental work to get to the answer that builds mental might. The brain benefits from doing work. Rewards for correct answers are nice but are nowhere as important as mental work in building brainpower.

1.   1 3 5 7 _

Ask questions. Asking yourself questions is the best approach to solving any problem. In what way are 1 and 3 similar to each other?

They are both numbers. They both are odd numbers.

In what way are 1 and 3 different from each other?

3 is 2 bigger than 1. If you add 2 to 1, you get 3.

What is the pattern? Now formulate a hypothesis about the sequence. In this case, the hypothesis might be that this is the sequence of odd numbers. Or that this is a sequence of progressively increasing numbers, starting at number 1, that are made bigger by adding 2?

Now test the hypothesis. If this is the sequence of odd numbers, then the next number after 3 should be 5, and the number after that should be 7. As 5 and 7 are, in fact, the next two numbers, the hypothesis appears to be confirmed, and the next number in the sequence should be 9. If we apply the add 2 to each number hypothesis, we get the same result. The answer is 9.

2.   AB CE CD EG EF G_

Remember the drill? Ask yourself questions. It is not enough to just stare at the problem and hope the answer will appear. You need to think. And you should think. What is this about, and why are we working out our brains? We are training our brains to think. So, ask yourself a question. How are AB and CD similar?

They both are groups of two capital letters. Both are in alphabetic order, with the second letter appearing later in the alphabet than the first letter.

How do the two groups of capital letters differ? The first two letters AB are in the exact sequence in the alphabet, with B following directly after the A. The second group of two letters, CE, is also in order, but the D, which is between C and E, has been left out.

How do the second two letters relate to the first? Answer: The first letter of the second group is the next letter in the alphabet after the last letter in the first group. Test this idea on the CD EG that follows. Does it work? Yes, E is the next letter after CD.

What is the pattern? Formulate a hypothesis, really a kind of guess about what's what, and then test the hypothesis. In this case, the hypothesis might be that this is a progression of capital letters that consists of two sets of two letters each. The first set is the exact order in the alphabet, and the second is the next letter after the last letter in the first set followed by the next letter plus one, that is, a skip is present. Test this hypothesis on CD EG. Does it work? Probably. EG has, in fact, skipped F.

Another hypothesis could be that this is a sequence of capital letters which consists of two letters in exact sequence followed by three letters in exact sequence from which the middle letter has been extracted. Because the middle letter has been extracted, it becomes necessary to make reparations by making the next two-letter sequence using the first letter of the second group of two letters and adding the omitted letter. This, of course, sounds stupid, but it is a possible narrative way of solving the problem if you don't immediately see the pattern presented. Such narrations will become necessary for you to solve some of the other sequences, so why not consider this narration among other explanations of the pattern? Always test the strength of the narrative solution against the actual data in the problem. If and when your narrations fails, go back and think of something different.

Another possible hypothesis is that the whole display is the exact order of letters in the alphabet in the odd number groups. Thus, group one is AB, group three is CD, and group five is EF. In the even number groups, the letter that usually follows the first letter in the group is omitted in favor of the next letter, and each even number group starts with the last letter of the preceding even group. Thus, the even number group CE would give rise to the next even group EG, which in turn would give rise to the last even group GI (remember to omit the letter that usually follows G). The answer to item 2 by systematic analysis turns out to be I. And not H!

Whatever works is OK.

My favorite for this item is to look at them as three separate groups of four letters. The first group is ABC skip D and get E, The second group is CDE skip F and get G, and therefore the last group has to be EFG skip H and get I. Sometimes just rearranging things and looking at the problem in a slightly different light will solve the item quite easily. Notice this last solution is easy to recall because it involves using the exact sequence of letters in the alphabet for the first three letters in the group of four and then just skips. If I gave you the next group as UVW_, you would have no trouble figuring that the next letter should be Y because you had to skip the X.

3.   blowhard hardhat hatcheck _____mate

How are blowhard and hardhat similar?

They both have the word hard.

How are they different?

The hard is the last part of blowhard and the first part of hardhat.

Any pattern?

The pattern could be: Extract an English word from the end of the first word and put that word in the front of something to make another English word to follow.

If that pattern is true, then we would predict that the end of word two (hardhat) would be the first part of word three.

Checking the hypothesis, we find that hat is the end of hardhat, and hat has becomes the first part of word three, which is hatcheck.

Applying the solution to the hatcheck _____mate, we find the end of hatcheck is an English word, namely "check," and putting check in front of mate gives us another English word checkmate. Check is the answer. Nothing else will do.

4.   toner tone ton __

How are toner and tone similar?

They both have the letters t-o-n-e in the same order.

How are toner and tone different?

Toner has one more letter, an r.

Any pattern?

One hypothesis might be to just remove the last letter of the preceding word to get the next word.

Testing: Removing the last letter of tone would give ton, which is, in fact, the next word in the sequence. Therefore, the hypothesis appears correct. Applying this idea, we remove the n from ton and get the answer to item 4: To. This looks like a nice arrangement (some would say sequence) of five letters, then four letters, then three letters, then two. Very satisfying! To is correct. Nothing else will do.

5.   stone tone ton ____

How are stone and tone similar?

Both share the letters t-o-n-e.

How are they different?

The tone has one less letter than the preceding word. In this case, the omitted letter was the first letter of the preceding word.

Any pattern?

The hypothesis is that removing the first letter of the preceding word will give the next word in the sequence.

Testing the hypothesis: We remove the t from tone and get one. But the next word in the sequence is not one. It is ton, so it appears that we must revise the hypothesis. Perhaps the hypothesis that we first remove the first letter and then remove the last letter. If that is true, then the second word would be tone, and the third word would be ton, which it is.

Now what? If we follow the sequence, the next word should have the first letter removed, and that would give us the answer as on.

Another way of looking at this is that the removal of the first or the last letter is a random event. In that case, the answer on or to would be acceptable with the on due to the removal of the first letter and the to being due to the removal of the

99

last letter. This last solution seems better to me as it reflects some of the entropy and chaos inherent in the universe, where random events often do play major roles. But I would bet whoever made up this item actually had on in mind as the desired answer.

6.   astray stray tray _____

This looks like the same problem as item 4. Therefore, the same reasoning might apply, in which case the answer is ray.

7.   snit in snot on prod or mode __

Similarities? Snit and in both have the letters in.

Differences? Snit has four letters. In has two letters. The order of the letters is reversed: It is n-i in snit and i-n in in.

Pattern? Looks like the pattern is a four-letter word followed by a two-letter word with the two letters in the two-letter word the reverse of the order in the four-letter word.

Test? If the hypothesis about the pattern is true then snot should be followed by on, which it is. And prod should be followed by or, which it is. Therefore, mode should be followed by do.

Note to you: It is my considered opinion that you will benefit greatly if you first think about the problem and try to get the answer yourself before looking at the answer displayed in the text. Your mental work builds brainpower. Mental laziness does not build brainpower.

8.   bib bib ton, not 399 993 pin ____

Similarities? Bib and bib are the same.

Differences? None

Pattern? Perhaps the exact repetition.

Test? Nope. This does not work. The exact repetition of ton should be ton. But it isn't. It is not. Ho ho. This is interesting and leads us to consider that the pattern is a reading backward of the first word. If that is the pattern, bib would still be bib, but ton would be not. Applying the alternative hypothesis to set three 399 read backward should be 993. Bingo. That is correct. Applying this to pin, we get nip. Nip is the answer.

9.   din don fan fen pep pip cod ____

Similarities? Din and don are three-letter words that share the letters d and n.

Differences? Din has an i, and don has an o.

Pattern? Take the middle letter out and substitute the next vowel in the alphabet.

Test? If the hypothesis works, fan should become fen, which it does. Pep should become pip, which it does, and therefore, cod had to become cud.

10.   289735 897352 973528 735289 _____

At first glance, this item looks difficult. Let's put on our thinking caps and stick to the program, examining similarities and differences. Try to detect a pattern, for that is what this gymnastic is trying to train you to do. The detection of a pattern greatly facilitates memory. So always do your best to detect a pattern. If you can't find a pattern based in some aspect of the real world, then use your imagination and make up a pattern that will exist (only) in the real world of your mind. For instance, memorize this number: 17761812186519191941. Unless you see the pattern, it will take some time to get this 20-digit number into your memory.

See the pattern? Even if you didn't see a pattern, even if a pattern doesn't exist exactly, imagine that this is a list of the years of major wars starting with the American Revolution of 1776 progressing to the War of 1812 and then the Civil War 1865, World War One 1919 and World War Two 1941. Study the numbers again for a minute and then write them on a sheet of paper. Pretty easy, right. I got them right even though the Civil War ended in 1865 and World War Two ended in 1945. When you have a pattern, associations that relate to the pattern, and can chunk a memory task, you are way, way ahead of the power curve. Later we will work on chunking techniques, and very soon, we will work on association techniques. For the nonce, let's stick to training our pattern recognition skills. We are looking for patterns, and we are working on finding similarities and differences that will help our understanding.

289735 897352

Similarities? Both are numbers, the exact same numbers.

Differences? The numbers are in the same order, except the second number of the number pair has the first digit of the first number placed at the end, thus making the eight the first digit of the second number.

Pattern? Take the first digit of the first number and put it at the end, and that will leave the second number.

Test? If that is true, then 897352 will become 973528, which it does; 973528 should become 735289, which it does. This means 735289 should become 352897.

11.   stops _____ top to

Similarities? All the words have letters that are present in stops.

Differences? Top has three letters and to has two. Stops has five letters, and the blank might have four to make a nice progression of loss of one letter each time we move to the right. So the problem devolves to finding what four-letter word is most appropriate. Not an easy problem.

Pattern? A reasonable hypothesis is that we lose a letter as we move to the right. If top to is the example, then it is the end letter that is eliminated.

Test? Take the end s from stops to get stop and then take the last letter from stop to get sto—ugh! The word we should get is top. So that hypothesis doesn't work. OK. How about we take the first letter from stops to get tops, then the last letter from tops to get top. Then the first letter again giving op. Ugh again! That doesn't work either. So maybe the idea is to eliminate the letter that allows the next word to be a real English word. Therefore, stops could go to stop or tops. But the s has to come off stop to get top, which is a given. And the p comes off the top to get to—also given. Conclusion: Correct word is not stop, but tops, and the correct sequence is stops→tops→top→to. Got any other ideas? Write me.

12. polygram 12345678 pray 1674 ploy _____

Similarities? Both the word polygram and the number displayed occupy 8 places or positions.

Differences? Polygram is a word with the letters not in alphabetic order; the other is a set of numbers in order from 1 to 8.

Pattern? Could the letters correspond to the numbers as a kind of code. If that were true, then p would be 1 and o would be 2 and so forth. Using such a code, we could translate letters to numbers and vice versa. When we get to the memory-heavy chapter wherein you will learn how to memorize a 50-digit number and all the presidents of the United States in or out of order, you will see how important the ability to convert numbers to letters is. Such a conversion table lets you convert the number to letters, and then you can convert the letters to words and the words to pictures and store the item to be remembered as a picture for easy recall. For instance, the 13th president of the United States is Millard Fillmore. There is no logical connection between the number 13 and Fillmore. That Millard Fillmore was the 13th president is an accident of history. It is not logical that his name is connected to 13. We need a way of connecting the two items (13 and Fillmore) in an illogical way. My idea is to take the 3 and turn it on its side, giving the 13 a 1m. The upright 1 reminds me of a t. The 3 turned down looks like an m. Therefore, I now have tm. That sound suggests a tomb. I see myself driving up to a gas station in a tomb and asking the boy to fill the tank—fill it more. Fill it more reminds me of Fillmore. All this may sound shockingly bizarre, but when we get to memory heavy and the Ancient Art of Memory it will be made clear and useful. Plus, this is the easy and sure-fire way of remembering Fillmore was the 13th president.

Therefore, the code

Polygram

12345678

To decode pray: p is 1; r is 6; a is 7; y is 4. So the number corresponding to pray should be 1674, which is correct. So ploy is 1324.

13. gum gun bar bat sun sup lip _____

Similarities? gum and gun both have three letters. They share the first two letters.

Differences? The last letter is different and makes a different word.

Pattern? There are lots of possibilities, but since n comes right after m, perhaps the process is to take off the last letter of the first word and add the next letter in the alphabet to the stem formed by the first two letters. That makes sense, and gum would become gun as given.

Test? Bar and bat. Taking the last letter off and adding the next letter after r, we get bas, which is wrong. So that hypothesis is wrong. The stem is ba, but the s has been skipped to get bat. The letter was t, so perhaps the pattern is in the second set to skip a letter. In that case, we would get bat, which is given. Applying the new hypothesis to sun sup gives skip o and the word suo, which is wrong. But skipping o would give sup, which is given. The pattern might be to gradually increase the skip. First no skip, then one skip, then one skip, and then? Skipping three letters (qrs), we get t, and the answer would be lit, a nice solid English word. Skipping just one letter assuming the pattern is no skip, skip one, skip one, skip one would give lir, which means "sea" in old Irish. This pattern is not as satisfying as the no skip, one skip, two skip, three skip progression, but what can we do? We have to go by the givens. Ugh! Not really satisfactory. Perhaps the pattern is more abstract or simpler. Perhaps the idea is just skip whatever doesn't make a good common solid English word and land on a letter that does make a good solid English word. Using this hypothesis, the answer would be lit, and the pair is lip lit.

14.   hole pit seed kick punt boat edge shore strengthen hurt _____clever

Similarities? All are words. They seem related to each other in groups of three because the middle word of each group of three has the same meaning or can have the same meaning as the word on either side of it. Thus, a pit can be a hole and a seed; a punt can be a boat or a kick (as in football). A shore is an edge, and shore also means to strengthen, as in the expression "shore up."

Problem: We have to have a word that can mean clever or hurt. The only word I can think of is smart. Sure enough, my dictionary lists smart as an intransitive verb meaning acutely painful, and it certainly can mean clever. Sharp probably won't do because although it can mean clever, its relation to hurt is not as direct as smart.

15.   bird crane stretch sprint run snag lozenge mint new note _____ beak

16.

17.   Wow! Is it my imagination, or are things getting more difficult?

Similarities? This looks similar to item 13, where there are groups of three words, and the middle word is OK to mean the word on the right or on the left.

Thus, crane can be a bird or the verb to stretch.

Run can be a sprint or a snag as a run in a stocking.

A mint can be a lozenge, or mint can mean new.

Problem: what word can mean note or beak?

Did you come up with bill, which can be a note as in negotiable instruments or the beak of a bird? If you have a different answer that makes sense, good for you.

18.   7913 992 488 569 72155 614_

Similarities? All are numbers. They appear in groups.

Differences? One number has four digits. One has five. The rest have three.

Pattern? The first five numbers all add up to 20. I can see this at a glance, and when you have finished with chapter six on mental math, you will see it at a glance also. Or perhaps, you see it without any special training. If so, good for you.

Test? All the numbers add to 20, so the last number must do the same. For that to happen, we must add a 9. Therefore, 9 is the missing digit. No other answer is correct.

19.   Q O M K I _

Similarities? All are letters.

Differences? All are different.

Pattern? They are in reverse sequence. Q comes after O, M after K, K after I. The intervening letter is omitted from the sequence. Working backward gives K (L) M (N) O (P) Q, with the letters in ( ) missing in action. Thus, the answer must be G because that would give the series the correct form of G (H) I working backward and Q O M K I G as printed in the item. Sometimes it is important to work problems backward. Those of you who took Organic Chemistry in College know about the train of reaction question where you are given a chain of chemical reactions, and you have to predict what the product is. Working trains backward works, even on the most complex trains. Thinking of complements helps sometimes. What is the chance of rolling a six on a die cube that has six sides. Answer: 1/6. What is the chance of not rolling a six. Answer: The complement: 1 − 1/6 = 5/6.

20.   A E I O _

Similarities? All are letters, and all are vowels.

Differences? All are different vowels with no repeats.

Pattern? This is the sequence of vowels in the English alphabet. E follows A, I follows E, and so forth. So the answer is (what else?) U.

21.   JK KJ LM IH NO G_

Similarities? All letters in groups of two. Set one repeats the K with KJ in the reverse order in the alphabet. All are adjacent a companion letter.

Differences? All different, except the repeated K.

Pattern? Looks like groups of twos so that JK and KJ go together. The second element of the group of two is the reverse alphabetic order. The first element is in alphabetic order.

Hypothesis: Patterns of two. The first two letters are in correct order, and the second two are in reverse order. Check this: LM is in correct order, and IH is reverse.

So NO is in correct order, and G_ should be reversed. Therefore, the answer is F.

22.   retire rite strafe fart inept pen peruse _____

Have you noticed something? Have you noticed that you are able to see the patterns now without as much mental work? If you have noticed that you are getting better, that is, of course, the desired effect. Congratulations! And more power to you!

Similarities? All words. Groups of two with the big word coming first. The second word in each group of two has letters that are also found in the first word.

Differences? The letters in group two of the sets appear in reverse order from the letters in the first word of the set of two and spell a real English word.

Pattern? Take the first and last letters off of word one, put the remaining letters in reverse order.

Test? If the hypothesis is right, retire should become etir, which when written backward, spells rite, which is given. Taking s and e from strafe gives traf, which spelled back is fart, which is given. Take i and t from inept and get nep which spelled backward is pen, which is given. Therefore, take p and e from peruse and get erus, which spelled backward is sure.

How did you do? Check your standing against the stated norms, which are reproduced here for your convenience.

Norms:

Age 20–39: 8–12 correct = average; 13–16 correct = above average; 17–18 correct = superior; 19–20 correct = gifted

Age 40–59 6–10 correct = average; 11–15 correct = above average; 16–18 correct = superior; 19–20 correct = gifted

Age 60–79 4–6 correct = average; 7–10 correct = above average; 11–17 correct = superior; 18–20 correct = gifted

Notice the older you are, the less you need to get right to be considered normal. The reason for this is the common age-related changes in mental horsepower. Sad but true. Mental abilities usually decline with age in most people. Usually decline, however, means sometimes mental ability does not decline with age.

Cognitive Functions Most Vulnerable to Aging

Age-related changes in the brain affect memory and related operations in different ways. The changes listed usually occur but do not happen in all older persons in the same way. In some older persons, they do not appear at all.

Vulnerable Functions

Working memory: Ability to hold and manipulate information in the mind is often reduced.

Processing speed: Thinking usually gets slow, which can affect retrieval of specific information like names or addresses. It becomes hard to follow a conversation if the speaker is talking faster than usual. Processing speed gets slower, so we get less and less complete encoding, which results in a weaker memory. Slow processing also shows up in driving, where response to emergency situations may be impaired. Slow processing makes it difficult to fully appreciate classical music played fast.

Attention to detail: Older people tend to forget the details in favor of getting the big picture or the general gist. A 20-year-old looking at a picture for five minutes will recall about 50% more details than a 75-year old looking at the same picture for the same amount of time. Sad, but true. Yes, attention to detail is or can be degraded that much, and that is why the older age group must concentrate more and pay more attention longer to compensate for this age-related change.

Declarative memory: Older people have more trouble forming and expressing verbal memories. Specifically, they have more trouble remembering verbal facts such as names of places, people, and objects. Special difficulties may occur with spatial orientation to place. That's the reason for the seniors getting lost in their cars so often and having trouble finding the way back home.

Reference memory: It becomes harder to recall when or where things happened. Time especially becomes jumbled. This is referred to as source memory in some psychology circles. Older people remember they parked their car but can't recall where they parked it. They remember dinners at their favorite Italian restaurant but can't actually tell when they dined there last. They may have trouble remembering the name of the restaurant, but chances are they will recall in vivid detail the atmosphere and the food and drinks.

Multitasking: This is a particular problem when driving. Older people have trouble paying attention to a passenger talking and at the same time paying attention to the road. Playing the radio while driving in the rain will be particularly difficult. Best bet is to shut down all distractions and concentrate on one important task at a time. Safety first! In the rain, slow down to a safe speed or pull over and wait until it stops.

Visual-spatial tasks: These may be quite simple for young people, but older have trouble figuring how to unlock their car or even replace the batteries in the smoke alarm or work the email on the iPhone or computer. Many have difficulty with the remote control of the TV and have to get formal instruction from children or grandchildren. My two granddaughters (Miranova and Arden) taught me how to take a selfie.

False Memory: The older age group tends to remember falsely. This can cause serious problems and must be guarded against. For instance, if they are asked to remember the following words: bed, night table, mattress, pillow, night light, blanket, dream. When asked to recall the list, almost all will "remember" the word *sleep,* which was not on the list. Even more troublesome: They will insist *sleep* was on the list even when assured it was not. They used the other words to organize a category of things that helps them remember the words on the list. But that grouping into the category *bedtime* made them vulnerable to the false memory. This is a robust finding, meaning it is a finding easy to repeat with different participants in different places and in different study situations. Older people tend to feel quite confident about their memories of past events. But when such memories are objectively checked, the memories often prove false. Sometimes there is a dangerous extrapolation of a memory slip where the older person has forgotten where they put their wallet or their stash of money, and they will accuse others of stealing. My mother-in-law swore her nurse stole her wallet. Subsequently, the wallet was found safe and sound in the refrigerator! How it got there is still a mystery. Probably she put it there instead of some other item (candy?) that belonged in the fridge.

Cognitive Functions That Are Age Resistant

Attention: The ability to focus attention is rarely impaired. Whether they do it or not is another question.

Spoken Language: Vocabulary and ingrained rules for meaningful linguistic structure are preserved, including correct syntax and diction. In fact, the older age group usually has a larger working vocabulary than the youth, and this continues to grow as they get older and continue to read, experience things, and think.

Procedural Memory: Skills for doing things like tying shoes, riding a bike, swimming, or playing the piano remain largely intact over the life span. In addition, the ability to learn a new procedural thing like social dance or cooking an apple pie is preserved to the end. No kidding! The older age group may have to spend more time and give greater application to learning the tasks, but the studies clearly show with the proper application of willpower, success is expected.

Reasoning: Aging has no effect on ability to make sense of what you know. Healthy older adults usually have solid judgment and the ability to construct and understand reasonable and logical arguments.

Will Power: Undiminished. The older group may have to make an extra effort, but if they have the will to do something, they will. After something is learned, the older group has no greater difficulty in recalling the learned material than the youth.

Creativity: Usually preserved and in some cases greatly increased because of more leisure time and more accumulated knowledge.

Wisdom: The hallmark of advancing years. Ancient and modern societies took advantage of this trait by having special advisory groups of older people. Our word "senate" comes from the Latin "senecta," meaning older. Experience, knowledge, and insight grow with age. It is not an accident that the average age of justices of the Supreme Court throughout American history was about 70.

Conclusion: About aging, much is taken, but much remains. To a large extent, how you age depends on your genes. But a large number of factors are within your control. You can reduce age-related changes in your brain with good habits, such as eating a healthy diet, getting regular physical exercise, adequate sleep, living in a pollution-free environment, avoiding head trauma (very important), and challenging your brain by learning new things.

Though much is taken, much abides; and though
We are not now that strength which in old days
Moved earth and heaven, that which we are we are,
One equal temper of heroic hearts,
Made weak by time and fate, but strong in will
To strive, to seek, to find, and not to yield.
Ulysses, Alfred, Lord Tennyson

Associations Facilitate Recall

Recognizing patterns is a gigantic tool to facilitate memory. Associations are the next great tool after pattern recognition and putting things into chunks, a process that the memory schools call chunking.

Our Doctor Ebbinghaus noted early in his studies that association facilitates recall. The reason for this is that once two items are associated in the human consciousness, each tends to recall the other. His idea is of great importance for those of us who want to memorize something, especially if that something is as abstract as music, for music exists in the ether. Music is not solid like a stone or a piece of wood. It is an abstract art form, probably the most abstract art form on this planet. For our minds to get a hold of it, we need to have some concrete hooks. Associations can provide such hooks. Much memorization of modern poetry requires association, as modern poetry tends to be abstract, much more abstract than poems like *In Flanders Fields,* where rhyme and rhythm and meter and images of poppies and crosses and the birds still singing fly clue and cue the memory.

How the Brain Does Its Work and How to Make It Work Better

We have already learned the human brain is a coincidence machine: When two items are viewed closely together in the consciousness, they recall each other, and they usually do so in the ordered sequence in which they were first associated, just as Aristotle said. Notice that I am repeating myself. Remember, repetition is an important tool of memory. Repetition, review, and rehearsal are closely related memory strategies. But here is a key point about review and rehearsal: When testing yourself to see what you remember and how well, never omit review of the things you know well or think you know well. The brain is programmed to forget the unimportant and remember the important. But how does it distinguish the important from the unimportant? Answer: it doesn't, and it can't. Instead, it is as if the brain considers what is important what is repeatedly experienced, and it is as if the brain considers what is not important is what is not repeatedly experienced. Thus, if you are reviewing for a test, cover what you know and what you think you know in addition to the things you don't know well. Failure to review what you know well will result in forgetting those items. No kidding! In psychological circles, this phenomenon is called retrieval-induced forgetting. We know that repeated self-testing is extremely effective in cementing memories, much more than simply studying materials or reading them over. But if you choose to retest only those items that you haven't yet mastered, you will run into the issue of retrieval-induced forgetting.

Human Brains Are Massively Parallel Processors

The parallel processing of the brain evolved as a survival mechanism, given the constraints imposed by the size and volume of the brain. Compared to a computer, the brain is slow, very slow. Electric impulses travel in the brain at about 80 meters per second, 100 meters per second maximum. That is about one-millionth of the speed of electric impulses in a computer. The brain compensates for this relative slowness by using many neurons at the same time and in parallel. The system is arranged in a roughly hierarchical order such that any activity activates a wide range of neuronal networks. Because of this fact, the brain is able to compare and contrast items presented to it at about the same time. These network interconnections power human memory.

In Human Memory, Sequence Counts

If we say A, most people will think B because A and B were associated in the consciousness early on and in that order. If we say B, most people will think C because they learned the alphabet forward, not backward, and C follows B. If you think this is not true, try reciting the alphabet backward. You will find it is harder, much harder, to recite the alphabet backward than to recite it forwards. It also follows that if you can recite the alphabet backward, you will be able to recite it forward for, if the harder task is possible, the easier is much more possible.

Lesson: Sequence is a great aid to memory.

Any previously learned sequence will do. The alphabet is a sequence we all know already, and therefore it is available to provide hooks to hang memory items. Ditto the number system. Ditto the loci of things on your body or in your home or the 12 images of the zodiac, the days of the week, the months of the year, the 14 stations of the cross—any organized and learned sequence will do.

Sequence Plays a Major Role in Remembering Events

If you have a fair idea of what will happen, you can use that sequence frame to help you remember the events. When the event is over, recalling sequence will facilitate exact recall.

Mental Gymnastic

Next time you go to a play or a movie, find out what's what by looking up that play or movie on the internet. Get an idea of the plot structure, the characters, and the narrative arc. This shouldn't take much time, say ten minutes. Then after you have viewed the play or movie, compare and contrast the details of what you remember with what the people who viewed the same play or movie with you remember. You will be amazed at how much you can recall compared to your friends, and in the process, you will look like a memory genius. The same preview technique applies to books. If you read about the war of 1812 in advance and the Russian resistance to the French invasion and who was who on each side, you will remember much more of *War and Peace* than you would have remembered under less-happy circumstances.

Most People Are Visual Thinkers, and Therefore, Visual Associations Are Best

Multimodal associations are best: visual, auditory, kinesthetic, the big V.A.K. of psychology texts. But, for good reason, commercial schools of memory training such as those run by Bruno Fürst and Harry Lorayne spend weeks training people how to make vivid visual image associations to facilitate recall. Using such association methods, it is possible to recall a 50-digit number or the presidents of the United States in or out of order or remember every card that has been played in a game of blackjack.

Try to master a variety of connecting links between memory items so that one link helps recall the other. When you try to master links, you are forced to pay attention to what you are trying to remember, so indirectly, the effort is helping you remember by requiring mindfulness and original awareness of the material.

My Introduction to the Art of Memory: History That Made History

In the Roosevelt Hotel in New York City in the cold month of December 1969, Harry Lorayne proved to me that it is possible to memorize the telephone numbers in the Manhattan telephone directory. He gave the directory to others interested in memory training, and eventually came my turn to tell him a name and ask the number. After about 20 successes from various parts of the directory, I decided to trick him. I gave him the number and asked for the name. To my astonishment, he got it right!

As a stunt, Lorayne memorized the Manhattan telephone book using visual association techniques called the ancient art of memory. Using this ancient art, Saint Augustine tells us that his friend Simplicius memorized and could recite Virgil's Aeneid backward. This is an amazing feat, as most of us can't recite Vigil's Aeneid forward.

Do you believe Saint Augustine?

I do. The Saint was quite sincere when he told us about this because he wanted us to understand the tremendous power of human memory.

Need another example of the power of these techniques? Scipio, the Roman general, knew by heart the three names (given name, family name, acquired name) of each of the 32,000 men in his army. That means he knew 3 x 32,000 = 96,000 individual names! It's a good thing he did. Because the effectiveness of his personally knowing his troops led them to defeat Carthage in the battle of Zama in 202 BC, ending the Second Punic War. If Rome had not defeated Carthage, this book would be written in Punic and not in a language based on Latin.

Themistocles knew the 21,000 citizens of Athens by sight and by name. This was no idle game. Think of how important this was in this little democratic city-state for each individual citizen to know he was personally acknowledged and recognized on every occasion by the leading statesman.

A similar story is told of Napoleon. He is said to have known by name most of his soldiers and to be acquainted with their personal histories.

Viviani tells us Galileo could recite at length and by heart from the works of Dante Alighieri, Ludovico Ariosto, and Torquato Tasso. This was not exaggerated adulation but a fact. Galileo was seriously interested in recitation throughout his life and paid tribute to that art by exact memorization of famous Italian poems.

General George C. Marshall had a press conference at the St. George Hotel in Algiers. According to the *Readers' Digest* report, about 60 reporters were present. Marshall opened the conference by saying, "To save time, I am going to ask each of you what question you have in mind." Every correspondent present asked his questions, and then Marshall began a talk that lasted 40 minutes. He answered each and every question that had been asked and directed his answer to the correspondent who asked that specific question. Frederick C. Painton, who related the story, concluded: All agreed on one thing: "That's the most brilliant interview I ever attended in my life." By the way, Marshall was 63 at the time. Painton emphasized that fact because there are some folks who use age as an excuse for a poor or failing memory. Later Marshall explained how he did it. He extracted a keyword from the given question, made a mental image out of the keyword, and attached that keyword's image to the reporter's face. The keyword image reminded Marshall of the question, and the face reminded him of who asked the question.

Historians agree some of our ancient ancestors recited the entire Iliad and the entire Aeneid from memory. How in the world did they do it? Answer: With visual images.

Here's a more modern example: We may not long remember that my friend Hank Ulrich lives at 8981 215 Place because there is very little to assist the memory in retaining those figures. But if we have observed the form and style of his house, the curving footpath strewn with shells, the evergreen pines that line the sidewalls, a peculiar climbing rose bush by the front door, or any other characteristic visual detail that produced an actual impression on us, we remember that house without apparent effort and the remembrance remains with us almost indefinitely.

Humans Are Visual Animals

What modality has the most sensory input to the human brain?

Remember?

Over 80% of the afferent input to the human brain is through the visual system. Our very ancient ancestors probably spent lots of time in trees swinging from branch to branch. To do that effectively, they evolved excellent visual equipment and wonderful hand-eye coordination.

We remember images much better than everything else. Did anyone ever have the experience of meeting a person and saying, "I don't remember your face, but I remember your name?"

Getting Hank's address right and the street is another story. That too can be done, but it requires a knowledge of the techniques of Memory Heavy, which will be explained in the chapter on Memory Heavy.

Stop now and make a mental picture of Hank's house. Visualize all the items mentioned and also see old Hank sitting on his stoop. What does he look like? Does it matter?

Our point: If our ancient ancestors could perform such gigantic memory feats with memory training, it shouldn't be difficult for you to memorize a little piece by Mozart or Beethoven, or a telephone number, or a poem by T.S. Eliot or whatever you want.

There Is Practically No Limit to the Memory Storage Capacity of the Brain

Amazing, right! And even more amazing is the fact that over 90% of the human brain is made of water. It's hard to imagine serious thinking and effective memory coming from something made mainly of water. But it does! Thus, our brains are a combination of meat (tissues) and water, a meat and water machine. As that is a fact, it is not hard to imagine that similar thinking machines can be made of other substances, including silicon or ceramic or fibers or gel. Machine intelligence and machine consciousness will be a fact at some future time.

For centuries, humans believed heavier-than-air flight was not possible despite the evidence that bats, birds, and insects (which are heavier than air) can fly and fly without much effort. Therefore, in light of the fact that there are 7.8 billion human meat and water machines out there on this planet that can think and are conscious, it has to be true that other machines will eventually be conscious and able to think and remember. When that happens, it is likely those machines will have memory systems as good or better than the human brain. They certainly will be faster.

Associations That Aid Memory Recall Need Not Be Logical

Because the brain is a coincidence machine, a logical association is not needed to facilitate recall. All that matters is the coincidence of the two items in the consciousness, that is, in stage one or the working memory. In fact, tasks that require associations that are not logical can have a kind of logic imposed on them that will force the brain to recall specific information. For instance, answer this question: Who was the 13th president of the United States? Do you remember?

Offhand, I would bet you don't know. You forgot already. But if you do remember—good for you!

I can't see you right now. But if I could see you, I would bet some of you are smiling. Right? Smiling because you do recall president 13 or smiling because you don't know who the 13th president was.

Relax. Most of the people you know don't know and don't care. And most of the people on your street don't know. I live close to Houston, Texas, the fourth largest city in the United States, but I would give odds that there aren't ten people in this fair city, history teachers excepted, who can name president 13. When I took a student-run tour of the University of the State of New York at Buffalo, the tour leader told the group as we approached the Millard Fillmore Building, "This building is named after Millard Fillmore."

When I asked, "Who was Millard Fillmore?" The student said, "He led an expedition to investigate the Northwest Territories."

Me: "That was Lewis and Clark. Millard Fillmore was the 13th president of the United States. He is buried near the University in Buffalo's Forest Lawn Cemetery."

The old grandmother-type woman who was standing next to me elbowed me in the ribs and said, "You should be ashamed of yourself for asking a question you knew the answer to."

The next day, I took the same tour led by a different student. I wanted to compare and contrast. I wanted to see if there was any enlightenment. This time, the answer was more honest: "Millard Fillmore? I don't know. I think he was a famous chemist."

How to recall that Millard was president 13?

First, recognize that there is no logical connection between the number 13 and the name Fillmore. The connection of 13 with Fillmore is an arbitrary event of history not in any manner, shape, or form related to the number 13.

OK, you grant that there is no logical connection between 13 and Fillmore. Therefore, we shall have to create a connection. The task is to associate the number 13 with the name and in that order. The task will be easily accomplished by association.

Repetition Is Good for Memory Training; Just as It Is Good for Memory

Don't be afraid of repetition. It is absolutely essential to memorize complex things, uninteresting facts, or large amounts of material.

Why are songs memorable? Answer: They repeat themselves, and the music cues the memory, and also there are rhymes and rhythm cues.

Mental Gymnastic: How Did We Connect Fillmore and 13?

Turn the number 3 so that it looks like an m. Now you have 1-m. Change the one to a t because 1 and t look similar as they both have a single vertical line. Now you have t-m. TM recalls the sounds tee em, which reminds us of the consonant sounds in the word *tomb*.

Pause and think. Can you now see in your mind's eye what came next in our imagining?

See yourself driving a tomb—yes, a tomb—you are driving the tomb up to a gas station and asking the man to fill your tank more. Your request to "fill more" reminds you of Fillmore, our 13th president. If someone asks what president was Fillmore, just work the sequence in reverse:

See the picture of the gas station. Recall asking to fill more. But strangely, you are not driving your car. You are driving the tomb. The tomb recalls TM, which reminds us of 13.

As most thoughts travel close to the speed of light (not really but fast), you will not notice a time-lapse between the 13 questions and your answer any more than anyone noticed a pause between people asking Harry Lorayne a telephone number in the Manhattan directory and his reply. When mastered, the systems seem to work instantly. And here is the topper: Once you get Fillmore, you will automatically recall his first name, which was what?

In a similar manner, if you wish, you will be able to recall all of the presidents in or out of order using these simple (and sometimes stupid) associations. You can do that if and only if you felt like encoding the information in your memory using the techniques to follow.

Make Your Own Personal Associations

Our ancient ancestors and the masters of the modern schools of memory, like Harry Lorayne, teach us that most associations work best when you yourself make the associations. The associations do not work as well when you are using some-one else's association. Also, it pays to build the new material, which you don't know and are trying to learn, on old material you do know and know well. In fact, the more you know, the more you can know by building new associations on what is already solidly in your mind.

In memorizing music, there will be as many associations and methods of associ-ation as there are individuals. There is no single way to approach a music task, and the one we choose may not be the only or even the best strategy despite our attempts to get the facts and completely encompass the data. But in general, the associations that will work best are those that are firmly based on what you know, recognizing similarities and differences between what you know already and what you are trying to learn. Thus, if you know your scales, chords, cadences, and rhythms, you will do better than if you didn't know them because your associa-tions will be richer and more numerous. How much easier is it to remember to play a C triad chord sequence than to try to remember to play C-E-G as individ-ual notes in that order.

Names and Labels, No Matter How Strange or Ridiculous, Help Encode Memory

There was a certain part of a Mozart piece that I had difficulty getting into my memory. When my teacher called this "the unusual chord," bingo! I now had a label and an association by which to recall this chord. In fact, the unusual chord now stands out in my memory as the landmark in the piece. My teacher pointed out the relation of this unusual chord to what was happening in my other hand and the fact that the chord appears nowhere else in the piece. The part of this mu-sic that used to give my memory trouble now had a local habitation, a name ("the unusual chord"), and a unique existence—plenty of reasons for me to remember it by multiple associations.

Notice the brain does not suffer from multiple associations. On the contrary, multiple associations, and multimodal associations (VAK = Visual, Auditory, Kin-esthetic), facilitate encoding and will subsequently facilitate recall.

Narrative, narrative, narrative—Tell yourself a story to help yourself remem-ber. Do it in your own words in your own way. If need be, make up your own words to go with a wordless piece that you are playing or make a story that

connects the main ideas of the poem you are working on. Use the narrative as a frame to recall specific items.

Sometimes illogical and imaginative stories can easily jog our memories. How this happens is that the items in the story are easier to recall than the items to be recalled, and it is the link in the story of the easy item with the hard item that facilitates the memory. Experts in education find that a powerful way to learn is from stories. We seem, as human beings, to respond profoundly to narratives and to extract from certain tales key items that are useful. A story is the narration of events in time. Even more helpful for memory is plot, which is the narration of events in time with a reason for the events. Whenever we have a reason, memory gets easier. "The king died, and then then the queen died." is a story. "The king died, and then the queen died of a broken heart." That's a story with a plot. The plotted story has more emotional impact and would be easier to recall.

Mental Gymnastic

For example, memorize this number:

76863572722

Not easy, right.

Now memorize this story with a map of Manhattan in mind.

Seventy-six trombones led the big parade across 86th street. When they reached 3rd Avenue, they turned left, and they met 57 clowns who were distributing 27 ice cream cones to 22 Dallas Cowboy Cheerleaders.

Read the story several times aloud until you feel confident you know the story. Those of you who can visualize a map of Manhattan will have an easier time of it. In my mind's eye, I see myself marching with the 76 trombones eastward to 3rd Avenue. At 3rd and 86th, I see one of my favorite restaurants, but in front of it is a waiter who is motioning me to turn left (that is, he wants the parade to head north). This waiter is laughing his head off because he knows I will soon see 57 clowns all dressed in vivid, colorful clown outfits that look like Heinz 57 Ketchup bottles. The clowns are distributing (WHAT?) 27 ice cream cones to 22 Dallas Cowboy Cheerleaders. So, five cheerleaders will get two cones.

Ridiculous story, right. But effective. Don't believe me? Try to memorize the number by rote, straight repetition, and sheer work and see how far you get and also, note how long it will take to get this number in the memory. Even if you do manage to memorize the number, chances are very good that in less than an hour, you will have forgotten more than half of it. Compare and contrast that performance with what happens with the narrative and visual image associations.

The images that work best are strange, ridiculous, oversized or undersized, in color, violent, and emotionally linked to our personal interests.

Mental Gymnastic Continued

Now turn aside and write the number by telling yourself the narration of the events in time. Check your answer. Note any mistakes and try to figure how to avoid the mistakes next time. Mistakes are good because they teach us what we need to correct. Was your visual image not vivid enough? Did you not recite the story aloud? Reciting aloud activates lots of muscle and cues the memory with words. The more associations, the easier will be recall from stage three memory.

Chances are people who live in Manhattan can do this easier than those people who do not live in Manhattan. The people who live there have a framework already learned to which they can more easily attach the images. They are natives there and to the manner born. Most New Yorkers have a map of Manhattan in their heads, the way some musicians have a picture of the Moonlight Sonata page by page in mind, or those London taxis drivers have a map of London in mind when they have to go from Charring-Cross to Westend. They make pictures of where they need to go as soon as the client tells them where.

Even if you don't know Manhattan, try to make pictures of 86th street and 3rd Avenue. You should have no trouble seeing clowns and those luscious Dallas Cowboy Cheerleaders. Dressing the clowns in Heinz 57 bottles helps recall the number. Don't just think 57; actually, visualize the clowns or try to. The associations are not logical, but they are my own, and thus I will have a further advantage. If you made up your own narration starting with the number 76 and your own images, your narration would work better for you than your narration would work for me.

Face It. You Were Probably Too Lazy to Do the Mental Gymnastic

Chances are you didn't even bother to make up a story. Chances are you were too eager to push ahead into something that was less work and easier. Most of you were too lazy! Having taught this stuff for 17 years, Doctor Patten knows people are lazy. Too bad! If you didn't do the story, you missed out on actually proving to yourself that a narrative technique helps recall of specific information. Mental laziness is the root cause of most memory failures. Don't let mental laziness set you back. Be eager, active, and energic. Approach memory problems with the interest, vigor, and energy of a child. Hold fast to the spirit of youth, for that spirit is likely to serve you best.

Sorry, This Book Is Not a Novel

Read a novel, as a novel moves along at a fast pace and does not require paying too much attention. Good! That is the way novels are meant to be read. While some novels are true artistic achievements, most are meant as entertainment merely. This book is not a novel and has to be read differently. This book has to be chewed and digested for you to get maximum benefit from it and for you to reach your goal of looking ten times smarter than you are.

MENTAL MAKING MIGHT

Narrative Notes

How about this? Memorize this sequence of notes:

C Eflat G Eflat C G Gflat F F#

Now try using a story. C, E flat, and G enter a bar. The place doesn't serve minors, so E flat leaves and C and G share a fifth of Irish whiskey. The fifth flattens G. F comes in and tries to augment the situation by looking sharp. Sound it out on the piano—presto, you have the sequence by a ridiculous narrative technique.

C Minor E Flat CG F#-F-F#

How about this? Same sequence using music knowledge and chunking: C minor arpeggio, then play E flat and take it out playing the ends of C minor, which are C and G. Then its F# (same tone as G flat) F F# (three Fs, the middle one natural; the ones on either side sharp). Sounding it on your piano—presto, you have learned the sequence by chunking and by asserting an intelligent musical narration. Try to memorize the same sequence the old rote way and notice the difficulties. Numerous studies show that simply repeating information over and over doesn't help us learn it very effectively.

Modern schools of memory training employ numbered peg lists of overly learned visual images onto which newly acquired information is pegged by association.

The Peg System

The great American mnemonist, Harry Lorayne, was (alas, he's dead) also big on peg lists. A peg list is a list of things we already know onto which we will peg the new items that we wish to recall.

Because you already know the numbers from one to infinity, you can usually organize your peg lists around numbers. Sometimes, to facilitate recall, you will also attach a visual image to the number, as we did with Fillmore and the number 13. The image, you will recall, was you driving a tomb. Because the image is weird, strange, in motion, and unusual, the brain is not likely to forget it. Our brains are naturally attracted to and interested in the unusual, weird, and bizarre. Seeing Jessie Ventura in a tutu and bright red lipstick painted on his lips would get more attention and be more memorable than seeing Donald John Trump reading a book, even though both scenes would be unusual enough to catch our attention.

Because you also know the alphabet by heart, you can use the alphabet as a peg to remember items. This system is also known as the abecederian system. Peg systems can be useful if employed at the right time in the right situation by the right people for the right reason. Usually, narrative works better when attached to pegs, and narrative with visual images and peg lists is usually particularly effective when there has been pattern recognition and chunking with notation of similarities and differences.

The New England Primer taught generations of kids the alphabet, helping them learn ABCs. Along the way, the kids got religious instructions by association of the letter with a bible thing. For example, A is Adam, and in Adam's fall, we sinned all. J was for Jesus in some editions and S for serpent, and so forth.

Lesson: Place images as pegs.

Ancient Memory Systems Used Peg Images in Places

In ancient Greece and in ancient Rome, the place system was the most famous of the techniques for remembering things. The places helped recall particular items in the narration and made it look like the poet had memorized the Iliad when he/ she had actually memorized the images associated with narrative items and used those images in sequence to fetch the story section from the memory. In many cases, the image recalled the gist of the section and not exactly word for word of what was to be recited. The same is true in public speaking. Cicero used the images in his villa to suggest the thought that would follow in his speech. Exact duplication of the exact words was not needed. In fact, (according to Cicero) exact duplication was avoided because it might sound artificial or stylized and off-putting. Reading a speech is a no-no for this same reason. Even if you look up frequently at the audience, your speech will lack vim and vigor. Never ever read a speech. Speak from memory naturally, or keep your mouth shut.

Images in Place as a Memory Aid

Aristotle mentions this technique four times, and (in Rome) Cicero used it routinely to recite his famous speeches in the Roman senate. In fact, Cicero made considerable claims about the systems and their effectiveness in his essay on oratory, *De. Oratore.* You were already told humans have a great memory for places, so this system takes advantage of a natural in-born talent.

Quintilian says that when using the place system, it was possible to witness a whole day's auctions, and at the end of the day, name all the articles sold, all the buyers, and the exact prices. Seneca claims he was able to repeat 2,000 names after a single hearing, or 200 disconnected lines of verse shouted out to him by members of an audience. He could repeat these lines in either the order given or in reverse order. Having seen Harry Lorayne and Bruno Fürst perform similar memory tricks, there is no doubt Seneca and Quintilian are telling the truth.

How about you? Do you believe these ancient authors and their claims?

I do, absolutely because I have taken many courses and seen many normal average people, myself included, do similar memory feats.

Place System

How does the place system work? In the Greek and Roman versions, there are two sets of images. First, one memorizes in advance a set of images. This is the laborious part of the method and the reason mnemonists prefer peg systems based on familiar numbers or letters of the alphabet or some personally well-known sequence. Cicero used the pictures in his villa and, in his imagination, walked through his house to view the images each in turn. He did this over and over again and checked the results with an actual walk until he could picture all the images in his mind in the correct sequence.

If you set your mind to it, you can make a mental set of ten place images by walking through your home. It will be a lot easier than you think because you are already familiar with your home and the items in it. It might help to also number the images. Example: #1 is the front door it is brown, and has no window, etc.

Next comes the second stage of the procedure. Supposing Cicero wanted to memorize the main points of a speech, he would form a second set of images symbolizing these points. The image symbolizing the first point would then be superimposed on the image of the first place, and his second major point would be mentally attached to the second place in his villa, and so on. When Cicero wants to recall what's next, or even what he was talking about at the moment, he will run through the set of places in his mind and find the superimposed images. He might even say, as he is recalling the images, "In the first place." And then, when he wished to recall the item or idea that was next, he would think and might even say to the Roman Senate, "In the second place" and so forth. He actually did say "in the second place" and then accused Cataline of treason, followed by the evidence. What his second place was, we don't know, but it may have been a fresco or a fountain on which Cicero had imagined the face of Cataline. Seeing the place image reminded Cicero it was time to accuse Cataline. Place three might have been the impluvium donating an image that reminded Cicero to talk about Cataline having killed his first wife and child or that Cataline had been accused of and tried for the capital crime of having had sex with a Vestal Virgin. Even ancient Rome had psychopathic politicians!

Using this system of recall, somewhat analogous to our PowerPoint where images suggest talking points, Cicero spoke for hours before the Roman Senate, convincing them of the conspiracy. Cataline fled the city to avoid arrest.

Cicero will not and cannot look at the whole panorama of images all at once but will review each in turn as if he were walking through his villa. Suddenly, says Cicero, the item to be recalled will be "donated" to him by the primary image to which the to-be-remembered item had been previously attached. Students should not be surprised by the effectiveness of the system when they realize how vividly the images are encoded with each other. The basic principle of human memory being, again, that once two items are connected with one another in the consciousness, each tends to recall the other and in that order.

Cicero and all the other ancient authors agree: "The more vivid, the more interesting, the more colorful, the more unusual, the more violent, the more tightly the items will be associated with each other in the mind and the more likely that each will recall the other."

The same set of images can be used to memorize a different speech or a poem or a set of the fifty names of the men in your army. Cicero considered the initial set of images a kind of wax tablet, Rome's scrap paper, which can be reused by merely blotting out the previous things written on the tablet and writing something new over it. Once one has made the effort to fix the original set of images in places in the home, one can reuse the same set of images any number of times.

It is possible to make a single sequence of images that link to each other. For example, a shopping list might consist of a giant loaf of bread that breaks apart, showing a can of bean soup. The can bursts open to reveal bananas inside and so on for an indefinite number of items. Thus, you need bread, a can of beans, and some bananas. That's OK. But two image lists are better, with one image list firmly in the memory to be used as pegs on which to hang the to-be-remembered items.

What Is the Point of Having Two Sets of Images? Why Not One?

Two sets have a number of advantages, including the ability to recall items in order or in reverse order or in any order whatsoever. This is why Seneca was able to recite the verses in reverse order: He just ran through his house backward. That's why Saint Augustine's friend could recite Vigil's poem backward. He went through his house backward. You can do the same. Why not get your wife, husband, friend, or partner to make a short shopping list. Then in your imagination, start somewhere in your place (home or apartment) and attach the item on the list to that place. Say, bread on the door, cabbage in the bathroom, ice cream in the bathtub. You have to do it. I can't do this for you. If you don't actually do the association, it will not work.

Lesson: You Have to Do It.

Then notice how easy it is to recall the items on the list. If you don't do this exercise, you will never know how powerful this simple task can be. It worked for Cicero, Saint Augustine, and Scipio, so why should it not work for you?

Using the place system, Cicero can not only recall the points in his speech but also the order he wanted them presented. He can also select an item and look to either side to see the point before that item and the point after. The background images also can supply a connection and association that might otherwise be difficult to recall, including specific facts and events that make for a more believable prosecution, story, argument, or appeal. Finding the relevant item and the images before and after will give additional information to answer questions that may come up from your audience.

It is easy to see how the place system could be used to remember a dozen items or twenty names. But how could it be used to remember two thousand?

Answer: Some of the ancients (believe it or not) had over 100,000 places to store items. Whatever we may think of this figure, Harry Lorayne had that many places and more to store the entire Manhattan telephone book. Quintilian mentions that Metrodorus had a set of 360 places probably for eristic arguments and could hang several items onto each place. *Rhetorica ad Herennium* tells us flatly that, if we want to remember many things, we shall have to prepare many places.

Matteo Ricki, an Italian Jesuit Priest and one of the founding figures of the Jesuit China mission, invented, using an image system with an imagined palace of place peg rooms, a remarkably effective system for learning Chinese. The Catholic Church lists Matteo as a "servant of God." His papers for Sainthood have been held up in the Vatican since 2014. The problem appears to be lack of miracles because to be a saint requires two proven miracles. Matteo's memory palace may not count as a miracle, but the use of it to learn Chinese was definitely miraculous for the candidates who wished to pass the imperial examinations in China. Want to know more? Take a look at a gem of historical writing, *The Memory Palace of Matteo Ricci* by Jonathan D. Spense.

Stations of the Cross Are an Example of Narration and Images Used to Jog Memories

Stations of the cross are a system of 14 places that recall the route Jesus took to get to the place he was killed. They are arranged in numerical order along a path the faithful travel to remember selected items from the passion of Jesus. In the case of stations of the cross, the images are usually already in place and ready to donate their information about when Jesus was condemned to death (station one) or when he fell for the first time (station three), or when Veronica wiped his face (station six), and so forth. The path followed reflects the Via Dolorosa in Jerusalem. Can anyone doubt the effectiveness of these images in recalling the specific events depicted? Stations of the cross are found in most Western Christian churches, Anglican, Lutheran, Methodist, Roman Catholic—for good reason. In some churches, specific narration about the image of the particular station is supplied under the image or in an accompanying booklet. The resemblance of PowerPoint to the stations of the cross is no accident. They are both based on the same brain principle: Images facilitate recall.

Narrative Sequence Can Be Illogical

Notice, we got from the number 13 to the image of riding up to the gas station by a sequence of imaginative but illogical steps: 13 → tm → tomb → driving a tomb to fill up more → Fillmore. That is how we did it. Others use abecedarian lists—lists that follow the order of letters in the alphabet. That's OK too. These people tell themselves this is part A of the musical piece or poem, this is part B, and now I am back on part A again with the variation that ends the piece, and so forth.

One of my friends just memorized Eric Satie's *First Gymnopedie*. But, of course, he didn't memorize it in the usual sense that most people think.

Instead, he knows it as a collection of patterns: A A' B C D A A' B C D '.

By recalling this pattern in order and by recalling the slight variations signaled by the A' and D', he plays the piece correctly. Notice the order. There is no way he would play C before B or D' before A because the sequence of the alphabet is so firmly fixed in in our minds by our culture. And when he does play *Gymnopedie,* people think he actually memorized it in some conventional sense. He didn't. What he memorized was an analytical pattern, the similarities and differences of the various parts. He reproduced that pattern on the piano in proper sequence with the (desired) effect so that it looks like he memorized the entire piece note for note.

Other people will use numbers and letters: This is part one of the two parts of the A section of the minuet and so forth. As for me, I use everything I can think of or imagine—numbers, letters, stories, whatever. Your mind is a channel for reaching worlds beyond the material objects of everyday life through imagination. The mind offers us a means of bringing an abstract world, such as the abstract world of music, into Technicolor reality. The Irish believe in three realities: The real world, the spirit world, and the world of the imagination. Of those three, the Irish think the world of imagination is the most important. Albert Einstein famously said, "Imagination is more powerful than the H-bomb." Why not develop and use your imagination? The trouble is most people have to force themselves to imagine anything. The average adult is way out of practice. Children do not have that problem. Imagination is one of their things. Most of the really cool inventions of our time first appeared in someone's imagination.

Break Time

Whew! That was a lot of info. So what? We already know we can't absorb much at the first go. There will plenty of review time and merciful repetition to cement the above ideas in your memory toolbox. Meanwhile, let's take a break and then come back and work out on some associations.

Mental Gymnastic

Study this group of couples for three minutes by the clock and remember what couples belong together:

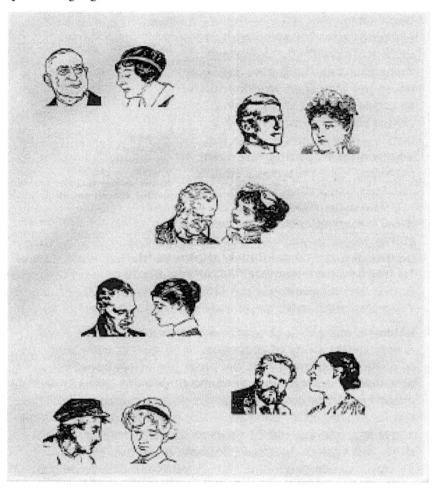

Fig3.1

OK? Got them all together? Now match them up. List the numbers one to six on a paper to represent the men, and next to each number, place the spouse's letter.

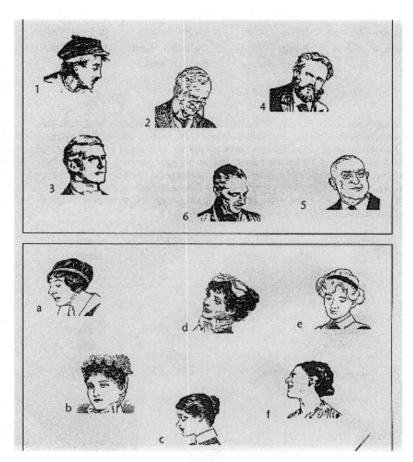

Fig3.2

Make sure you have recorded your answers on paper. It is very easy, too easy, to fool yourself into thinking you know something when you don't.

Answers: 1e 2d 3b 4f 5a 6c

Normal is two right. Anyone reading this book is unlikely to be normal. Else why would you be reading it? Most people reading this book are superior. Don't be surprised if you did better than normal. But note this: I have not viewed this panel in over three years, nor did I study the panel before testing myself. Yet, I got them all right. The reason? I encoded the couples three years ago with visual associations to a narrative. The association-narrative encoding is strong, and therefore, I had no trouble recalling what man goes with what woman. Follow along with me and use my narrative to encode couples. It is much better if you do your own associations and narration, but for the sake of illustration and to help you learn the method, use my associations this time. Just read the associations once. Be sure to pass the information directly into your consciousness. Make a mental image also, if you can. Then forget it, if you can.

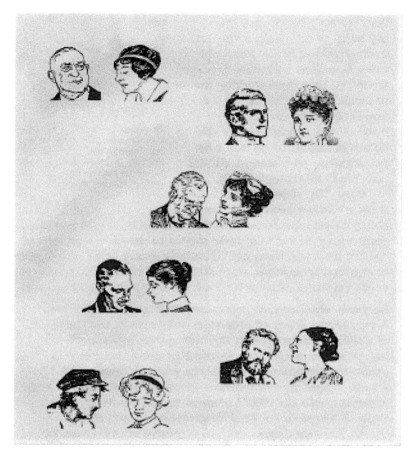

Fig3.3

Top couple: He lacks hair, and she has abundant hair. This couple complements each other by one making up for the lack of the other.

Second couple from top: Well-groomed both, and she has a nice doily hat that looks Victorian. Hence, this is a nice, respectable, well-groomed Victorian couple. Note that I multiply images, ideas, and narration to fix the association in my memory. The brain is not bothered or confused by multiple associations. The more, the better.

Third couple from top: I am going to do this in a flash. He has glasses with two lenses, and she has a hair decoration with two big bows. This couple matches by glasses and bows.

Forth couple: Both quiet and respectful and very well-groomed. A perfect match in beauty.

Fifth couple: She looks a lot like Madame Curie, and he looks like Pierre, her husband.

The more you know, the more associations you can make. But by the way, it doesn't make a hill of beans difference whether or not she looks like Madame Curie or not. The image I make in my mind will work regardless. Associations you make need not be logical or true. They are just tags to facilitate retrieval of information from memory.

Sixth couple: This is hard because I am having trouble coming up with a visual clue in the picture that will trigger the memory. So, I will just make up a story based on a pretend (imagined) emotional event. The man is a fisherman (see the fisherman's cap) who has returned empty-handed. He is reluctantly explaining to his saddened wife that he has caught no fish and she, he, and the kids will have nothing to eat.

OK? Did you do the gymnastic?

Now let's test the system to see if it helps us recall the couples.

Same drill. Write the numbers one to six on a paper and put the letter of the spouse next to the appropriate number. In each case, look at the man's face first and then search the women for the match while trying to recall the narrative, peg tag, or image association.

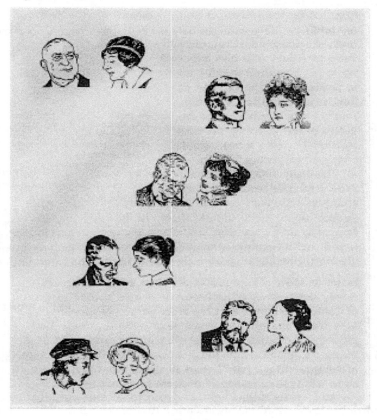

Fig3.4

Here's my answers, which come to me in a flash. I hope they do the same for you.

1. Fisherman matches with e—both sad.
2. Glasses match bow d.
3. Victorian correctness matches Victorian correctness c
4. Pierre with Marie f.
5. Bald complemented by full hair a.
6. Well-groomed matches well-groomed c

Oh no! There can't be two men attached to c wife. That would be polyandry. One of the c's has to match with another man. I was moving too fast and failed to note the give-away doily on b. So, three must match with b.

When you miss, review the item to see why you missed it. Perhaps you didn't make a vivid enough image, or the narration was not enough. In this case, I don't know what my problem was. My memory simply failed. No big deal. I am used to it. I am a failure in many things. Anyway, we all know that forgetting is the default mode of human memory.

How did you do? Don't judge yourself too harshly. Remember, only two correct is normal. If you did that, good. If you did better than two, great.

Explicit Memory and Implicit Memory

Let's talk about this topic. Books on memory make a big deal of it, so we should at least be familiar with the concepts of explicit and implicit memory.

Explicit memory is memory under conscious control, and implicit memory is not under conscious control. Explicit memory is very dependent on language, and implicit memory is not. The dependence of explicit memory on language is not a mere coincidence, for language and conscious, focused awareness are closely linked phenomena. We use explicit memory when we are explaining how to play a C triad. We use implicit memory when we play that chord without consciously thinking about it. We use implicit memory when we ride a bike or do anything automatically. We use explicit memory when we try to explain (hint: both explicit and explain begin with ex) how to ride a bike.

There's no question that most human cognitive processes use implicit memory in the absence of language or even self-aware focused consciousness. Any physical activity, such as playing tennis, or walking, running, dancing, eating, drinking, tying shoes, ice skating, driving a car, etc., goes on largely automatically—without a verbal running commentary on what to do next. Yesterday, I drove to Galveston, a distance of 52 miles. The car arrived safely, so I presume I drove safely and, yet, I don't recall much of the mechanics of driving. I can't tell you when I braked, passed, accelerated, stopped for a light, dodged that pickup truck that cut me off, and so forth because I wasn't paying attention to those trivial things. Correction: I do remember the pick-up truck because it missed by only inches. Do people with pick-up trucks have an ego problem?

All my driving was pretty much automatic or semiautomatic and based on implicit memories of past driving experiences and procedures. It was automatic and did not command my personal attention. So, I can't tell you much about it because I don't remember much about it. What I can tell you about is the CD lecture by professor Bob Brier of Long Island University on the history of Egypt that I listened to on the way down. That is what I was paying attention to, and that is what I may talk about tonight at dinner.

Subconscious Thinking Is Real

Have you ever had a solution to a problem pop into your head, the way that Irish proverb popped into mine? That's a clear example that thinking about that problem took place at a level other than self-aware consciousness. Indeed, most neuroscientists believe spoken language is merely an afterthought, so to speak, of more fundamental cognition that is preconscious. Follow the majority and agree. The majority usually gets things right, especially if they are scientists.

Watch yourself next time you buy an ice cream cone. Usually, you will know what flavor you want before the word for that flavor appears in your mind. Therefore, the decision on flavor was preconscious. The preconscious decision was then consciously expressed in words and actions. And usually, you will know in advance as soon as you see the vendor that you want an ice cream, and if you have the money and you feel like it, you will make the purchase without much thought. Do you think Jackie Robinson at-bat has any conscious thought about that baseball that is hurling toward him? His swing, eye-arm-hand coordination, and whatever else is needed to hit the ball is all subconscious and pretty automatic based on years of practice. In fact, truth be told, if he hit a homer, he will be just as surprised and just as happy as his fans.

Decision System One

In psychological circles, this brain mechanism that is fast to respond and largely unconscious is called system one. The other system is slower and more analytical and looks at evidence, draws on experience, reason, and insight before making a decision or reaching a conclusion. Scientists believe system one evolved to protect humans from immediate dangers. The problem with system one is that gut hunches or shoot-from-the-hip decisions are often wrong when applied to non-emergent situations or long-term, complicated problems. Donald John Trump, unfortunately, is locked into system one with disastrous consequences. The history of his multiple failures is too well known to be reviewed here.

Decision System Two

In the evolution of mankind, system two came later when our ancient ancestors were safe in the cave and trying to figure out how to kill the animals they needed for food. System two is much more useful to solve complex modern problems. System two (rational thought) is essential for real progress in science, art, literature, and government.

Explicit Memory and Implicit Memory—Use Them Both

The key task in music memory is to get the piece into the implicit memory while using explicit memory to keep on track, recover from implicit memory failure, and give overall shape to the performance. Reminder: Yes, that is the key task of music memory, but the key task of the performance of music is an overall sense of musicality (feelings and emotions) without which none of the masterpieces can be played well.

The key task in reciting a poem is to get the poem into implicit memory while using explicit memory to get it into implicit memory and then during read-out to keep on track, recover from implicit memory failures using rhythm, rhyme, and other clues, and give an overall emotional shape (emotion is what poetry is about or should be about) to the performance. Reminder: Good poetry recitation must be automatic so that you can give the proper emotional coloring to the rendition. People will be bored to tears with a technically correct but essentially lifeless recitation, especially if it is read from a book or paper with or without looking at the audience. Never ever read a poem before an audience. Always do your poem from memory. Nothing else will make you look good or smarter than you are.

In the same way, the key task in dancing the waltz is to get the mechanics of the dance into implicit memory while using explicit memory to get it into the implicit motor memory. In other words, you must do the work to learn the dance. Then during dancing, most of the dance will be automatic, like driving a car or riding a bike. Because it is automatic, you will be able to use your conscious working memory to talk to your dance partner or to create an artistic individual dance style that reflects your individual personality and style of beauty. Isadora Duncan famously remarked, "If I could say it in words, I wouldn't have to dance it." Psychologists sometimes talk about closed and open motor tasks and the memory requirements of both. Social dance is considered mainly closed because the rules are set and do not change much. Social dancers know how they are supposed to move (counter-clockwise looking down from the ceiling) around the room in Foxtrot. Social dancers understand they can't go clockwise without crashing into other dancers. They understand the distances that must be observed between couples. They understand slower couples should stay closer to the center of the dance floor. All these rules are fixed, and that's why social dance is considered a closed motor task. Driving a car or piloting a plane, on the other hand, is considered an open motor task and is considered more complex and therefore more difficult to learn because the environment in which the motor response is required is not fixed and will change depending on circumstances. To better understand the difference between closed and open motor tasks, take a one-hour lesson in foxtrot and a one-hour lesson in flying a helicopter. Then compare and contrast the two experiences.

Use Language to Help Memory, Thought, and Performance

Use language to shape elements of thought and performance in a way that the mute mind cannot. Use both explicit and implicit memory in performance. Use both in trying to memorize. But never forget your first duty is to be human and show the human touch. That is the best way to neutralize our too modern, too technical environment.

Motor Memory

Whew! That was a lot of info about memory.

Let's take a breather. But before the breather and before we get to the next part, the part that deals with techniques to encode and retrieve memory, before we get to that, and lots of other specific advice about memory, there is one more key general point about human memory you should know about—motor memory, also known as kinesthetic memory, also known as muscle memory—an aspect of memory not studied by Ebbinghaus.

Some people refer to this type of memory modality as finger memory. We saved the discussion of this aspect of memory for last because, in many ways, it is the most important since it does the most work in any performance from memory, and it does most of the work in the performance of almost all routine everyday tasks.

Motor memory is mainly unconscious. That is the advantage. Motor memory can run things like driving, riding a bike, dancing, fencing, swimming, drinking, eating, talking, and so forth almost automatically without much conscious control. That frees our minds to pay attention to our spouse while we are driving and allows us to multitask.

The trouble is that unconscious motor memory is unreliable and is made less reliable by directing our attention to the way it works. And thus, we can foul our motor memory by thinking too much about it. Those of you who play a sport know what this is about. Think too much about that easy putt and the motor programs previously in place to make that easy putt may fail. Many of you have seen that scene during a championship golf tournament. It is the last hole and a two-foot-put. The pressure is on. Lots of money is at stake, and lots of paid endorsements. And he misses! He missed a put he could probably do in his sleep or certainly do without much thought, just as Jackie hit a homer without real conscious thought.

Time for a Break

Do you have to take a pee? All right, you know best. Taking a break is good for the body and for the mind.

After your break and breather, come back and learn about the most powerful form of human memory and how it may be applied to memorizing tasks that have a motor component like performance sports, music, and speech making.

Pause Here and Take a Break

As for me, I don't have to pee, so I will get a drink of water, and I will check my email. Also, I will see if I recall that note sequence I made up. It started with C minor entering a bar. Also, how about the number that starts with a parade of trombones? Come back when you are rested and ready to learn about motor memory. And you, too, test yourself to see if the note sequence is or is not in your memory. Test yourself on the number. Write down the answer and try to figure why you got it right and why you didn't. What the devil was Cicero's place memory system about? How did the ancients use place images to remember facts exactly? How did Saint Augustine's friend recite Vergil's Aeneid backward? What was Saint Augustine's friend's name? What number president was Millard Fillmore, and where is he buried?

Motor Memory, Kinesthetic Memory, Muscle Memory, and Finger Memory

O.K. We're back. Did you get the note sequence? If you didn't get the note sequence, go back and memorize the narrative and then proceed to the discussion of finger memory. Same drill—ditto the number.

As for me, I tried, but I didn't get the note sequence correct even though I was the one who made it up. I forgot that when E flat left the bar that E flat was supposed to be played, not omitted. When I tried the sequence at the piano, the correct sequence was obvious. My experience confirms the importance of review in the form of self-test to make sure that you have things correct and also confirms the important way that playing the notes on the piano can clue the memory. The touch, the pitch sequences, the tones themselves, the way my fingers and hands looked on the keyboard—all helped cue the memory. Again, thinking while doing is the best for memory, and encoding in multimodalities (VAK) is best.

The number did arrive correct. Probably, I am better at numbers and narration, and there wasn't any hesitation about recalling the number. The map of Manhattan helped, and so did the ridiculous colorful visual images. The clowns with the Heinz 57 suits were cool, and so were the Dallas Cowboy Cheerleaders.

Original Emotional Significance Plays a Major Role in Encoding Memory

Most of you out there will not remember even reading about the sequence of notes, but you may have a vague notion about people entering a bar. Why didn't you remember? Think about this. Probably you didn't care. You probably were not interested. Another reason is that you just didn't think it was important enough to come up again. So why bother remembering? You didn't think anyone would ever quiz you on the item. But the major reason is you had no emotional interest or connection in the notes or the story. Emotional interest is a great motivator of memory. On the other hand, if you thought you might use the bar jokes to look entertaining at the next dinner party, you probably did pay attention to the joke, and you may be able to pull it off now. Lawyers probably remember the joke about a lawyer being an asshole. Which reminds me. At the annual meeting of the American Bar Association, this joke had them rolling in the aisles:

"Sandra Day O'Connor sat with the other justices in a restaurant and ordered a steak. The waiter asked, 'And what about the other vegetables?' She said, 'Oh, they'll have the same.'"

Who Remembers What and Why?

Patients tell in exact detail where they lived in Eaton's Neck, Long Island in 1942 and what they did there (mainly fished, dug clams, and water skied). But those people could not recall that at the time the United States was at War nor when they were informed about the war, could many of them recall who was fighting whom and for what reason.

Lesson: Personal life is usually way more important and much more memorable!

In the memory clinic at Columbia Presbyterian Medical Center in 1969, many older people were asked about historical events they lived through. They remembered a million (useless?) things, a quarrel with a boss, the hunt for a lost wedding ring, the expression on a long-dead father's face, the swirls of dust and papers on 168th street on a windy winter morning 70 years ago; but in many cases, the relevant facts and events happening in the nation and the world were outside their memory.

And the shocker at the time was that detailed investigation of the things these old folks said they remembered quite well were actually false, at least in part. Their memory of the layout of their apartment, even the memory of the location, size, and situation of the church they got married in, was defective and often completely missing or completely wrong.

Conclusion: Memories of old people are not reliable even though they think they are. The idea that older people remember the past better than they remember the present is simply not true. The memory power of older people is very low and defective for both past and recent events. This is sad to say, but it is true. The hope is that this book will improve the situation. But that, sorry to say, is a slim hope if memory work is not done.

Family Pictures and Written Records Are Important and Help Clue the Memories of Old Folks

Pictures and written records are much more reliable, and when these older adults were confronted with the pictures and written records, they were truly puzzled that their memories, which they thought were so good, were actually so bad.

Why? Their own lives were much more emotionally important to them than the war known as World War II. Hence, there was a tendency to think they remembered personal memories, and some did, but those personal memories faded with time and, in many cases, were rearranged and even falsified.

Someone who was at Omaha Beach or a gold-star mother would have a different memory of World War II. To them, the war would loom large in their memories because of their personal emotional connection with what was happening and what happened.

Think back on your life. Some of the most vivid memories will be charged with emotion. Do you recall your first sexual experience in detail? How about when you broke your arm? Was it ice skating? Did you cry for days when your friend or your son died? What's the point? The point is simply that we tend to recall events charged with personal emotions. We remember what we want to remember in the same way we believe what we want to believe. These are significant grave faults of the human brain and the human experience, which we must try to overcome by constructive energy and reasoned thought, and mental force!

Knowing about the influence of emotion on memory gives us ideas on how to use emotion to advantage: First, don't try to memorize anything you are really not interested in. That is pushing memory uphill and mainly a waste of time and life. Second, stick to what is emotionally important to you, the things you really want to learn, or need to learn, the things you really want to know. Arrange your courses in college on the basis of your real interests. Don't go to law school if you want to be a movie star. Don't be a businessman if you want to be a doctor.

For example: Later, we will cover the old bugaboo about memorizing names. It is a fact that if you are not interested in the person, if you don't have a personal reason to remember their name, or if you just don't care about them, the chance of remembering their name and the chance of remembering them goes way down.

On the other hand, if you resolve that you will remember the name because you need to or because you want to remember the name, you will be way ahead. Repeat the name so that you are sure you got it right. Later, review the name so that it gets fixed in your memory. Linking the name with some association will help. Put the face and the name in the place where you met; link them with the good food or drink or the current topic of conversation. The more associations and the better the links, the more likely you will recall the name next time you meet, even if you don't meet them for decades. Some people even write the name down and review it later just before they hit the hay. Whatever is the last thing you review before sleep, usually will stick. Did we have a mental gymnastic on face-face problems? Did we learn to use bizarre images and unusual narratives to cement the faces of wives and husbands? Did we have a face to name exercise? Why can't you remember?

Soon we will do a face-name problem where we will practice making associations to help recall names.

Meanwhile, back to motor memory.

Finger Memory

Fingers have no memory. The memory is in the brain, without which the fingers cannot function. "Finger memory" is but a name for whatever the hands have been trained in advance to execute, be it knitting, playing a musical instrument, taking out a brain tumor, shuffling cards, tying shoes, riding your motorcycle, or scrambling an egg.

The fingers may acquire a muscular habit of performing feats and evolutions, but the fingers have no memory. You can prove this by cutting the nerves to your fingers. The fingers will instantly become useless and will have no memory whatsoever. (Only kidding. For heaven's sake, please don't do that. Cutting the nerves to your fingers will result in disaster.)

Kinesthetic Motor Memory Is Hard to Beat

Motor memories are mainly non-verbal, non-visual memory programs stored initially in special regions of the brain (first in medial structures and then basal ganglia and cerebellum). The physical basis of these memories is well known to neuroscientists and consists initially of visual, tactile, auditory, (occasional olfactory and gustatory) and kinesthetic inputs, which, when overlearned, are then delocalized and stored diffusely throughout the brain and in the aforementioned special areas in a kind of hologram of neuronal networks. Because these motor programs are delocalized and stored diffusely, these overlearned motor memories are virtually indestructible. Thus, these motor memories are the best and most powerful memory encoding systems we have. The human brain devotes trillions of bites of storage capacity to these memories. Motor memory is what enables us to ride a bike long after our childhood experiences with biking. Motor memory also allows us to ride the bike without consciously thinking about the task. The motor program for bike riding has essentially become subconscious and non-verbal. Don't believe me? Try explaining to someone how to ride a bike. Try explaining it to yourself. See? It's not easy. It is much easier to get on the bike and ride away. We learn bike riding by doing. We teach bike riding by showing and then making the student ride.

No normal person has to use his intellect consciously to walk: we walk without mental effort. An effort of will is necessary to start walking, but it is the subconscious non-verbal habitual motor programs of the brain that keep us going.

In fact, much of the brain's work is done automatically, including the mainte-nance of heart rate, blood pressure, chemical content of the blood, and so forth. To be conscious of your breathing is to breathe irregularly: to be conscious of our walking is to walk—well, self-consciously. In the same way, we learn how to do tasks (driving, swimming, playing music) by repeatedly doing the tasks so that we can do them without conscious effort. That is, in fact, the effect we are seeking in our music memory, our poetry memory, our tennis memory, and so forth, an effect I call AUTOMATICITY. Ultimately, we would like to play our pieces that way—automatically, without much conscious thought, just the way we ride our bikes without much conscious thought. Just the way, we would like to recite Longfellow's poem *Evangeline* without much conscious thought. My generation can drive a clutch car without much effort, but it took a great deal of concentrated attention to learn that skill and to not stall out. Why is human motor memory so good? The short answer to that question is no one knows. Probably it evolved to automatically manipulate weapons and allow the conscious mind to simulta-neously plan and execute the attack on animals for food and to effectively fight enemies for conquest or defense.

Warning! Motor Memory Can Betray You

As I am typing this book, I am not giving conscious thought to what letter keys to press. In fact, if I think about the keys too much, I will foul up. That's another point: Because motor memory is usually undirected by the intellect, it is often traitorous when you try to direct it. Consequently, in performance, a single wrong note may throw a player out, and she will break down (if she lets herself). Nor can she usually pick up the piece a bar or two farther on. She may often have to begin again or go on to the section she reserved as her lifesaver.

Remember: No normal person would have trouble walking a plank 18 feet long and a foot wide. But if that plank were suspended over a cliff, there would be much hesitation, clumsiness, and perhaps a fall because the conscious mind wouldn't let the unconscious mind run that task by itself for fear of death from a fall.

The good news is that the overlearned motor program is so deeply embedded in the brain that it usually functions automatically. The bad news is the programs are such that they often will fail if interrupted or if the mind is switched from unconscious control to conscious control. That happens a lot. If you have had any recital experience, it has happened to you. Usually, the thing that interrupts is your own thought about something other than the task at hand. A failure of attention breaks the motor program. Even though the thought is just an idle mo-ment, it sometimes has the power to derail the performance.

Remedy: Get better at focusing attention on the performance and avoid distract-ing thoughts. Consequently, your performances will break down less often. Re-cently, the thought that throws me off is, "Gee, Mickey, you are playing better than usual." As soon as that thought enters my mind, the motor program goes awry, and mistakes are made.

Because I have typed so many books, I don't have to think about typing any more than I have to think much about driving my car or flying an airplane or reciting Shakespeare. Someday my piano playing will be as automatic if I keep at it.

Things must happen that way as that is the way the human brain works, your brain works, our brains work. Sooner or later, you will be able to find and play the right keys on the piano without thinking much about them. Sooner or later, with sufficient practice, you will become a great public speaker or a great whatever. Just keep working, and see. Sooner or later, you will master the task or tasks you want to master. Just keep working! There is an old Irish motto: "It's the holding that counts." Meaning: Persist! Persistence counts! Persistence is the key to success.

Some Startling Examples of the Strengths of Motor Memory

Example: Demented patients who do not know their own name or where they are, when a bicycle is placed in their hands, will say they don't know what the bicycle is or what it does. They can't even name it, and when told it is a bicycle, they are puzzled about what it is that it does. And yet, those demented patients, without apparent effort, can get right on the bike and drive that bike away. A demented patient who had a career as a nightclub pianist can play on the piano quite well, including *Sidewalks of New York* and *Give My Regard to Broadway*. And yet, he is unable to tell what those songs are about, and he is unable to explain what or how he is playing. The motor memory is preserved even though the other memories (verbal, visual) are gone, completely and long gone. YouTube has startling examples of this phenomenon where a poor suffering demented woman or man sits at a piano, looks all around dazed and befuddled, announces she doesn't know what the piano is or what it is for, and then suddenly, marvelously and without apparent effort plays Chopin's *Nocturne Nine*.

Mental Gymnastic: Why Is Motor Memory the Strongest Modality of Human Memory?

Stop! This was explained to you. Tell the reason.

Answer: Motor memory systems probably evolved to enable humans to automatically manipulate weapons while consciously planning hunting or fighting strategies. Brain system one used in conjunction with brain system two put humans in charge of this planet. Trouble does occur with the exclusive use of only one of the systems. If you rely solely on system one as your policy (what to do), you will fail to benefit from the reasoned benefits of system two. Politicians, like Donald John Trump who routinely rely solely on system one, will routinely produce disasters.

Musicians can take advantage of the same motor memory capabilities of the brain by encoding their pieces not so much in verbal or visual modalities of memory but in the motor (kinesthetic) memory itself. This might create psychological problems because you might not think you know a music piece. And let's face it, you probably don't know that piece—not consciously. And yet, you do know it—unconsciously. You know it in the non-verbal realm—the motor modality of human memory. A good treatment for that problem is to make sure you know how to begin your piece and the exact right note and beginning sequence to start. Once started in the right direction, motor memory should take over and keep going unless interrupted. Similar strategy applies to poetry recitation and to public speaking, sky diving, ice skating, target shooting, shoe tying, and so forth.

No Interruptions

Aye, there's the rub. As every real performer knows, if a motor sequence is interrupted, the program may fail. Don't believe it? While you are playing a piece you know by heart, have a friend turn on the radio or hum or talk to you or even just look over your shoulder. Or while playing a piece, momentarily shift your consciousness to something else, even something silly like "Gee, I am playing this piece very well."

How true! In fact, congratulating yourself on how well you are doing is one of the usual distractions that cause foul-up. The same situation applies to professional golfers and gymnasts. Interrupt the routine, and you may get disaster. Ever notice in the championship tennis match the player in the lead may, at the last easy two serves, completely foul up and fail entirely? Tony Fauci, our United States infectious disease champion, threw the baseball to first base and not home when he opened the baseball season. What the devil was he thinking? What the devil fouled him up? He says he doesn't know, but he thinks he may have been **distracted** by a pain in his shoulder. Distracted is the right word here because the throw to the catcher at home base would have been automatic, should have been automatic, to Tony, who had lots of sports experience at Regis High School.

Mental Gymnastic

A law student was a double amputee and was 6 feet 9 inches tall. The prosthetic technicians had trouble with his prosthetic legs and needed to shorten them two inches until they could get a proper replacement for him to use.

Question: Based on your knowledge of motor memory and its frailties, predict what difficulties the law student would be expected to encounter now that he was 2 inches shorter.

Answer: He was so accustomed to being 6' 9" that when he went to 6' 7", he had trouble reaching for doorknobs and handles and stair railings and so forth due to his motor memory being used to reaching at a certain height. Fascinating stuff! Really!

Question: What solutions would you propose?

Answer: Solution 1. Go back to the original height.

Solution 2. Retrain motor memory to operate at 6' 7". The retraining will be long and hard because once motor habits are firmly fixed, they are extremely difficult to change.

How to handle distractions that foul motor memory and how to cope with loss of sequence, and how to compensate for this performance problem posed by the defects in motor memory will be covered later. Meanwhile, consider the interesting case of Oscar Levant.

The Story of Oscar Levant

Oscar Levant, one of the great pianists of all time, a friend of George Gershwin, stopped in the middle of *Rhapsody in Blue* that he was playing in Lewiston Stadium circa 1944. Levant had played *Rhapsody* many, many times. But this time, he momentarily thought of something else (his paycheck) and lost it.

Ugh! What did Levant do? He scratched his head and, for the life of him, didn't know how to continue.

STOP! Explain why he who had played *Rhapsody* many, many times didn't know how to continue.

Answer: He was working his routine, which consisted entirely of unconscious motor memory. The unconscious motor program was suddenly derailed by a conscious thought about his paycheck.

Oscar did an unusual thing: he and the orchestra started back at the beginning. And from that new beginning, Oscar kept going without apparent difficulty because he concentrated on the piece and didn't think about the paycheck until the performance was over. The whole instructive story of this event is featured in Levant's delightful autobiography, *Memoirs of an Amnesiac*.

Levant could have used some other tricks besides going back to the beginning. He could have asked himself not what was needed but where he had played the piece last. He could have then visualized the room and the piano where he practiced. As that image flashed across the slate of his consciousness, the forgotten item should have a high probability of being recalled. Cicero used this type of place clue during his speeches before the Roman Senate. The visual items that helped recall were always items in his own villa, a statue, a fresco, the impluvium, and so forth. Place clues (as they are called in the memory schools) helped Cicero recall what he wanted to talk about next. In fact, the word topic comes from the Greek work topoi, which means—you guessed it—place. Next time you can't think of a name, think of a place where that name was learned. Thinking of the place and the events, sights, sounds, smells, tastes, emotional state, and any other thing at the time you previously heard the name should clue the memory.

Remembrance of Things Past

Proust recalled his whole past life and wrote a nine-volume novel *(A la recherché du temp perdu)* on the basis of the associations triggered by the taste of that madeleine cookie after it was dipped in tea. Strictly speaking, this was an involuntary memory in which the taste of the madeleine summoned forth images of his aunt's house and his happy childhood. The same mechanism can be used to voluntarily recall items temporarily out of the consciousness. The recapture of past times, the making of time stand still, is one of the blessed benefits of literature and memory. We can read *The Naked and the Dead* and actually experience vicariously fighting those yellow devils for control of an island in the Pacific whose name nobody knows anymore.

How to Recall Things You Know but Can't Quite Remember

Just think of items that are close to the needed item—close in either time or place or both, putting or trying to put the needed memory in context.

Right now, I don't know what I ate at the Hotel Roanoke last Friday. But if I visualize the Regency Room, the people at the table, the seating arrangements, it might come back.

Yes, it did come back, popped right into my consciousness without any great effort! Lamb chops. They were delicious. And as expected, the lamb chops triggered other memories. Not only do I now "see" the meal, I see the people (my daughter's family) at the table, and I hear the head waiter ask me to play *Blues in the Night* on the piano, which I did after the main course. All that came rushing back into consciousness the way the madeleine made Proust recall the events at his aunt's country home.

Another illustration to help you understand memory in general and your memory in particular: I just came from a lecture on dystopias. And now I am trying to recall the one that was based on a quote from Shakespeare. Still trying but not getting it. So, I decide to think about the two dystopic novels I do remember—*Animal Farm* and 1984 and bingo! *Brave New World* popped into my head.

If you get stuck, ask where not what. And think about the items around what you want to recall. Also, remember the state-dependent problem. If you are stuck, keep calm. The tenser you get, the worse your chance of recall. If putting the memory in context does not work, you might have to go back to the last place in the poem that you recall. Restarting is usually considered déclassé, but what can you do? Desperate people do desperate things. Or why not skip ahead to your rescue spot and recite from there? Sometimes I lose it while reciting the Gettysburg Address. What I have done is skip ahead and continue from there. This has gone over well, and I would bet not a soul in the audience knew what was missing. That's what happens. No one (except the teachers and the real history aficionados) notices.

BERNARD MICHAEL PATTEN, M.D.

Mental Gymnastic

Recall the height of Mount Fuji. If you have trouble, does the number 12 help you remember?

12,365 feet. Have you any recall that this was mentioned? That you were told to remember the height by association with the 12 months of the year and the fact that there are 365 days in the year. Remember now?

Answer: If you thought you recalled this item, you are wrong. It was not mentioned. That's another problem with memory. Many memories are fake. They are what we would like to recall, or they have been suggested to us, and we have latched on to them. At class at Rice, two students staged a fake fight and then left the room. When asked what happened, there were as many different stories as there were respondents, proving both memories and observations were defective. This phenomenon is known in psychology circles as the Rashomon effect based on the movie by that name wherein four individuals witnessed the rape of Masako and the murder of her samurai husband, but each had a different memory of what happened. The lesson here is eye witness accounts are not entirely trustworthy. My father, who was the chief homicide prosecutor in Queens for decades, used to dress up for the lineups. Because he was in a trench coat and looked shady, eye witnesses often picked him out as the perpetrator of the crime. A black man in a lineup has a very good probability of being fingered as the rapist even though he was the law clerk that year. If old people are asked to recall a list of bed, night table, dream, pillow, they will almost always say the word "sleep" was on the list when it was not. We all have to be careful of false memories. This is particularly true when we are told a lie by a highly placed politician. Initially, we may know the lie is a lie, but eventually, we forget the source was known to be unreliable, and eventually, not able to recall the source, we may begin to believe the lie. This is a known brain defect. Immediately after hearing a message, the credibility of a source matters. However, over time the low-credibility source message becomes more persuasive. This is what is called the sleeper effect (I am not making this up) because it is as though the not-very-credible message is just slumbering in your brain until it suddenly pops up as influential. The sleeper effect is used in advertising where someone endorses a product, let's say, a movie star who really knows nothing about soap or windows or the right medicine for arthritis. Eventually, the source of the recommendation is forgotten, but the message is not. Our brains are not good at remembering exactly where, when, and from whom we learned a piece of information. The low-credibility source information fades in time and makes space for the message to stick around and influence us.

The lesson is to watch out for false memories. Verify sources and information. Don't pass on misinformation or any information you are not sure about. Reference: Kumkale, GT and D. Abarracin. "The Sleeper Effect on Persuasion: A Meta-Analytic Review." Psychological Bulletin, 130 (2004) 143–172.

Repeat Discussion of Rescue Techniques

Instead of restarting, a better trick (as mentioned) might be to have a place forward. Call those places rescue spots because they really are lifesavers. If you are stuck, you don't go back; you don't repeat; you just skip ahead to the place you have already designated as your lifesaver. Few in the audience will notice. Most of the audience will be doing the time-honored thing most audiences do—thinking of something else or daydreaming. Some, alas, will be sleeping.

Emotions, Positive and Negative—Good, Bad, and Ugly Encode Memories

Emotional significance often determines what we remember and what we choose to forget. Human memory works best when the thing we are trying to remember has a personal emotional significance for us and when we are in a positive good mood. Think back on your own life. You'll see that this is true. We remember what is emotionally important to us, and we tend to forget what is not emotionally important to us.

I recall my childhood battle with measles (72 years ago), in which I almost died. That situation is pictured in my mind in great vivid detail, including my bedroom, the window, the blue wallpaper, Doctor Mellisy looming over me, the tea with whiskey given to me by my mother as a treatment, etc. Yet, I can't recall what I had for lunch last Wednesday or even what color socks I have on right now. From which follows, we are better off trying to memorize things we connect with on an emotional level than something we don't connect with. But that does raise the question of how to approach a memory task or a learning task that you don't like but must do. The answer is to give it a try, and you may find, as many people do, that you warm up to the project, and after you have made significant progress, you actually enjoy it.

If you like fast jazzy pieces, it would be hard to memorize a slow, romantic piece and vice versa. For this reason, do not try to memorize a musical piece that you don't like. And do not bother with a piece you hate. Drop, without regret, any course of study you honestly dislike. In college, I dropped with a sigh of relief an utterly boring course in medical statistics. Life is short. There are better things to do like reading this book and doing the mental gymnastics:

Mental Gymnastic

Read over the comic. Then answer the questions. Probably better read aloud.

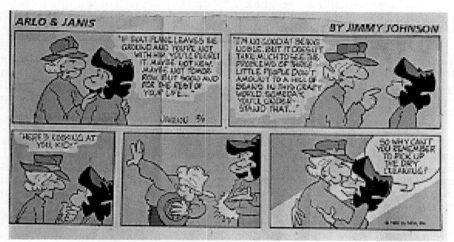

Fig3.5

Questions: Why can he recite from memory (with some errors that are unapparent to his listener) the famous speech at the end of the movie Casablanca? And yet, he can't remember to pick up the dry cleaning? Think about this for five minutes. Make notes about your answers. Compare your answers with the ones at the end of this chapter. Remember, the answer doesn't count as much as the mental work to get the answer. So almost any reasonably considered answer will do.

Whew!

That was a lot to learn about the facts of memory. In the chapters on memory light and memory heavy, we apply what we learned to various memory tasks. The applications are more important than anything else because memory is a performance art.

Before we get to techniques, review the summary list below on human memory principles. Review these several times until they are part of your memory repertoire. A good time to review is just before you hit the hay. Believe it or not, the brain will work on encoding the items while you sleep. Even if it doesn't, review time is never wasted.

You will know you know the principles when you can successfully explain what the principle is and how it applies to memory. Challenge yourself on these items. Don't think you know something. Prove you do! No one is watching. Prove you know this stuff to yourself. The unexamined life is not worth living, said someone famous, and he was right. Self-testing is a key technique for making yourself look ten times smarter.

How To Make Sure You Know Anything

Ask yourself questions. Quiz yourself right now, for instance, on state-dependent learning. Give yourself time to think. Explain state-dependent learning to yourself. This is a pain and will seem pedantic, but it is the right thing to do if you wish to actually know a subject, any subject, well.

You are testing yourself to see if you really know it. In most situations, it is better for you to be the first to learn that you don't know something rather than your teacher or your boss. It is better for you to know now that you will fail the French test (unless you study more) than to learn the hard way tomorrow after the test is over.

After you have given yourself your answers, go back to that section in this book and see how many items and examples you recalled and how many you missed. Imagine how you can apply the principle to memorizing what you want to remember. If you can't think of anything that you want to remember, how about memorizing the first ten amendments to the Constitution of the United States or at least the preamble.

Again, repeat: There is a gigantic difference between thinking you know something and actually knowing it. Prove to yourself that you know this stuff. Make at least three intelligent points about each of the following topics. When you can make at least three intelligent points about each of the principles of memory, go on to chapter four—Memory Lite.

Summary of the Chapter's Memory Topics and Review

Consider the following questions and requests:

What general activities benefit the brain?

What techniques would you use to recall something on the tip of your tongue?

Explain why lost opportunities are opportunities lost.

How do we know that forgetting is the default mode of human memory?

How much of a perfectly memorized poem will be recalled in two weeks if there has been no interim review or rehearsal or associations?

How does review time affect memory?

How do sickness and boredom affect memory?

Why do associations produce recall?

What associations are best?

What's VAK, and how does it help encode memory?

If you are learning a language, why is it better to see and hear the new word at the same time?

What is the advantage of spacing your learning?

What roles do active attention and active mental engagement play in memory?

Why is cramming not the best way of memorizing anything?

What mechanisms control stage fright, and how does stage fright affect memory?

What is meant by modality-specific memories?

Name the six modalities of human memory.

Which of the six modalities of human memory is the strongest?

Do emotions play a role in encoding memories?

Extra Credit:

Explain why neurologists think TV is bad for your brain.

Arrange the following activities in terms of what is best (number 1) and what is worst for the brain's health:

a. Thinking and doing

b. Doing

c. Thinking

d. Watching without thinking or doing.

Explain why a positive mental attitude is important.

Some psychologists call motor memory "procedural memory." Why?

Some psychologists call explicit memory "declarative memory." Why?

What are the other names for declarative and procedural memory?

Extra extra credit

What is the best way to develop your knitting ability?

(Give yourself a big pat on the back if you immediately said to yourself: "The best way to develop knitting ability is to knit.")

More extra credit

Explain what happens when neurons fire together. Recite the poem that cements the memory.

Why do we need to forget almost everything we experience?

What is the serial position effect, and how does it influence memory of lists?

What techniques can be used to compensate for the serial position effect in a shopping list?

Why is social dance considered a closed motor task?

Explain the recency effect on memory. How can you take advantage of this effect?

Why would knowing the historical perspectives help your performance attain the correct stylistic, musical, and technical result in the performance of a classic tap dance?

Explain brain system one.

Explain brain system two.

What activities does system one support?

What activities does system two support?

What is the Rashomon effect? What lesson does it teach us?

Why does previewing help cement memories of plays and movies?

Put a checkmark here _____ if you think you learned one useful thing from reading this book so far.

Answer to the Arlo & Janis comic question: Give yourself a pat on the back if you said Arlo had more emotional interest and energy invested in reciting the speech than he had in picking up the dry cleaning. Part of that emotional interest includes trying to impress Janis that he has a good memory and that he understands romance and is romantic. He is a show-off. Many people are. How about you?

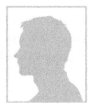

CHAPTER FOUR
MEMORY LITE

CHAPTER FOUR: MEMORY LITE

◆ ◆ ◆

Summary of This Chapter:

This chapter covers memory lite, simple ways to encode and read out memories. Most of the techniques will be familiar. They include thinking (very important and often omitted), paying attention (very important and often omitted), studying the outline of the task, making up your mind to do the memory task in the shortest, most efficient way, looking for and consciously noting chunks, clusters, repeats, patterns, sequences, memory hooks, memorable phases, simple mnemonics, interesting narrative possibilities, scripts, schemata, and emotional connections.

Making up questions about the material that you will try to answer after your study will help you confirm you have mastered the task. The chapter tells you to consider how you might apply rhythm, rhyme, numbers and number lists, alphabet lists, first-letter clues, color fields, ideas, emotions, eidetic, and other images (anything really) to specific memory problems. To help you apply this knowledge, the chapter gives mental gymnastic exercises that might develop your own memory techniques to help you memorize things like English language vocabulary, foreign language vocabulary, literary structures, movie plots, faces, legal definitions, dance routines, names, chemical formulae and what have you.

Your best results will come from daily practice where progress and lack of progress is reviewed (on videotape preferably), with mistakes corrected until AUTOMATICIY is reached. Automatic or semiautomatic rendition of the memory task is the desired effect. It is possible to dance tango while thinking about every step and move, but you are not going to look like a Valentino. You are going to look like a tyro. Effective tango would only come from an automatic knowledge of the basic steps and procedures. After you mastered the basic steps and ideas of Tango, you can then be artistic and put your own spin on the performance.

Despite these high standards, please manage your expectations. Progress may be slower than you think and, in some cases, a lot slower than you think. Despite the difficulties, hang in there. Be patient! Persistence counts!

How to Approach a Memory Task

Start by making up your mind that you want to do the memory task. Doing things you don't want to do is hard, an uphill battle. Unless something is required for school or the job or you are just trying to prove something to yourself or others, your best results will obtain from doing the things you want to do, memorizing the things that are important to you, or fun. Yes, it is that simple: Where there is fun, there is a way.

Recent research suggests that while mental exercise does delay the onset of dementia, it may be the case that once dementia starts in those who have benefited from a delay, the dementia will progress more rapidly than expected. This finding seems counter to what we know about cognitive reserve and how and why mental activity protects the brain. But even if this research result were true, the overall benefit of mental exercise would still remain and be a good thing in general for everyone.

But suppose the results are true. Then they would suggest that whatever mental exercise you decide to do should be more fun than work. In general, if you find yourself straining on anything, you will be better off in the long run by cutting back and giving yourself some slack. Use it and improve it. Have fun with it just in case you might lose it. All work and no play make Jack a dull boy. Jill too.

Think about What You Are Doing; Don't Just Rush In

Next, think. Think about the task. Develop a habit of original awareness. Think about how you might accomplish the task. In a normal human, things just keep popping into the mind. You have to learn to ignore them and develop focus. Begin by studying the overall outline of what needs to be done. Try to organize a program of learning that is reasonable and doable. Time is more precious than most people think. It is a non-renewable resource. Bill Gates and Warren Buffett, who have bank accounts that resemble the national debt, cannot buy a single second of time. Nor can you.

Time is the real enemy of mankind and the real enemy of perfect memory and automaticity. Time is needed to memorize, and time itself erodes memory. Save considerable time and energy by planning a tactic and organizing a strategy. General George S. Patton said, "Time spent in RECONNAISSANCE is never wasted." Time spent in thinking about simple, easy, and efficient ways of getting the task done will pay off. This means if you are intent on memorizing *To a Wild Rose* by MacDowell, you would be much better off in the long run actually looking at the score for 15 whole minutes, trying to see the overall structure, the repeats, the actual rhythms. The same for a poem.

At Columbia College, we students were not permitted to discuss a poem in class unless we certified to the instructor and our classmates that we had actually read that poem at least 13 times. Why 13? I don't know. But the general idea was to spend considerable time with the poem in view of the fact that the poet spent considerable time composing the poem.

Look at the lines, the diction, the syntax, the tone, the rhymes, the repeats, and so forth before you start your memory work on any poem. Listen to expert recitations at conferences, poetry slams, or on YouTube. Get the feel for the work by researching some information about the poet, the poem, and the historical context. Knowing background makes you look smarter and makes you perform better. Your goal should be to be able to speak intelligently about the poem or music piece or whatever for three minutes. That will be especially impressive because most people cannot speak intelligently about anything.

Time Is Needed for Any Substantial Memory Task

If the task is to study for the New York Bar examination and you have only two days left and have not yet memorized the rules of evidence or the law of bailment, you are not going to make it this time around—the task is too big and too complex to master in the available time. Complex things like the law of bailment need to be practiced and reviewed over a longer time to make them part of your mental set. You will need to know the three types of bailment and the legal principles and duties applied to each and so forth.

If the task is to memorize and play correctly Chopin's *Waltz in B Minor*, and recital is tomorrow afternoon, you are not going to make that either. That waltz is too big and too complex and too difficult to master in the available time. You will need to break it down to easy, digestible pieces and patterns and work at fingering, rhythm, tempo, and so forth. After weeks of work, you may be OK.

Rome Wasn't Built in a Day

Complex memory tasks require plenty of work, time, and repetition. The diligent application of the memory techniques that you pick up in this book and elsewhere will help speed and ease the process. In fact, application of the techniques to be discussed actually saves time. Jerry Lucas, in his excellent *The Memory Book* claims applications of memory techniques got him excellent grades in college with study times about 10% of the times spent by fellow students. This claim sounds outrageous, but those who have completed memory courses know it is well within the range of the possible, and most of us, myself included, expect it.

About expectations: But don't expect too much, especially in the beginning. Chances are, you won't make fast progress on any complex memory project. Go easy on yourself. Give yourself plenty of time to get the task done. Manage your expectation as much as you manage the memory task itself. But know this, just trying a memory task develops brainpower, focuses attention, and develops powers of concentration. The effort itself produces results even if the effort doesn't produce the desired results exactly.

Understanding the Task and Your Goal Before You Start Is Key

Memory is modality- and task-specific. When you travel to France, you should bone up on your French so that you can easily ask directions, order a tuna burger, and understand the insults and innuendoes they are leveling against you during the elevator ride to the Jules Verne Restaurant on the second floor of the Eiffel tower. The time to start your work on learning French is not two days before the trip starts. Two days is not enough time to master French.

In your memory work, it's not only advisable but critical to understand what the task requires in terms of material to be mastered and the time needed to master it. That is what it is all about. After that, after you have done these, the preliminaries, put on your thinking cap and apply the tips and tricks about memorization.

Before getting to tips and tricks, let's answer the two important questions that come up:

1. **How long will it take for me to complete this memory task?**
2. **How long will the memorized item remain in my memory once I have completely mastered it?**

Most people don't ask these questions, but some do. When they do, they usually get an answer that sounds like this:

"As long as necessary" or "Much longer than you think."

Such answers, while true, do tend to beg the question. They certainly are not scientific, as they do not lend themselves to experimental verification. They are not scientific because they have not been answered in quantitative terms.

Qualitative and vague answers need to be replaced by something quantitative and definite. What is needed to answer these two questions is some actual data from actual experience or experiments designed to find out how long it takes you to memorize something, a piece of music or a poem or your speech before The Lion's Club or a page of French and how long (once it is memorized) that piece will remain in the memory. In a sense, in memory work, unlike in investments, past performance is a good indication of future performance. Keep track of the time you spend on given tasks and use that time as an estimate of what time you will need to do that task again or to master similar tasks.

Do You Want to Swing on a Star, Be Better off Than You Are, or Do You Want to Be a Fish?

You have a choice. What you select to do is up to you. If you concentrate your attention on building an English language vocabulary, that's what you get. Concentrate on math and music; that's what you get. Concentrate on golf. Ditto. Song styling—you bet. Concentrate on song styling, and your golf will not improve, but your song styling will.

Into its form and functions, the brain is programmed to incorporate the activities you do. That is the neuroplasticity thing about the brain. You can and do modify your brain by the habits you develop. The brain makes no distinction about what is worthwhile or not worthwhile. That's up to you. If you decide to just hang out, or spend your time mindlessly gossiping on your cell phone, or working on your Facebook page, or (God forbid) watching TV, the brain will make circuits for these activities. If you practice getting up from a chair like an old man, you will soon look like an old man when you get up from a chair. Aristotle said, "We are what we do habitually." If you habitually climb stairs like an old person, then you will eventually actually look like an old person climbing stairs. Repetition cements brain motor programs for better or for worse.

Repeat after me: I am the master of my fate. I am the captain of my soul. I choose what brain circuits and what neurons will function well on the basis of the activities that I myself choose. I make myself. I make my brain.

What You Should Not Do: Don't Waste Time, and Don't Watch TV

Why, Doctor Patten, if TV is so bad for the brain and for health in general, do so many people watch it?

Doctor Patten answers: The short answer to that question is I don't know, and for the life of me, I don't understand it. But part of the long answer is that mental passivity is a lot less work than self-reliance and action. The easy path is tempting even when we are repeatedly disappointed in where it takes us and where it leaves us. To accept responsibility and to achieve and maintain honest appraisals of self-worth, capability, and achievement requires mental energy, focus, and, above all, courage.

Watch out for Fake Things

My more abstract answer why TV is bad involves the fact that TV often shows a fake view of reality. The emotions displayed are often fake, the interpersonal relations are often fake, and the situations and solutions to problems are fake. When your brain sees so much stuff that isn't real, so much that is fake, you begin to have a fake view of reality. Why is that bad? Because reality is what we humans have to deal with. The reality of our physical existence: the fact we need food, clothing, shelter, love, freedom from infections, a lot of things. If we don't deal realistically with reality, then reality will deal with us, and sometimes it will deal with us rather harshly.

For example: You are flying your airplane, and the fuel gauge approaches empty. What should you do? Pick from the following list the appropriate management of the reality:

1. Assume the gauge is wrong and keep flying.
2. Pray to the Virgin Mary, and rest assured she will help.
3. Assume your plane, when it runs out of fuel, will keep flying and not fall out of the sky.
4. Know that because you are a very special person, the law of gravity will not apply to you or your plane, and therefore you will remain aloft.
5. Talk with President Trump, who will assure you there is nothing to be concerned about.
6. Land and refuel.

Solutions 1 to 5 will cause you and the plane to fall out of the sky, and you may actually crash. But don't worry. There will be no fire because there is no fuel.

The solid world exists; its laws do not change. Stones are hard, water is wet, and objects unsupported are pulled toward the center of the earth. Physical facts cannot be ignored. Two and two make four now and forever, and in constructing a ship or an airplane, they have to make four, otherwise disaster. You can think whatever you wish and say what you want, but cold hard facts speak for themselves. In the above example, the cold hard fact is the internal combustion engine will not work without fuel. Many people have learned that lesson directly.

You Are Unique; There Is No One Else Like You, Says Mr. Rogers

Every person on this planet is an individual, no exceptions. What is easy for you might be hard for me and vice versa. "Know thyself" was inscribed on the Temple of Apollo at Delphi. That's good advice. Work at your memory tasks and see how much time and effort is needed for the particular tasks you work on. Super performers often concentrate their attention on the things they do better than others. Igor Stravinsky gave up law because he didn't like it. When he switched to music composition, he became a star, famous, and he delighted audiences worldwide. Galileo, one of the most scientific men in all history, left the University of Pisa in 1585 after having dropped out of medicine and not having any degree. He quit med school to study math. Look where that got him.

Keep a written record of your times and record the difficulties you encounter. This is the database from which you can get estimates of how much time will be required. For instance, to become a skilled neurosurgeon, you will need over 10,000 hours of diligent application and study. To learn how to effectively tell a joke in public, you will need about 50 hours. (Yes, 50!) Most people are terrible joke tellers and don't know it. Most people are terrible storytellers and don't know it. Telling jokes or telling stories are performance arts that must be mastered by long hard work and practice.

Most people underestimate the amount of time and effort needed to achieve automaticity and look natural. Psychologists call this well-known phenomenon the illusion of confidence, the tendencies to overestimate our own abilities.

Surveys show Americans outrank people from all other countries in one thing and one thing only: Self-confidence. It's a pity that, in most cases, this over-blown American self-confidence is not justified by any reasonable analysis of the facts.

The illusion of confidence is one of the many ways that our intuitions deceive us. This illusion, like the other illusions that afflict our mental life (inattentional blindness), illusion of control (dangerous when texting while driving or crossing the street), continuity errors in narration memory (common in recent movies), and so forth are brain hoaxes, the consequence of how our brains work and sometimes trick us. The confidence illusion is a brain failure that probably derives from the inability to realistically deal with the idea that our brains are weak, so weak that we routinely often wrongly overestimate our capabilities and underestimate our limitations. Our brains are the end product of millions of years of evolution and were designed to function in an environment quite different from our modern life. Our brain is seriously behind the times and is like a model T Ford at the raceway, unable to keep up with the modern cars. That's fact, and that's the reality. And we must deal with this reality effectively so that it doesn't deal effectively with us.

The Brain Is Easily Tricked

It is easy for experimental psychologists to show how the brain can be tricked. A startling illustration is how they can create false memories, whereby people are intuitively certain they did hear or see some item that was in fact suggested and then imagined. Imagining that you perform a particular action if the mental image is repeated often enough may create the illusion that you actually performed it.

Much pain and suffering have been caused by well-meaning social workers and child protective agents in suggesting to children that they have been abused. Leading questions do exactly that—lead and often mislead. Such leading questions are not allowed in a court of law under certain conditions for the reason that they tend to lead away from truth toward error. You can ask leading questions but not of your own client. You can ask leading questions if the court declares the witness hostile. You can ask leading questions of opposition's expert witness but can't ask leading questions of your own expert witness. And, of course, you can ask all the leading questions you wish if opposing counsel is sleeping and doesn't object.

The brain tends to believe what is repeated to it. Thus, if you pretend you are happy when you are blue, it is likely that you will get happy. If you, as a politician, keep telling people on the campaign circuit that you are a Vietnam veteran and a war hero, sooner or later, you may actually believe your own misstatement. How else are we to explain the common occurrence of a prominent politician being called to task about an exaggerated biography of himself?

One prominent politician (Donald John Trump) stated in public he knows more about medicine than medical doctors! He considered this pretty remarkable in view of the fact he did not attend medical school. He said his uncle was a doctor, and some of it may have rubbed off on him! His uncle was a doctor, but not a medical doctor. John Trump held an ScD from M.I.T. in electrical engineering. Electrical engineering has little to do with medicine, so Trump was misleading us again.

President Trump's medical advice subsequently caused problems among those who actually believed him. He famously said he knows more about military matters than five-star generals, even though he never served. This politician has made so many misstatements and told so many lies, I call him agent orange because he is that dangerous.

Hamlet kept pretending he was mad, and then toward the end of the play, he actually became mad. Practice makes perfect. And the perfect practice of acting crazy makes perfect craziness. It has been proven that in certain legal cases, a molestation was repeatedly suggested by the investigating psychologist, and eventually, the person involved actually believed that they were molested even though they were not.

Cryptomnesia

In 1952, Morey Bernstein using hypnosis, regressed Virginia Tighe passed her birth and into what she felt was a previous life as Bridey Murphy. Virginia even claimed she remembered her own funeral as Bridey and watched it from above. After publication of Bernstein's book, many people "remembered" their previous lives as soldiers in Caesar's army or as workers who built the pyramids in Egypt and so forth.

"Brainwashing" is another notable example and explains why people confess to crimes they couldn't have possibly committed or previously patriotic soldiers denounce their country in videotapes made by an enemy that has captured them and "reeducated" them.

The Illusion of Memory

Because the world is fairly consistent and fairly predictable most of the time, we rely on our past experiences to fill in the proverbial blanks of what was actually seen with what we think we saw. For instance, in a scene reminiscent of Candid Camera, a shill pretending he is a lost tourist holds out a map and asks for directions while secretly the event is recorded on a video. As the pedestrian is trying to help by studying the map, two men carrying a large door walk between the interlocutors, disrupting the face-to-face. Behind the door and out of sight, one of the doormen changes places with the shill (lost tourist). More than half of the pedestrians failed to notice that they were now talking to someone new.

Some of you readers out there have seen the movie where you are asked to keep an eye on a basketball as it moves along the court. Many are shocked after seeing the movie that while their full attention was on the ball, an unnoticed man in a gorilla outfit walked among the players.

A Human Failing: Sometimes in Error but Never in Doubt

Watch out! There is an enormous fallibility of our intuitions about what we see, remember, know, think, predict, and believe. The lesson is clear: When in doubt, fall back on cognitive modesty: Think long and hard before you think you know. When in doubt, prove you know it or don't know it by self-test or consultation with a reliable source. For heaven's sake, don't pass on anything that you are not sure is true. Do not contribute to the vast pile of misinformation on the internet. Share only that which you are sure is true. That is critical today when indisputable facts are labeled "fake news" or a "hoax."

BERNARD MICHAEL PATTEN, M.D.

Misinformation as a Public Health Crisis

Misinformation has accelerated the spread of COVID-19 by fragmenting and influencing the response to prevention strategies like wearing a mask and physical distancing. Misinformation was spread about nearly every aspect of the pandemic, including the origins of the virus (e.g., it was manufactured in a laboratory in China), treatments (e.g., bleach, alcohol, anti-malarial drugs), and vaccine safety (e.g., vaccines include embedded microchips, cause autism). Because misinformation is not labeled as such, distinguishing it from real information can be difficult, particularly when highly politicized and opposing views are categorized as fake news. A gigantic problem has been misinformation from irresponsible leaders in the United States like Donald John Trump and from highly organized groups in Russia. Lewis Carroll advised in his book *Alice's Adventures in Wonderland* not to exercise the believing muscles of the brain too much. In other words, be skeptical and doubt until something is proven true.

Most People Don't Know What They Are Talking About

Long ago, I used to carry a notebook. When one of my friends told me something they thought was true, I wrote that in the notebook. Say it was a tip on the stock market, or a prediction about the weather, or who would win an election. Then months later, I would look over the notes and see what was what. Almost 99% of what I was told was, at least in part, wrong! Misinformation—the plague of modern society. In fact, the level of bullshit in the current media is so high, we have to stand on our tip toes to avoid suffocation.

Mental Gymnastic

Go to your local library and read newspapers from a year ago or two years ago and then compare and contrast what was printed there with what actually happened. Start with the financial sections because they have quantitative data. See how wrong the experts were and how wrong they can be. Knowing how little you know and how little others know is a big step forward in becoming a genius. Follow Socrates! He said he knew nothing.

Do Not Accept Expert Advice on Faith Alone. Verify.

Even experts often don't know what they are talking about. Here in Houston, we have a well-known political pundit named Murray who made the solemn prediction that a bald man whose ears stick out would never be elected mayor of our fair city. Guess what? Bill White won the election. He was elected mayor. His bald plate and ears are still in evidence, as he ran against Perry for the Texas governorship.

Still don't believe me that most people don't know what they are talking about? Obviously, you did not do the last mental gymnastic. Why not go read last year's newspapers? Why not read the financial section from two years ago? Why not have your eyes open? Why not arm yourself against believing every little thing? Thomas Jefferson said, "The man who doesn't read the papers is better off because his head is not filled with stuff that isn't true. And Mark Twain said, "It isn't what I don't know that hurts; it's all that stuff I think I know that ain't true."

I am paraphrasing these two men because I am too lazy to look up the exact quotes. You get the gist. If you want an exact quote, look it up.

Advice from Arthur Schopenhauer (1788-1860)

"If we have made obvious mistakes, we should not try, as we generally do, to gloss them over, or to find something to excuse...them; we should admit to ourselves that we have committed faults, and open our eyes wide to all their enormity, in order that we may firmly resolve to avoid them in the time to come."

Prove or Disprove Your Investment Actions

When you make an investment, write a full page of reasons why you made that investment. Every year review the page to see where you went right and where you went wrong. That technique will be a gigantic humbling experience and a gigantic learning experience. You live the future ahead, but you must evaluate your actions by looking back. Learn from the past and try not to repeat the mistakes.

For more information on cognitive illusions, how our brains fool us, consult the excellent book by Chabris and Simons, *The Invisible Gorilla: And Other Ways Our Intuitions Deceive Us,* Crown, New York, 2010.

Work from Your Database

You need to collect data on your own memory and use that data to predict how much time will be needed for a memory task. My forte is memorizing poetry. As I have been doing this for over 50 years, I am native in poetry land and to the manner born. I get it. Therefore, I can get it in my memory quickly. With poetry, I understand rhyme and meter, alliteration, assonance, caesura, poetic imagery, how to manage sequence, and so forth. That knowledge and more than 50 years of experience give me the chunking tools for quick memorization. Experience is a great teacher.

Example: Recently, I decided to memorize *Evangeline*, the famous poem by Henry Wadsworth Longfellow. Looking at the introduction to that great poem, we see 35 lines, with each line about six words long—about 200 words. From my previous experience, I estimate it will take me one-half hour to get this in the memory.

So, I read the first paragraph over, close the book, and try to recite the first paragraph. Then I review and see how I did. I am pretty good at deceiving myself into believing I did something right when actually I made mistakes. That's why for me, it is crucial to test myself and prove that I did it right. If the test shows that I need correction, then at least I know what's wrong. It's hard to correct what's wrong when you don't know what's wrong. So, I tested myself on that first paragraph.

Result: Not bad, but I messed up on "Loud from its rocky caverns." Instead of rocky, I said rock. I note the mistake and repeat the lines, then check my progress, and bingo! Correct in detail.

Note that I work on this task in pieces. Divide and conquer—that's the ticket. Time cost: Seven minutes. Accomplishment: Introduction memorized.

On to the next paragraph. Review again. Instead of leaped, I said leapt. I did say roe correctly but, come to think on it, I don't know what a roe is. That's probably why I said rue—pure ignorance. When you come across a word that you don't know the meaning of, you quite literally don't know what you are thinking about or talking about or memorizing.

Also important is using words clearly understood by the person you are talking to. Failure to understand where the listener is coming from can cause trouble. For instance, at the reunion of my wife's high school, Curtis, in Staten Island, the dinner conversation bored me, so I went to the bar for a drink. At the bar, seated on a stool, was an old man nursing a beer. He said, "Curtis High School is having a reunion." I replied, "Yes, it is a very cohesive group." Suddenly he got off the stool, raised his fists, squinted his eyes, and said, "I don't know who you are, buddy, but no one says cohesive about Curtis High School." Another time at a dinner party, I asked the hostess what condiments she used, and she replied, "I'm Catholic. I don't believe in birth control."

Understanding an intellectual grasp of the memory material is a great help. Knowing the meaning of words facilitates understanding. Therefore, what should I do if I don't know the meaning of the word roe?

Exactly right!

Look it up. The Oxford English Dictionary says a roe is a small species of deer. Repeat—correct except missed the part about men whose lives glided on like rivers that water the woodlands. I had said, "Men whose lives glide like the rivers that water the woodlands." "Glide on" does sound better and is probably more realistic. But "glided like" sounds more poetic.

Next—repeat to check.

The line that follows is so beautiful and has such a startling image that I shall never forget it: Darkened by shadows of earth, but reflecting an image of heaven. Get it? The image is applied both to the rivers and to the men. The men and the rivers are darkened and yet reflect images of heaven. Review and check—OK; so on to the next. And so forth. The actual time to recite this introduction correctly took me 28 minutes. Notice my estimate was close—30 minutes versus the actual

28 minutes. You may take longer or shorter. Why not give it a try as a mental gymnastic?

Memorizing Poetry Is a Lost Art

My poetry memory skills are outstanding because I trained up to it. I am not bragging. I am just stating a fact, and the fact occurred only because I love poetry and have devoted lots of time to memorizing lots of poems. This is nothing special. You could do the same if you felt the same about poetry. But I have a feeling that modern education forgets to teach young people how to remember. As a child, I memorized and recited by heart many times in elementary school; it was part and parcel of the curriculum. In school, we even memorized and recited words we didn't know. In reciting the Hail Mary, for instance, there was a long, long time that I knew the prayer by heart, could recite it perfectly, and yet didn't know what was meant by "fruit of thy womb." At age six, I could recite the Apostle's Creed without knowing what was meant by the phrase "conceived by the Holy Ghost."

Too bad oration and recitation, staples of the school system that trained me, where almost everything was memorized, not just poetry, have largely been phased out. Consequently, Britney Spears forgot the words she meant to lip-sync at the MTV Video Music Awards. Thus, Britney joins the absent-minded ranks of Katharine McPhee (American Idol runner-up), who dropped a whole line from "Hound Dog," and President Bush, who couldn't recall the punch line of the "Fool me once" aphorism: Fool me once, shame on thee; fool me twice, er…????????"

Help President Bush by filling in the blank.

Answer: "Shame on me."

Jenny Lyn Bader reported in her article *Britney? That's All She Rote* (sic) (The New York Times, September 16, 2007) that Miss Teen South Carolina Lauren Caitlin Upton completely forgot what she was saying in a pageant interview in a clip that became a viral hit on the website YouTube.

Why blame them? Memory is just not their thing. Distraction also probably played a role in their poor performances and stress and "nerves." And maybe stage fright put their brains in a different state. The excuses are legion. But the real reason probably relates to how their brains were trained in their youth. They are products of a culture that does not enforce the development of memory skills or serious thinking. The older heritage in American education, where recitation was the standard pedagogical mode, has gone the way of the buggy whip. No one even knows phone numbers anymore. Why bother? The numbers are encoded already in the iPhone. Many people don't even know their own phone number. Do you?

All that's gone in this age of multitasking, except for poetry memorization, which held on in some cultural backwaters because it sounded good, and a small group loves it. And a small group of classic music players and lovers have held on to classical music.

Then there were slews of claims that poetry developed the mind, followed by slews of psychological tests that showed that memorizing poetry doesn't do much more than help you memorize poetry. Still, poetry held on. More recent neurobic science says poetry memory may help stave off dementia and that memory needs a workout as much as abs do. Furthermore, as mentioned, poetry recitation aloud restores verbal fluency by exercising a gigantic amount of brain and muscle. Decline in verbal fluency is common in the senior population. Recitation aloud corrects the defect. Try it! The scientific studies show it works, and science is usually right.

Good Memory for One Thing Doesn't Imply Good Memory for Everything

My poetry memory is good. My memory for sports statistics is terrible, mainly because I don't give a damn about professional sports. My next-door neighbor, Steve Greenley, knows this for sure. He knows I know nothing about professional sports. He told me I don't know who LeBron James is, and Steve is right. I don't. When I was interviewed at Cornell Medical School, the three doctors doing the interview thought it was very funny that I didn't know how many points you get for a touchdown. At the time, I didn't even know what a touchdown was. As I write this, it is Superbowl Sunday. Needless to say, I don't know who is playing, nor do I care. It is not my thing. Not my bag. What's your bag? What's not your thing?

On the other hand, my music memory is lousy, and I do care about it, and I do work on it. I have been memorizing music for about 12 years. Thus, my experience and knowledge are far less for this art form than they are for poetry. Consequently, progress is slower. In fact, it will take about an hour to memorize four measures of a Chopin waltz (53 notes). Within a few weeks of working on music memory, I decided I needed some real data on how long it takes me to memorize some music so that I could reasonably predict how long it would take me to memorize some music. Review what I did so that you can get some ideas on how to approach the estimation of work required for the memory project that you have in mind. Note that keeping track of the time was not much labor. The real labor was in the memory work itself.

Preliminary Results of Experimental Studies of Music Memory

In order to study music memory quantitatively, I followed the protocol of Hermann Ebbinghaus, except I didn't memorize meaningless words, and I didn't lock myself in my room. I memorized (what else?) music and sat (where else?) at the piano. I recorded the time spent in the process. When I was able to play the piece twice without an error, I considered the piece in my memory. Then, just as Ebbinghaus did, I tested myself at periodic intervals to see how much of the piece remained in the memory over time. My aim was to get forgetting curves for music so that those curves for music memory could be compared and contrasted with the classical forgetting curves for unassociated verbal material (those three-letter non-words like CYK or WZF), as first discovered by Ebbinghaus.

Unlike Ebbinghaus, I had the physical means of recording my performances and followed the playback with the score. If there was a single wrong note in a measure, that measure was counted as an error. The percent measures correct was the percent of correct measures in the whole piece that were played note-perfect. Thus, even if there were only one false note in a measure, I counted the whole measure as an error. Thus, the percent retention is a worst-case estimate of retained music because usually, there was only one wrong note in the measures that were graded wrong. In most cases, such wrong notes would not be detected by the usual audience under the usual circumstances or the usual performance.

The data on some of the pieces that I memorized is presented below. Right now, before giving you the data, I want to talk about the results. In the results, there is good news, and there is bad news. First, the good news:

The Good News about Music Memory

Music memory, like poetry memory, is solid and decays only slightly with time. It certainly does not decay anywhere near as much or as quickly as verbal memory, as shown in the forgetting curve first published by Ebbinghaus. Remember Ebbinghaus's work avoided associations. In music memory and in poetry memory, associations are there all the time to help us, and besides, the music and the poem are much more interesting than unassociated, meaningless three-letter combinations. Music memory and poetry memory are also aided by sequence and pattern recognition. Dendrites of neurons are sensitive to the sequence of synaptic activation and can thereby implement recall. Why this is the case is not known. That is, we don't know why the brain is so keen on handling sequences. But the data is unequivocal on this fact. This means once you have learned to play your piece from memory or recite your poem from memory, it is highly likely that that piece or poem will remain in your memory more or less intact and in the right sequence for at least a week. The magnetic resonance images of the brain done on practice memory do show the same considerable savings of memory tracts. Only at about two weeks do we see significant loss of memory if there is no rehearsal. Rehearsal renews the memory by freshening and reconfirming the synapses in the brain. Therefore, if you wish to keep your repertoire in your memory, it is a good idea to actually play your repertoire once a week or recite your poems once a week. Experts might get away with a review once every two weeks, but for real security, once a week is best. Review the poems and music pieces you know well in addition to the ones you don't know so well. Avoid retrieval-induced forgetting.

My practice has been to play part of my repertoire every Sunday. If there is trouble or hesitations or mistakes, I consult the score and review the notes after I have gone through the piece as best I could. If a piece is not played correctly, I work on it until it is played correctly. The amount of time involved is minimal compared to the amount of time that was needed to get the piece in the memory in the first place. Once learned, pieces can be polished quickly, even if not played for years. Which brings us to some bad news.

BERNARD MICHAEL PATTEN, M.D.

The Bad News about Music Memory

To get music in the memory requires a great deal of skill, hard work, and time. The experience with memory tasks has been that the longer the piece, the more complicated the piece, the fewer the repeats and the greater the note density (that is, the average number of notes per measure), the more unique measures, the faster the piece is to be played are all items that increase the time and work needed to get the piece firmly into the memory.

In general, you will not be able to predict exactly how long it will take to memorize a given piece. Two rules of thumb that work for me might also work for you. Rule one is a guesstimation based on the Fermi equations for guessing. (Yes, these come from the same atomic scientist whose name you know so well. His hobby was predicting events by sophisticated guessing, and the technique is called Fermi guesstimation.)

Fermi Guesstimation

Look at your piece (or poem or this week's reading assignment in social work or whatnot) and estimate the minimal amount of time you think you will need to get the item firmly in your memory. After you have quantitative data on your own experience with many memory tasks, your estimate of this minimal time will be more accurate. Then estimate the maximal time that you think it will take to learn the piece. Multiply minimal time by maximal time and then take the square root of the answer. This is the geometric mean which Fermi has discovered is a more accurate predictor than the arithmetic mean.

For example: I am looking at a poem by Langston Hughes titled *"The Negro Speaks of Rivers."* It has 13 lines and 103 words. The structure and syntax look reasonable, and lines 4 and 13 repeat, so I estimate it will take, at minimum, 20 minutes to memorize this poem and recite it perfectly twice on my video recorder. Furthermore, I think the maximum time would be 120 minutes for the same result. Thus, my Fermi estimate will be 20 x 120 minutes = 2,400, the square root of which is 48.98 minutes.

Actual result: 42 minutes. Fermi estimation was pretty close.

Fermi guesstimation may be applied to any memory task. For example, looking over the 35 lines in the introduction to *Evangeline,* I Fermiguessed that the maximum time for me to commit all of them to perfect memory would be 60 minutes, and the minimum time would be about 20 minutes. Multiplying 60 by 20 gives 1,200. The square root of 1,200 is about 35. The time the task actually took was pretty close.

This week, my teacher told me to memorize a piece called *Carnival Rag* by Mona Rejino. Looking over the piece and doing an analysis of the repeats and organization, I estimate it will take a minimum of three hours and a maximum of five hours to memorize. Thus, the Fermi guesstimation would be 3 x 5 = 15, and the square root of 15 is 3.87 hours or 3 hours and 52 minutes. On the *Morning*

Song by Cornelius Gurlitt (1820–1901) (see data below), the minimum was three hours, and the max was also five. But, stupid me did not see the ABABA structure initially which turned out to be a great chunking tool and a repeat, so the estimate had to be revised to one hour minimum and three maximum for an estimate of square root of three or 1.73 hours or 1 hour and 44 minutes. This estimate came in under the actual time, which was one hour and 22 minutes.

Patten Guesstimation in Music Memory

Experience is a great teacher. My experience is that the time to complete memorization is not linearly related to the length of the music piece or to the number of measures, but it is strongly correlated with the number of unique measures and less strongly correlated with the average number of notes per measure, which I call note density. Empirically multiplying the number of unique measures by two and then multiplying the result by the note density will give an estimation of the number of minutes needed to memorize the piece. Thus, *Morning Song* has only 11 unique measures and a note density of eight, giving a Patten guesstimation of 2 x 11 = 22 x 8 = 176 minutes as the time needed to get the piece into the memory. The actual time that it took to memorize this piece was 82 minutes. Applying the same formula to *Scarborough Fair*, we get 44 x 5 = 220 minutes, which matches the 217 minutes actually needed. *Blues in the Night* had 34 unique measures and a note density of 10, so the estimation was 680 minutes. The actual time to memorize this classic blues piece was 745 minutes. Yes, it took that long! But once in the memory, it stays there with only brief reviews on Sundays. *Swing Low Sweet Chariot* (arr. by Bill Messenger) has 13 unique measures and an average note density of 4.9. Hence, the estimation was 127 minutes. The actual time was pretty close at 132 minutes.

How to Calculate the Number of Unique Measures and the Note Density

Copy the piece. Start at the beginning and look at each measure. When you come to a measure that is exactly the same as a measure that you have already seen, put an X through the duplicate measure. Do this for the entire piece and then count the number of measures that have no X. On the note density, just eyeball the first page and estimate the average number of notes per measure. If you are the obsessive-compulsive type, count the number of notes in each measure and divide by the total number of measures.

Here's some data from memory studies on Student Patten. Recall that the criterion was perfect performance twice. Time to less-than-perfect performance would be less, in some cases much less:

Morning Song **By Cornelius Gurlitt (1820–1901): Total time to criterion: 82 minutes**

Key: F Major

Study time breakdown: five sessions on five separate days over a seven-day period, average session 16.4 minutes, range seven to 22 minutes:

40 measures

307 notes

11 unique measures

Average notes per measure: Eight (calculated value 7.675)

Comment: ABABA form makes for easy organization. First two measures of A exactly repeat as measures 4 and 5 of A. First two measures of B exactly repeat as measures 4 and 5 of B.

Memory retention (time values are after the piece has been played perfectly twice):

At criterion 100% twice

One hour—90% (36 measures correct out of 40)

24 hours—90%

48 hours—90%

72 hours—not tested

96 hours—95%

120 hours—not tested

144 hours—not tested

168 hours—90%

Scarborough Fair by Anonymous circa 1625: Total time to criterion: 217 minutes

Key listed as d minor, but actually probably is the dorian mode.

Study time breakdown: 14 sessions on 14 separate days over a 22-day period, average session 15.5 minutes, range three to 20 minutes.

42 measures

229 notes

22 unique measures

Average notes per measure: five (calculated value 5.452)

Comment: Middle part repeats exactly, but the treble is an octave higher in the second repeat.

Memory retention:

At criterion 100% twice

24 hours—93% (39 measures correct out of 42)

48 hours—not tested

72 hours—not tested

96 hours—93%

120 hours—93%

144 hours—100% (note-perfect!)

168 hours—95%

Nine days post criterion—100% after a 22-minute review at the piano

Blues in the Night by Harold Arlen (words by Johnny Mercer): Total time to criterion: 745 minutes

Key: C Major

Study time breakdown: 40 sessions over a 53-day period, average session 18.6 minutes, range four to 50 minutes. Usually, there was only one session per day, but on 9/8/2008, there were two sessions: 10–10:10 AM & 10:10–10:30 PM; there were two sessions on 9/14: 2:00–2:30 & 4:00–4:50; two sessions on 9/20 2:06–2:36 & 9:30–9:40; there was one mental review on 9/22 lasting 8 minutes, and there were three sessions on 9/23 4:07–4:20, 7:57–8:01, and 8:10–8:18

53 measures

525 notes

34 unique measures

Average notes per measure: ten (calculated value 9.906)

Comment: Memorization started on September 5, 2008 and actually reached only two wrong notes on September 23. So the piece was pretty much in the memory after 494 minutes of work. The bulk of the rest of memory training time was thus spent trying to reach the criterion of note-perfection.

Memory retention

At criterion 100% twice

24 hours—96%

48 hours—not tested

72 hours—98% (left out D on page 3)

96 hours—not tested

120 hours—not tested

144 hours—92%

168 hours—90%

192 hours—100% after a 13-minute review at the piano

Minuet in G Major from the Notebook of Anna Magdalena Bach (1725)

Study time breakdown and other data were stolen with Doctor Patten's car on 11/30/2008, but a copy of the memory retention data was left at home.

Memory retention

At criterion 100% twice

One hour—98%

24 hours—not tested

46 hours—98%

72 hours—not tested

96 hours—not tested

120 hours—not tested

144 hours—not tested

168 hours—80%

192 hours (that is eight days post criteria)—80%

192 hours after a ten-minute review of the piece—100% (note-perfect)

Comment: Perhaps the absence of the testing on days three, four, five, and six led to a degradation in the memory. On day eight (192 hours), the performance that immediately followed a ten-minute review at the piano was 100% note-perfect.

How about Dance Memory?

How would you estimate how long it would take you to memorize to the point of automaticity a dance routine?

The answer is, of course, more time than you think.

The Silver Star Tappers of Pasadena, Texas, have over 30 tap dance routines. The usual routine is memorized by the dancers and performed before multiple audiences at nursing homes, hospitals, churches, retirement parties, Japanese tourists (once), CNN (twice), and so forth. The age of the dancers ranges from 54 to 96, with the average age coming in at 78 years. How do these people do it?

By now, your answer should be something like this: "Hard work, multiple repetitions, reviews, self-tests, and memory tricks." If you want to look like a memory genius, you have to work at it.

Consider the groups' tap routine called *Chicago Medley*. This has an introduction consisting of a wait while the music plays, a shuffle-ball change, a pivot turn, a step, a walk, another step, and then a repeat of the whole sequence followed by eight flaps forward. Thus, the intro alone has 32 beats and 19 steps. The ending of this dance has 16 beats and 13 steps. In between the intro and ending, there are 11 separate sections, usually consisting of 32 beats, each with multiple steps. Yet, the group was able to memorize and perform this dance automatically after only 47 hours of practice and study!

As for me, it took me three hours to get the introduction down correctly and about three hours to get the ending. That's six hours. I figured I would need three hours per each other section making 3 x 11 = 33 hours. Thus, the whole thing would be predicted to come into the memory in 33 + 6 = 39 hours of work. And that, friends, is how you might estimate the time needed to memorize a dance routine—take a part as a sample, record the time required, and calculate the time needed on the basis of what remains to be memorized.

Apply the same methods of estimation to any task you want to do. The basic idea is to have a realistic estimate of the time needed to master the task. That way, you will not be disappointed when the task is not memorized in the blinking of an eye. Remember, when making your estimates take into account your personal experience with the task at hand. Considering that I have never attempted tightrope walking, my estimate for the time to master that skill would probably exceed my available lifespan.

My pool man pounded on the window when he heard me playing *Fur Elise.*

"How long would it take me to learn to play *Fur Elise* from memory?" he asked. "Have you had any piano lessons?"

"No."

"Ten years."

How about Memory for a Foreign Language?

Chinese, for instance. Ho ho ho. You already know the score. Attack the estimation of this kind of memory task as you would attack the estimation of dance or music memory or any other learning task, flying an airplane, getting a driver's license, and so forth. Second languages are difficult for adults to learn, and most adults will never come close to being a native speaker. The more the new language differs from the language of your youth, the harder the task.

Routine Tasks

Estimate the time for routine tasks the same way. Time required to mail a book at the Nassau Bay post office: Estimated time there—15 minutes and back 15, and in the office in line, 15 minutes. Total estimate: 45 minutes. Fermi guess: Max 60 minutes, min 25, so Fermi estimation is 25 x 60 = 1,500. Square root is 38.72 minutes. Actual time: nine there, nine back, and five in office for a total of 23. Conclusion: My estimates were way off, and so was Fermi. Next time, I shall estimate better based on my experience.

How to Memorize English Language Vocabulary

Keep a notebook. Write words that you come across down and look them up in the evening. Memorize the word, the pronunciation, the word history, and the spelling. All those are associations that will help recall the word and its meaning. Elaborative encoding is very useful. The Oxford English Dictionary is the best. It comes on a CD so that you can have all 700,000+ words in English at your fingertips. The more words you know, the better, as words are the food and material of complex thought.

But what if you actually have trouble keeping the word and its meaning in your mind?

Answer: Apply the usual solutions.

Follow the rules:

- Understand the problem
- Make associations that help link the word to the meaning
- The best associations are visual images
- Review and test yourself
- Practice using the new word, preferably aloud
- Sometimes a word history will suggest a meaning and help recall the word's meaning. Advanced dictionaries like the Oxford English dictionary give multiple examples of how the word is used, so you might profit by reading the examples.
- If you have had a classical education in Latin or Greek or both, you will be a step ahead in figuring out the meaning. For example: What is the meaning of sinecure? If you know it comes from the Latin sine cura, you might figure it means without a cure. That's the meaning, alright! A sinecure is a church appointed or other appointed benefit during which you don't have to take care of or "cure" anything or anybody, nor do you need to do any required work. That sounds like an ideal job. No work, but you get paid anyway.

Case Study

A patient (mentioned already) lost his English language vocabulary to a severe herpes simplex viral infection of the left hemisphere of his brain. The left hemisphere is the brain structure specialized for language. This man was not entirely unhappy about the loss, for he had discovered his ability to make mental images had increased remarkably after his illness. The reason for this improvement in the ability to make mental images is not clear, but it probably relates to a release of the right hemisphere from left hemisphere inhibition and control. The right hemisphere is the brain structure specialized for non-language and visual-spatial tasks. This newly acquired skill in making mental images was of distinct advantage in the patient's work, as he was a movie director. He could now envision the scenes in his head without having to put the actors and crew through the scenes, a gigantic savings in time, energy, and money. Interestingly, the patient also claimed an improvement in his creativity, which some neurologists think is centered in the right hemisphere.

Creative impulses are present in all of us. Many of these impulses are suppressed by the school system and by parents. The suppression is probably mediated by the left hemisphere. If the left hemisphere is damaged, as was the case with our movie director, the suppression might have been relieved, and the embedded creative impulses permitted to flourish. Sudden acquisition of creative abilities has been reported in patients who have specific brain diseases. The usual report is about an aged person, who has never been particularly creative prior to the onset of a dementia, who may take up painting after little or no instruction and produce original works of art. The same has been reported for the sudden acquisition of musical talent, both composition and performance. Check out the movie *Maudie* based on the true story of late acquisition of artistic talent.

OK, He Was More Creative and Could Think Better in Images

But still, it was a pain for our movie director to be so limited in his English language vocabulary that he sounded like he never made it past seventh grade. So, he consulted Doctor Patten to see if we could get a program going that would rebuild his English language vocabulary. Treatment of this condition presents a gigantic problem. Can you guess what that problem is? Think about this for two minutes. If you were the doctor, what would be the obvious impediment to this movie director learning English words?

The problem in treatment would be that his left hemisphere was damaged by the virus, and therefore much of his language abilities in the verbal realm would be impaired. The way around the problem would be to encode the meaning of words in the visual modality, which was functioning above normal, and to teach the patient to read out the meanings of words by visual associations. That is exactly what neurologists are trained to do: Look, in handicapped people, for the abilities and develop them.

Examples

Do you recall how he remembered "olfactory"? Pause and think!

The patient couldn't recall the meaning of the word "olfactory." He was taught to take the word apart and make a visual image that would associate the meaning of the word with the image. Thus, he saw in his mind's eye an old factory. From the factory, a jet of smoke carrying a foul odor hits his nose. The idea of a jet of smoke hitting the nose reminds the patient that olfactory relates to the sense of smell.

Summary of Doctor Patten's instructions to learn the meaning of olfactory:

- Olfactory—no obvious connection between the word and its meaning, unless you have a classical education and know the Latin word for to smell, olfacere.
- Classical education? Olfacere, make the association.
- Non-classical? Make associations that remind you of the word. The best associations will be weird, in color, larger than life, somewhat aggressive, and visual. For a movie director, the meaning of the word might be better recalled if it was studied and encoded as a short movie: E.g., an old factory in which you see yourself and a stream of smoke that floats through the

air and hits and offends your nose with an ugly stench. When you see the word or hear the word, you will see the old factory and the smoke, which represents the stink. That smoke and the stink reminds you of smell. From the idea of smell, you deduce the meaning of olfactory.

Piebald

The patient couldn't recall the meaning of the word "piebald." He was taught to take the word apart and make a visual image that would associate the meaning of the word with the image. Thus, he saw in his mind's eye a pie that had on its surface black and white patches. The visual image reminds him that piebald refers to patches of black and white.

Summary of Doctor Patten's instructions on how to learn the meaning of piebald:
- Piebald
- No obvious connection between the word and its meaning.
- So we must make a connection.
- How about: A bald Pie? See that in your mind's eye and make the pie have two contrasting patches of black and white.
- Then when you hear piebald, you will "see" the bald pie, which will suggest the meaning.

So what?

So, a lot!

The application of visual images enabled this movie director to augment his English language vocabulary by over 50 new words a week. The application of the same technique can help you recall the meanings of some English words that might be difficult to learn. For example: What is the meaning of the word "pankration?"

Are you scratching your head? You don't know what pankration means. And that, dear reader, is why pankration was selected. It was selected because it was likely you wouldn't know its meaning. In fact, until I visited a museum in Athens in 2001, I didn't know the meaning of pankration either, but I see that my Microsoft spellchecker does recognize pankration as a word, whereas my Oxford English Dictionary does not. Most dictionaries do not list it, yet I assure you it is a solid English word.

Pankration comes from the Latin pancratium, which means all-powerful. The Latin meaning evidently derives from the Greek words Pan Kratos, meaning (guess what?) all-powerful. The Olympic game of pankration was a fight in which contestants used both arms and legs to box and wrestle at the same time. The event was quite brutal as a result, and the winner was considered to have achieved pankration. Ancient judges sometimes had trouble deciding who actually won the pankration because both of the contestants were dead. Usually, the dead man who did not have his eyes gouged out was declared the winner. You need to have criteria and standards for things, and the gouged eyes was the criteria in ancient time that identified the loser of the pankration. Intact eyes identified the winner, even if he were as dead as a doornail, as dead as his opponent.

Whew! Now that we know the meaning of pankration, let's try to make associations that will help us recall the meaning when we wish to show off.

Humm. This is difficult. Unless you knew Latin or Greek for the word, there is no obvious connection between the word and its meaning. Wait a second; there is a painting of Christ in a church in Istanbul. In gold letters on the statue were written Christ, the Pancrator of the Universe. That should have suggested power, but at the time, it didn't register. Now I can use it to help me recall the meaning. But I really should follow the rules and make an association that will be vivid, visual, somewhat aggressive, in color, and capable of reminding me and you of the meaning of the word.

Remember, the best mnemonic images are those that you imagine for yourself. Try to make one now by yourself and for yourself, then examine my narration and image and compare and contrast what I thought up with what you thought up. There is no right answer. See if your pankration mnemonic matches or exceeds mine for weirdness and memorability.

Pan suggests a frying pan. Cration suggests a crate. So, I see a frying pan hitting a crate. The crate breaks open, and boxing gloves fall out. But they are not ordinary boxing gloves: They are made of wrestling trunks. The boxing gloves and trunks remind me of Ancient Olympic combat sports: Boxing and Wrestling. Therefore, pankration is the ancient fight game of boxing combined with wrestling. The winner of this brutal contest was considered all-powerful by the ancient Greeks. Therefore, by extrapolation, pankration means all-powerful.

What Is the Meaning of Tergiversation?

- If you know that tergum tergi n. means back in Latin and verso versare means to turn about, then the meaning of the word is clear
- If you don't know the word's origin, you either look up and memorize the origin or the meaning or both, or you impose your own visual association. Do not turn your back on this task.

Mental Gymnastic

Look up and memorize the meaning of the word tergiversation. Make it your word for the day. Make sure you understand the word's meaning and color and how to use it and say it. Then make an image that connects the word to the meaning.

Want to learn a word a day? If you don't run across a new word, then use the Google word of the day, which gives the definition, and so forth. The CD of the Oxford English Dictionary has a similar feature and calls up a random word for you to view and learn. Wordsmith.org ditto—has the same feature.

Words are the food of thought and provide nuanced ways of looking at the world and the events you see in your life. Learning a new word every day enriches your understanding of the reality we have to deal with. But even more important to your personal advancement is looking up words you encounter in your daily activities and adding that word to your working vocabulary.

Advice: Whenever you encounter a new word, and you are not sure of the pronunciation, the meaning, the color of the meaning, the denotation, the connotation, the word atmosphere, the word usage, and its proper place in diction and syntax, look up the word, write out the meaning, recite the meaning, memorize the word's origin, and use the word, if you can, as soon as you can.

If you are really into this word business, you should keep a word journal with all the words you didn't know that are now transferred to long-term memory. Over fifty years ago, as a freshman at Columbia College, Doctor Patten overheard a conversation in the dorm elevator. One student said to the other: "What he did was an opprobrious, contumelious insult."

Can you guess what two words had not been heard before? That afternoon, while rounding the first turn in a 440 race at Bakersfield, Doctor Patten resolved to write down and look up each evening every new word that came his way. That evening, he looked up contumelious and tried to find opprobrious but hadn't spelled it well enough to find it.

Now he doesn't write words down but should to help store them in long-term memory. When he reads, he circles the words that he is not fully familiar with and looks them up after he had finished reading the book.

This method of acquiring knowledge (daytime notes, night look-up) was also quite effective in medical school. Each day, Doctor Patten would write down the words or ideas or diseases or operations that were mentioned on rounds and would look them up that night. He looked up the items, whether they were new to him or old hat. After a while, he looked like he had a textbook knowledge of the subjects broached on rounds, which incidentally was just about all he did have and all he did know.

The amazing thing was that the same things kept coming up time and time again on rounds and in conferences. Doctor Patten began to look like he really knew a lot of medicine when what he knew was merely the stuff that was repeated often. He looked like a memory genius on the subject of the side effects of Dilantin because he had re-read the side effects at least ten times that month. When the next attending physician asked, "What are the side effects of Dilantin?" he reeled off the answer without hesitation.

Thus, his medical education did not reflect textbook knowledge of whole areas of medicine, just the items that turned up frequently on rounds. About syphilis and tuberculosis, and rheumatic heart disease, he was an encyclopedia because those three conditions were just about the only diseases medical students saw in the hospital and in the clinics. A similar method could be applied to other trades besides medicine—shoe repair, for instance, or air conditioning maintenance. Let us know your experience.

Mental Gymnastic

Tell how a person should approach the task of memorizing a poem for recitation. List the items you think are important, and then compare your list with this:

How to learn to correctly recite:

- Aloud with mind and heart, actively engaged
- Multiple times
- In front of a mirror or video camera
- Recording your performance
- Using body language, facial expression, and gesture
- The best way to make a poem your own is to memorize it cold. The way to memorize it cold is to practice it several hundred times.
- Use association tools, memory pegs, images as discussed in the following pages to facilitate recall.

Mental Gymnastic

Tell what benefits are expected from learning to recite a poem. List the items you think are important, and then compare your list with this:

- Greater oral presentation skills—includes more fluent speech, larger vocabulary, greater intellectual range, and a greater emotional range.
- A decreased chance of getting Alzheimer's disease or other forms of dementia. A remarkably improved memory for verbal and visual items.
- A greater awareness of the multiple realities of life and on this planet and their complexities.
- Another item that can be used to show off at dinner parties, cocktail parties, or for the grandchildren.

BERNARD MICHAEL PATTEN, M.D.

Memory Lite

Repetition while in a state of focused attention is a key (one of the many keys) to lite memory. Repeat to yourself what you want to recall. Deliberately pause for a moment and focus your attention on the to-be-remembered item. Then try to forget it. You can't.

Example: How to Remember Where You Parked Your Car

"This is where I parked my car, the eighth floor of terminal B in this section called Easter Island."

Houston Bush International Airport actually names the sections to help you make associations that will facilitate recall. The airport also has the parking sections color-coded. Last time I parked there, I was in the purple section on the roof, the sixth floor of terminal C. Here, I paused for just a moment to tell myself, "If I get sea-sick (C6—get it?), I might turn purple. That little idea will help me recall C6 and the purple section. But that might not be enough, so I shall make some more associations. Sitting in the car from here, I can clearly see the airport hotel on my right, elevator B close by, and the control tower up ahead. I am parked in section C, even though I am going on an airplane in the air and not a ship in the sea."

Notice, multiple associations, not just one, are made. Elaborative encoding! The brain benefits and is not discouraged, annoyed, or confused by multiple associations. Once the associations are made, try to forget it. You can't. Time spent: less than a minute. Time saved? That depends. Plenty of people forget where they parked and have to spend hours trying to find the car.

When you get back from Chile, it is unlikely that you will not recall where you parked. With me when I got back, I suddenly thought of parking, and just the idea of parking summoned the sea-sick business. It wasn't until I actually got in the purple elevator that the purple had anything to do with my recall. Seeing that I was again in the purple reassured me that I was on the right track and gave me confidence that I would find my car without any difficulty.

The above method works because you are forced to pay attention to where you parked. But there are other methods that also work. At a racetrack, airport, shopping center, etc., if you forget where you parked your car, you can always wait until everyone else has driven away. The car remaining is yours!

Other Traditional Methods That Are Not So Good

The old memory books talk about the displaced object trick. If you wish to remember that you put the roast in the oven, place a frying pan on the kitchen floor. When you see it or trip over it, you will recall that it was put there to remind you of something. One woman objected and said, "What good is that? After I put the roast in the oven, I go watch TV in the other room." In that case, the advice was "put the frying pan on the TV set."

Instead of a frying pan, you can use anything that looks out of place on the TV or on the floor, a potholder, a plate, a mustard jar. These simple ideas are based on the standard rule of memory—one thing reminds you of another. It is like tying a string around your finger, putting your watch in your pocket instead of on your wrist, or turning your pinky ring the wrong way. Out of place, things are supposed to remind you of something you want to remember. All that is not helpful if you can't recall what that something was. Therefore, when you put the out-of-place object in its out-of-place place, you had best consciously tell yourself what it is there for and what it is to remind you of.

How to Not Forget Why You Went into Another Room

Before you go into that other room, deliberately tell yourself why you are going there. Focus attention on the item to be remembered. "I am going into the kitchen to get the scissors." Then no matter what distractions (including your own thoughts) should intervene between your present position and your arrival in the kitchen, it is unlikely that you will not recall why you went into the kitchen.

When desperate, go back to the room where you had the idea. That usually triggers the memory, but don't forget to tell yourself not to forget again.

Repetition Helps in Memorizing Anything

Usually, if you can repeat something five times correctly, you won't forget it. Example: The Chinese word for power (the energy force of nature) is chi. The Chinese word for power is chi. Chi is the Chinese word for power. Chi is power in Chinese. Chi = power. Power = chi.

What is the Chinese word for power?

Chi, of course. Also spelled Qi.

While learning Chi, it is a good idea to shout it out. That will help firm up the memory because it will give an auditory association to the idea. How about telling yourself that you have good chi. That might help by making chi personal. "My teacher said I have plenty of Qi."

Hermann Ebbinghaus discovered that the number of repetitions was more important in cementing the memory than the time spent in repetition, so don't be afraid to repeat a number of times. It's not your fault that that is the way human memory is structured. One-step learning for complex tasks is just not compatible with the way our brains work. So, despite the high standards, please manage your expectations.

Directions

You drive into a gas station to ask directions. The first thing you hear is the famous, "You can't miss it." Then you know you are in trouble. But you don't have to be. Make sure you hear and get the directions correctly by actually repeating them to the gas guy so that he can amend or correct your view of the instructions. Pay particular attention to left or right turns as the correct turn or the wrong turn can make all the difference. Some books recommend visual aids by picturing a red (communist) flag for left and a punch with the right uppercut for right. Go three lights, and turn left. See three red lights, and know the turn is left.

Memory Lite—Rhyme

These things are trivial, but even trivial pieces of information may be life-saving: Red on yellow kills a fellow; red on black venom lack. That's a good way to remember the coral snake that has red on yellow is poisonous.

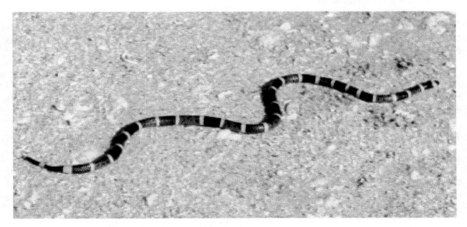

Fig4.1

177

These things are trivial, but even trivial pieces of information may help you on your spelling test:

I before e, except after c or when sounding like a, as in neighbor or weigh.

That's a good way to remember how to spell receive, die, pieces, laddie, deity, and freight. Siege is an exception, and seize has a different meaning. Weird is, well, just weird. In elementary school, teacher said I should remember how to spell piece because piece has a pie in it. Don't believe a lie, recognizing lie is in the word believe.

More trivia: At night, a boater must know which way another boat is moving and what side is what. The positions also determine right of way. Boats must display lights on their sides. The red is on the left or port side, and the green on the right or starboard side. But how to remember that fact? Port wine is red, and the word port and the word left both have four letters. Starboard has two letter r's; therefore, starboard is on the right side.

An old salt died. When they were preparing him for the funeral, they turned the lapel of his jacket. It read, "Red right returning." That alliterative RRR was the way he remembers the red buoys should be on the right when coming back to port. If the red buoys are on your left, you are not in the channel and are likely to run aground. The system is the exact reverse in some other parts of the world, so watch out.

Mnemonics Help Recall

Mnemonics (ne mon' ics- the m is silent) is the art of assisting recall by using artificial associations. The mother of all the nine muses (can you name them?) was Mnemosyne, the goddess of memory.

Rhyme, rhythm, rules, symmetry, alliteration, phrases, acronyms, and so forth were used by our ancient ancestors, so why not use them yourself? If you can put a rhyme on the thing to be remembered, recall is strengthened.

In 1492, Columbus set out on the ocean blue.

That helps us recall the date of the supposed discovery of America. But how in the world could a world be discovered when there were people already here when Columbus arrived? What does a stitch in time save? Most of us would almost automatically reply NINE.

Use it or lose it!

That is good advice and is what this book is about.

At sundown, an evening sky appears red in the west when thin high clouds are present. Such clouds usually indicate a dry night and no rain the next day. Hence:

Red sky at night
Sailor's delight
Red sky in morning
Sailor's warning

In Many Fields, There Is an Enormous Amount of Material to Memorize

Early in their medical career, medical students realize that there is an enormous amount of material to memorize, and most of it doesn't make much sense because the human body is a gigantic chaotic mess—a collection of evolutionary fixes and stand-in solutions. In view of the situation, medical students resort to medical memory tricks.

Mental Gymnastic

For two minutes, try to memorize the twelve cranial nerves.

One: Olfactory
Two: Optic
Three: Oculomotor
Four: Trochlear
Five: Trigeminal
Six: Abducens
Seven: Facial
Eight: Auditory
Nine: Glossopharyngeal
Ten: Vagus
Eleven: Spinal accessory
Twelve: Hypoglossal

Medical mnemonic for cranial nerves: "On Old Olympus Towering Tops A Finn And German Viewed Some Hops."

Spend another two minutes on the same task. This time use the poem to trigger recall, where each word in the poem starts with a letter corresponding to the cranial nerve. Use part of the time to memorize the poem and part of the time to review what the first letters of the words refer to. Example: O O O (On Old Olympus) means olfactory, optic, oculomotor, the first three cranial nerves. T and T (Towering Tops) remind us of trochlear and trigeminal. A = abducens, F = facial, A of And is auditory, G—you tell. V—vagus S—spinal accessory. H of Hops recalls hypoglossal.

"On Old Olympus Towering Tops A Finn And German Viewed Some Hops."

Those of you who went to medical school know there were also a host of obscene poems to remember basic anatomy. "O O O to touch and feel a girl's vagina, some happiness."

Mental Gymnastic

How about the holes in the bottom of the skull through which these nerves travel? Looking at a skull and trying to figure this out can be, as a memory task, quite daunting. But if doctors and dentists don't know this stuff, who is going to know it?

1. olfactory—cribriform plate
2. optic—optic foramen (note foramen is window in Latin)
3. oculomotor—superior orbital fissure
4. trochlear—superior orbital fissure
5. trigeminal—Ugh! Trigeminal implies three twin branches: ophthalmic goes through the superior orbital fissure; the maxillary through the foramen rotundum; the mandibular through the foramen ovale. The mandibular motor nerve also goes through ovale, as does the lesser petrosal branch of cranial nerve 9.
6. abducens—superior orbital fissure
7. facial—internal auditory meatus
8. auditory—internal auditory meatus
9. glossopharyngeal—jugular foramen
10. vagus—jugular foramen
11. spinal accessory—jugular foramen
12. hypoglossal—hypoglossal canal

Believe it or not, the medical mnemonic for this mess of medical facts is

"Cocks Out Spurt Some Spunk Right Over Sexy Isabel's Incredible Jingling Jizz Jet Hole."

It is important to keep loose and not get stuck on any one trick to memorize material.

In the case of the skull holes, it is difficult to remember the mnemonic poem. Instead, just reorganize the data into smaller bite-sized quantities. Olfactory goes into the cribriform plate, as seen many times in dissections. And optic has its own hole. That leaves cranial nerves 3 and 4 going through the superior orbital fissure with the first branch of nerve 5 and with nerve 6. Nerves 7 and 8 go through the auditory meatus. Nerves 9, 10, and 11 go through the jugular foramen, and 12 has its own hole, the hypoglossal canal. Now list the numbers 1–12 and test to see if you really know it.

But whoa! When I did this, I left out the second and third branches of 5. They go through foramen rotundum and ovale with the second branch (maxillary) rotundum and the third branch ovale.

Self-test:

1. cribriform plate
2. optic foramen
3. superior orbital fissure
4. same as 4
5. first branch same as 4, then rotuntdum and ovale
6. superior orbital fissure with 3 and 4
7. auditory meatus
8. auditory meatus
9. jugular foramen
10. same as 9
11. same as 9
12. hypoglossal

Reviewing the list, I got them all right, except I spelled rotundum wrong. Next time around, I will spell it right without the extra t. Notice how my reorganization of the material made the memory task more memorable and easier. Organized patterns facilitate recall, and the best patterns are the ones you make for yourself.

Mental Gymnastic

Name all the cranial nerves. Tell what holes in the skull they travel through. In doing this gymnastic, rely heavily on the mnemonic hook of the order of numbers 1 to 12, correlating the numbers, if needed, with the first letters in one of the sentences used by medical students.

How to remember the numbers 1 to 12, I can't tell you. Chances are you already can count to 12 without difficulty. That well-learned sequence will provide the memory hooks to hang the cranial nerves in your memory closet. Review your answers and correct what you did wrong. If you have trouble, look up the pictures on the internet. Visual aids help some people. Most medical texts list the cranial nerves in Roman Numerals I–XII (Why? Probably to make the subject matter look more scientific than it is), so don't get confused by that convention.

Doctors, of course, don't use any mnemonics for stuff like this. They know it cold. They don't need it any more than an electrical engineer would need a mnemonic to recall Ohm's law (V = A x R), or a chemist would need a mnemonic to recall what happens with the electrolysis of water: $2H2O \rightarrow 2H2 + O2$.

Warning! With Most Memory Tasks, the More You Understand, the Easier the Task

Beware! Sometimes, the mnemonics get in the way with material like this that is well-learned and understood by specialists. In fact, although I had no trouble recalling the cranial nerves and their function and the holes in the skull that the cranial nerves go through, I did have trouble recalling the mnemonics themselves. My first thought was that the poem ended "A Finn and German shared some hops." But that had to be wrong because shared has to start with a v to remind me of cranial nerve ten, the vagus nerve. The points here are clear: What works serves you best. The more you understand about what you are trying to memorize, the better. Aim for an intellectual understanding, for that will help you remember better than any cheap memory tricks. When desperate, use rote memory. Reserve rote memory for those things you truly don't understand or can't keep straight. Most professionals know their own field automatically and do not need or use memory tricks.

Visualizing Helps

Doctor Patten: With me and most (old school) doctors, there is, in my mind's eye, a clear picture of the skull and the organization of the nerves that go through the skull. Recalling the image first and then reading the nerves from the image is what works because I have done the dissections, and I saw the nerves in situ and traced where they went. Experience, preferably personal experience, is a great teacher. Also, the experience of actual dissection gives a great lift to the memory. Foramen ovale not only has motor V and sensory mandibular V but also the accessory meningeal artery, the lesser petrosal nerve of IX, and the emissary vein. I know this in a flash because I saw it and can visualize it at will. How come? Because neurology is my profession. The things you absolutely need you should know cold.

First-Letter Mnemonics

The poem about the Finn and German uses first letters as the clue to retrieve the memories. Offhand, can you name all the great lakes? HOMES reminds us of H = Huron, O = Ontario, M = Michigan, E = Eire, S = Superior. How about the colors of the rainbow? ROY G. BIV reminds us of R = Red, O = Orange, Y = Yellow, G = Green (the middle of the visible spectrum), B = Blue, I = Indigo, V = Violet. What were the four elements the ancients believed in? In those days, there were only AFEW elements—air, fire, earth, water.

Small poems help recall large ideas:

> Spring ahead
> Fall back

That poem plays on the two meanings of two words. Spring can mean jumping forward, and spring can mean the season. Ditto fall—fall can mean a sudden drop down, and fall can mean the season. So, the poem reminds us what to do with the clock when we are following daylight savings time. Set the clock ahead an hour in springtime and set it back in the fall.

Pure-Letter Mnemonics

FACE reminds us of the notes in the four spaces on the treble staff: Starting with the first space—the note is F; second space is A; third is C, and the top space is E. Treble clef lines (E-G-B-D-F) are traditionally recalled by the sexist Every Good Boy Does Fine. Bass clef spaces are bottom-up (A-C-E-G): American Composers Envy Gershwin. Bass clef lines (G-B-D-F-A): Great Beethoven's Deafness Frustrated All.

These rules are for beginners only. Real musicians automatically read the notes from the score without thinking. They have to because music, in general, moves faster than life.

Mental Gymnastic

Using the FACE mnemonic, tell what note is circled red with a little 5 above it.

Answer: E

Using the FACE mnemonic, tell what note is indicated by the green arrow.

Answer: B. The first space is F, the second A, the third space is C, the last space E. As the note at the arrow is in between A and C, it must be B.

Again, the better system for remembering is the one you derive for yourself. In sight-reading music, know the notes are organized alphabetically, going up in pitch A-B-C-D-E-F-G, followed by a repeat of the same sequence again and again until the keys run out. Therefore, if you know the alphabet and the position of just one note, say middle C, on the staff, you can deduce all the other notes. By the same token, it is easy to play any major or minor scale by knowing the formula of the scales. A major scale is whole note, whole note, half note, whole note, whole note, whole note, half note, and back to the original letter note only an octave higher. How much easier is this to recall and play than memorizing all 14 major scales. The natural minor scales, harmonic minor, and melodic minor also have each their own formula reducing over 36 scales to simple patterns.

Understanding the overall pattern of any memory task can save lots of drudge work. There are many ways to skin a cat. There are many ways to memorize. Remain open-minded, flexible, and practical. In time the mnemonics become unimportant because you will know the material automatically. A real musician just looks at the score and reads the notes directly without having to go through any mental acrobatics.

Real Story from Harry Lorayne's Course in Memory Isometrics

Do you want a good laugh? Get Harry's book *Super Memory Super Student: How to raise your grades in 30 days.* Turn to page 124, chapter 18 on music memory. Harry is all at sea, making up complicated mnemonics to memorize how to read key signatures. He actually admits he knows nothing about music. What a waste of time! And note this: Here's how he memorizes the components of the D major chord: *a dean holds half a knife and fights an ape.* Where (we guess) Dean reminds us of D, half (we guess) is supposed to remind us of F as the word half ends in the letter F, and the knife reminds us that that F is sharp and leads to an A (the ape). Aren't you glad you learned the diatonic scale (whole tone, whole tone, half tone, whole tone, whole tone, whole tone, half tone) and can instantly play any major chord without thinking much about it? Every major chord is just the same pattern with note one, note three, and note five of the scale.

See if you roll off your chair on this: Harry memorizes the position of the keys on the piano:

"All the G and A keys

Are between the black threes

And 'tween the twos are all the D's

Then on the right side of the threes

Will be found the B's and C's

But on the left side of the threes

Are all the F's and all the E's"

Harry, evidently, didn't get that the keys are organized in the exact sequence of the letters of the alphabet, and all you had to know is where any one key was, and you could easily deduce where the others lay. Thank the gods that the sequence of keys is ABCDEFG. If you know where middle C is (it's right under the manufacturer's name on the piano), every other key follows logically. ABCDEFG—That sequence is easier to recall than the complicated mnemonic proposed by Harry Lorayne, an illustration that the proper recognition of important patterns are worth ten thousand mnemonics. The middle note of every major chord is two whole tones up from the lower note that starts the chord (called the tonic—note one of the chord), and one and a half tones up again from the middle note gets to the third note of the major chord. Thus, D Major is D F# A. Easy as pie.

An intellectual understanding makes memory much easier, so try to understand your memory task before you try to memorize it. When in doubt, consult a teacher or someone in the know who might give you some help with discovering the patterns involved. In music, the items that make for good chunking are the scales and chords. All that is pretty simple once you understand how it is based on the ABC system. Which brings us to Abecedarian systems in general.

Abecedarian Systems

Just as you can use numbers as memory hooks to hang memory items on, you can use letters. You can make a word with the letters of the items you wish to recall the way HOMES recalls the names of the great lakes, and AFEW recites the four ancient elements. You can make a narrative stream with the first letter of each word reminding you of an item to be recalled, as we saw in those stupid mnemonics for the cranial nerves. We can attach the item to be recalled directly to the letter. And recall the list by starting at A and working down the list.

The *New England Primer,* the principal textbook of colonial America, taught kids how to read by using the alphabet with pictures and poems. Here are pictures from the 1784 edition.

Other editions had different religious ideas associated with the letters. For instance, J was Jesus, and S was Serpent. The most famous poem from this book was the one that starts "Now I lay me down to sleep." Fill in the rest. Most people can.

Z did not associate with zebra. Z was Zacchaeus, chief tax-collector of Jericho, who climbed a sycamore tree to see Jesus. The story is found in the Gospel of Luke.

Z's picture is a tree, and his poem is:

Zacchaeus did climb the Tree,
His Lord to see.

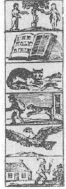
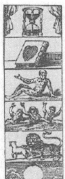

Fig4.2

MENTAL MAKING MIGHT

In the United States, government officials use first letters as a kind of abbreviation of a particular thing or concept. Do you know what FLOTUS is? Did you know the FLOTUS staffers in the Oval presented their versions of the FLOTUS Africa trip? According to Bolton's memoir (page 243) *The Room Where It Happened,* "Ricardel tried to keep from going off the rails due to the ignorance and insensitivity of the First Lady's staffers." How about INF? ABM? ZTE? SCOTUS? POTUS? CIA? USKBN1GX09K? Ugh! We are surrounded by this stuff.

Mental Gymnastic

Take three minutes to memorize this list: jail, face of evil, delphinium, beam of light, egg, horse, of course, India, candle, apple, grandchildren

Now get a piece of paper and write all the items you recall. Record the result. A normal person will get two correct. If you did better than two, congratulations!

People reading this book are not normal, so we will expect a better result. If a large group of normal people are tested, the correct items will tend to be the first items in the list and the last items in the list. This phenomenon, in which we tend to recall the beginning and end and forget the middle, is called the serial position effect. Musically, we must compensate for this serial position effect by special attention to the middle of our piece, as we will tend to better recall the end and the beginning of a piece than the middle. By the same token, the middle of a poem will usually give the most trouble, so we had better pay more attention to it than to the ends. The plot structure of a novel ditto: People will better recall the beginning and the end but have trouble with the middle. Think of movies. Go over in your mind the most recent Hollywood movie you viewed. Notice that you usually recall the end and the beginning better than the middle. Think of the last lecture you attended. The beginning will probably be pretty clear, and you probably recall the end, but you might just be hazy on the middle, especially if you fell asleep.

Usually, the beginning of a memory task gets the most practice, so that usually beats the end. But some people are really into endings and will recall the end better than the beginning. There is a class of people who routinely start their memorization project at the end, in the which case they know the end better than the beginning. As for me, and this is an individual preference, the priorities in the usual memory task would usually be study the middle more than the end and the end more than the beginning.

Now memorize the same list for one minute by encoding the items according to the first letter of the item. There are ten items, and each starts with a letter A to J. Tell yourself, out loud, A is apple, B is beam of light, C is candle, etc. Don't worry about encoding, and don't make mental images; just say the item with the letter that starts that item. Go through the entire list. Remember, you are trying to prove something to yourself. You are trying to prove that having a mental hook like a letter will facilitate recall and improve memory performance.

A is apple

B is beam of light

C is candle

D is delphinium

E is egg

F is face of evil (it might help to visualize an evil face with this item)

G is grandchildren (see a grandchild in your mind's eye)

H is horse, of course (note that the rhyme helps recall of the complete item)

I is India (picture it)

J is jail (picture yourself in jail)

Now turn away again and write what you recall. Your score should improve because you are now attaching the new information (the items) to a systematic set of pegs that you already know (the letters A, B, C, etc.). If you have trouble doing this, remember to be systematic. The letters of the alphabet are your memory places, just as the pictures in Cicero's home were his memory places. Pegs help memory the way a peg holds up a picture. Try to hang a picture on a bare wall. It will fall to the floor. Put a peg in the wall, and the picture will hang in place. Here the memory pegs are the letters A to J.

Say to yourself what's A? Apple should then spring to mind. Using the letter clues, most people will get eight items correct. Eight of ten; that's not bad. Furthermore, the serial position effect will not be present. That is, using the system, each item will have an equal probability of recall. Not using the system, the beginning and end of the list will have the highest probability of recall.

Don't look. Tell me, what's the G word? The H word? The F word? You should be able to recall the items in or out of order. Most people have trouble with item F. Something about face of evil might be off-putting. Recall in or out of order is an additional benefit of hooking to-be-recalled items onto well-learned material like the alphabet or the number system.

Mental Gymnastic: How about This?

Memorize and be prepared to recite the following letters in sequence. Take only 15 seconds for this task and write your answer:

Llew derepmet reivalc

Now recognize the pattern and chunk it.

Did you get the pattern? I don't blame you if you didn't. I didn't get it either when I first saw it. Hint: It is words written in reverse order.

MENTAL MAKING MIGHT

This is well-tempered clavier with each word spelled backward. *The Well-Tempered Clavier* is a collection of keyboard music by Johann Sebastian Bach. Now write the sequence by thinking of the keywords and reading the words backward. You should have no trouble with llew (well spelled backward), but most people will have to break the second sequence into two parts, dere and pmet because stage one of human memory can usually only hold seven items, not eight. Most people will be able to read the reivalc directly out of the memory by thinking of clavier backward. Some will need to break clavier into two pieces and recall the rei and then the valc. The point is that it is easier to memorize something if you can chunk it, and it is easier to chunk it if you recognize a pattern.

Mental Gymnastic

Recognize the pattern, chunk, and recite in order:

DOGSSELBACTIREMA

Try it. Break it down to component parts and link the parts to get the whole item. If need be, see the dogs selling bacteria that are in the blood. You out there who suffer dyslexia will probably read this as God bless America with an extra "T" between I and C.

Memory Lite—Storytelling

Narrative, narrative, narrative. There's lots of narrative out there, and for good reason. Humans love stories. The stories that they love the best are causal stories: Sequences of events distributed in time where each event follows the one before for a reason. The king died, and then the queen died. That's a story: The narration of events in time. The king died, and then the queen died of a broken heart. That is a causal story because the plot of the story explains the cause of the queen's death. It is easier to remember a story if the story has a plot because the plot gives us additional associations on which to hang our memory. A plotted story is a causal story. A story is just the narration of events in time. But a plot fills out the narration by giving us the reasons for the events. Sometimes the plot is not reasonable, in which case we can remember it precisely because it didn't make causal sense at that plot point. The logical plot point makes sense, so we remember it. The defective plot point doesn't make sense, so we remember it. Either way, we get a peg, something to hang the memory on to facilitate recall.

Remembering a causal story is easier than remembering a sequence of unrelated events because a causal story is logical; it makes sense because the events told make sense; they follow for reasons that can be understood or, if not understood, at least recalled because they were not understood. In our memory work, we have learned that the brain doesn't need a strictly logical connection between events to connect them together and to remember them both. Therefore, when there is a logical connection, use that to facilitate recall. When there is no apparent logical connection, make one up to facilitate recall.

People everywhere make up stories for lots of reasons. They are fun. They teach lessons about life and emotions. They entertain us. They (you fill in some reasons).

But the narrative drive goes deeper. It is embedded in our mental representation of what happens around us and what will happen around us, given a set of circumstances. My guess is that long ago, in a time out of mind, in a time older than the time of chronometers, our ancient ancestors sat in a cave around a campfire and listened to stories. No one knows what their stories were about, but we can guess. If the paintings on the walls of Paleolithic caves like those at Lascaux (c. 17,000 BC) are an indication, the stories were about humans and animals. Perhaps included in the stories were pieces of advice about how to herd the buffalos or auks into a narrow blind canyon and kill the animals en mass or how to herd the animals off a cliff and kill them that way. Or perhaps the pictures in the caves are places of worship, their cathedrals, and the animals are the sacred things venerated. Whatever. The people, our ancient ancestors, who paid attention and learned the lessons the stories taught may have had the advantage, better survival skills, and their survival may explain why we, their inheritors, love stories and remember the main points of the stories we hear or see.

Whatever the true evolutionary reason, the fact is that narration is a powerful tool in augmenting human memory. Use it whenever you need to. Use it whenever you can.

Reading as a Memory Task

Speed reading is a common term, but it doesn't really work. People who speed read are not really reading. They are culling ideas from the text. When advertisement claims you can be trained to read 1,500 words per minute, remember this: neurophysiologists have found it is impossible to read faster than 800 words a minute. The problem with the so-called speed readers is they don't remember what they read. There are ways to improve reading speed by practice and attention to detail. But the key thing is to remember what you read. On the SAT (note the letter mnemonic), there will be a paragraph for you to read, followed by questions. If you read through once and remark and remember the key points, you will answer the questions without having to go back and reread. That is the ticket to success. Read at your normal rate, but remember what you read. The goal is to read only once and know it. How? Apply concentrated attention to the material and make mental notes about what you are reading. Quiz yourself about key points and review. Facts in written materials are usually sequential, so you can apply linked words or images to get things in order and to get them right. Whispering to yourself what you are reading on the SAT will cement the memory and give you a giant heads up on the questions that follow. Circling the key points might help call attention to them. Don't believe me? Take the sample SAT on the internet using your old method and then apply the new methods and ideas. Prediction: Your final score will go up at least 50 points.

Event Memory

Let's pretend that you just witnessed a hit-and-run traffic accident. You saw the license plate of the car that fled. It was NM120F. How will you remember that?

If you said write it down, you get some credit but not much. Writing stuff down is not memory. That is a way of avoiding memory. When the great Egyptian god Thoth invented writing, the other gods (Amun included) thought this invention would have an adverse effect on human ability to remember. Those gods were right. Writing something down is a good way to cast the item out of mind. Another disadvantage is that the paper you wrote on could get lost or wet in the rain, or you might have the same trouble that my son, Craig, has: he can't read his own writing. In the case of the above-mentioned accident, you might not have a pen and paper handy.

No, friends, the answer was not to write it down. The answer was to memorize the plate number so that you can tell the police the exact number.

How about constructing a narrative? NM120F—New Mexico has temperatures of 120 degrees Fahrenheit. This narration may or may not be true. New Mexico probably does have some places where the temperature goes that high. Who knows? And who cares? The idea is we have made up a story that has a semi-logical premise (seems to make sense on some level) because New Mexico is, relatively speaking, a state where the average temperatures exceed the average temperatures of other states, and that story that we made up will help us recall the license plate number exactly.

My take: in New Mexico, the temperature is 120F degrees. Hence, the plate number was NM120F.

By the way, if you think we made up this plate number as a special case so it would be easy to remember. You're wrong. This is a plate Mickey saw this morning. You can do the same thing for any plate number. Try it. It's fun. Plates are easy to remember. In fact, they are designed that way so people can recall who ran them over and left the scene of the accident.

It is fun just to memorize things for the fun of it. Sometimes I do this at a store. Recently, the memory thing came in handy. I bought a pound of shrimp and handed a $50 dollar bill. The clerk gave me change of $20 and insisted I had tendered a 20.

"OK," I said. "Call the cops. There is a $50 dollar bill in the till, and I will recite for them its serial number, which I memorized just before I handed the 50 to you."

The clerk frowned, shook his head, and looked at me as if I had sprouted two heads, and one head had green hair and the other had red hair. Then, he admitted he had lied and admitted he tried to cheat me. He handed me the 50 after verifying my number. And I got a pound of shrimp free. Of course, I will think twice about shopping there. Any time someone is dishonest with you or lies about anything, watch out! If someone has lied to you, do not trust them. Even if the liar is the president of the United States, do not trust him.

Mental Gymnastic

What was the 12-digit number that starts with 76?

What are the colors of the rainbow?

Name the great lakes.

What were the four elements our ancient ancestors believed in?

What was the license plate of the hit-and-run driver?

What kind of weather usually follows a red sky at night?

Explain (again?) why Arlo can recall most of Humphrey Bogart's speech at the end of the movie *Casablanca* and yet can't remember to pick up the dry cleaning:

Remembering Names and Faces

Follow the rules. Decide that you want to remember the person's name. Repeat the name during the introduction to make sure you got it right. Make associations that might help recall the name at some time in the future. The associations need not be logical. Weird, unusual, colored, violent, improbable images are best, but your own personal associations are what count. What works is what you should use. Pay attention to details. Make associations that will help recall like the person's occupation, political beliefs, business interests, and so forth. Anything will do as long as you look at that face with interest, attention, and concentration.

My associations are good for me. Here's an example: I remember a man I met in the lounge in a hotel in Washington, DC. His name was Cornfield. He was a psychiatrist. When I met him, I imagined seeing a large corn plant growing out of his large forehead. Around the corn plant was wrapped a stethoscope. If I want to recall this doctor and his name, I think of the lounge and actually, see myself sitting there. Place is much more powerful a peg item than time, so this place, the subdued light, the brown leather soft chairs, the relaxed atmosphere, my cognac on the table in front of me—all that helped me see him, his face, the cornstalk, and all that recalled the event and conversation. Unfortunately, I can't even recall what year it was. Probably 1995. But that is just a guess. Our memories for time are far less powerful than our memories for place and person.

Test yourself: Review the name after a while to make sure you got it. If you didn't get it or are not sure, ask the hostess of the party (or someone) to tell you.

Mental Gymnastic

Memorize the names and faces. Be prepared to tell what name connects with what face.

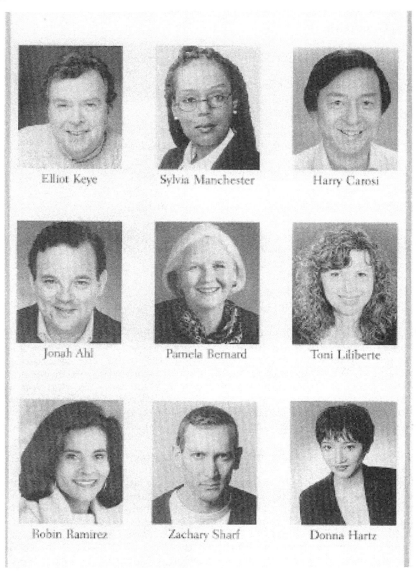

Fig4.3

Quiz time. Now without looking at the names and faces, just looking at the faces, write the names on a sheet of paper.

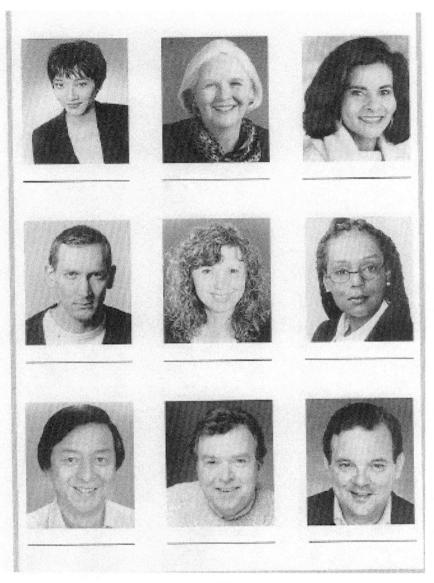

Fig4.4

Now go back and check your answers. How did you do? If you did OK, then pass on to the next chapter on memory heavy. If you didn't like your performance and are still interested in learning how to remember names and face, follow my associations and see if my associations improve your performance.

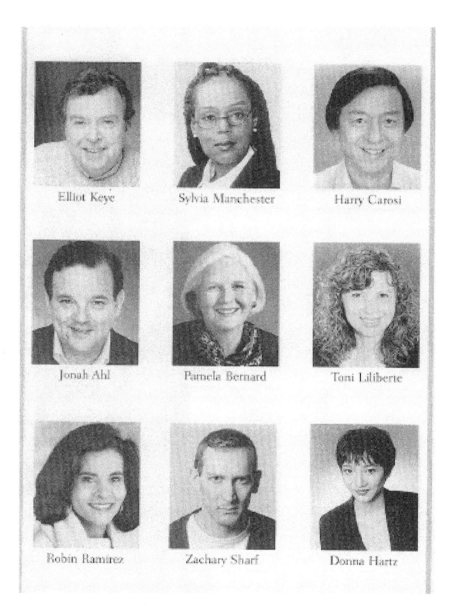

Fig4.5

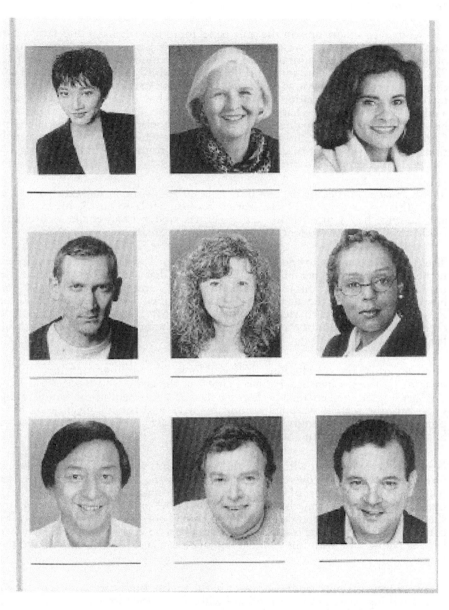

Fig4.6

Let's start at the top left corner and work right, then drop to the second section of faces and work right, and then finish the project with the bottom section working again from left to right.

The woman in square one on the quiz panel looks like she has a bird face. Going back to the name panel, we note that her name is Donna Hartz. That reminds of bird food—Hartz Mountain Bird food. That reminds that her name is Hartz. She might want to donate some bird feed to some bird feeding organization and, therefore, her name is Donna as Donna and donate start with the same three letters. An additional association that might attach to her image is the idea that she is a gift to birds because the Latin word for gift is done. Our recall of her name will be strengthened, not impaired by the multiple associations. Elaborate encoding! Concentrate on her face and name for an instance while thinking of the associations. Then try to forget her. Yes, dismiss Donna from your mind and forget all that stuff about birds and bird feed.

The next face (middle of the top line) belongs to a woman named Pamela Bernard. This one is easy for Doctor Patten because her last name is his first name, and he once had a nice friend named Pamela who worked at the Neurological Institute as a medical student. If you need more associations, make them.

The next face belongs to the Hispanic beauty. So, I will associate her Hispanic name (Ramirez) with her Hispanic beauty, and that should be sufficient. Men may have significant trouble remembering men's names, but men usually don't have difficulty with the names of beautiful women. What about the Robin? Ramirez and Robin start with the same letter R. See a Robin red-breast perched on her head. Think about the name and the associations, for an instant, and then forget her.

Now we are at the middle line. This guy looks like an angry marine. But let's imagine he is not a marine. He is a general in the army who is a descendant of Zachary Taylor, the general who became the 12th president of the United States. Oh, yeah, the scarf is wrapped around his neck and is choking him—a fitting punishment for being angry. Thus, his name is Zachary Scarf—almost. Zachary Sharf because of Sharf and Scarf rhyme.

Next, we have a woman with curls, and she reminds some older folks of the hair product that used to advertise "Which one has the Toni." Therefore, her first name is Toni, and she is, of course, a liberated woman, which will recall her last name is Liliberti. No way that when I talk with her and mention her name, that she will hear Liberberti and not Liliberte. But if she does hear a difference and corrects me, so what. She is soft and delicate like a flower, a lily in fact. That's why her last name starts with Lili. Look at her face and make the associations and then forget her, if you can.

Next, we have the only woman of color in the group. But I can't connect her color with anything related to her name, so I will try for other associations. To me, she looks like she is English, an English person from the midlands of England. In the midlands of England stands a town from which my ancestors moved to America. The name of that town is Manchester. Manchester is also her name. Around Manchester is a dense forest (this might be true or not, but who cares), and that forest reminds me of the Latin for forest, which is Sylva, -ae f. Hence, I shall recall her name: Sylvia Manchester. Make associations and then pass on to the next.

By now, you are getting the idea and can build your own associations, which will probably serve you well—better than any associations other people make for you. But for heuristic sake, continue to follow my associations in the last line of faces. The first man has dense hair, so I consider him hairy, which will remind me that his first name is Harry. Harry is a singer, of course, but he never reached the exalted heights of Caruso. So, he is not a Caruso; he is a Carosi. Right away, I know this is not going to work so well, so I must figure how to convert a Caruso to a Carosi. I shall think of Caruso and say that the u needs to be replaced by a different vowel, an o, and the o at the end has to be replaced by an i. Those are my ideas. Not too good, I admit. But we shall see if they hold up during the review before the quiz. Remember, review time is never wasted. Review is the way you prove to yourself that you actually know it. When you get it right, it's wonderful. When you get it wrong, it's wonderful. Getting it wrong teaches you where you need to do more work to get it right.

The next man has a gold key stuck in his forehead. The bright red blood is oozing down onto his face. His first name is Elliot, and his last name is Key, which will be close enough to Keye, close enough for government work.

Whew! At last, we come to the last face. Do him fast. He has an awl (looks like ahl) stuck in his head. Yes, some blood is dripping down, and he spent some time in the whale, so his name is Jonah Ahl. Here we rely on similar sounds to jog the memory.

Now take the quiz. I will too. Ready, set, go.

I got them all right, but one. How about you?

Recall was fast and easy and occurred at the speed of light. Well, not quite that fast, but very fast. There was a hesitation on Zachary because I called him Zachary Taylor. Then I realized that was the mnemonic, and that made me look at the face more intensely. The scarf did not appear before my mind, but the idea of Scarf did enter my head. Then I tried to figure out what the name really was because I knew Scarf wasn't exactly right. Another brief moment and Scarf still popped into my head, so I gave up on that one. On review, I find his name is Zachary Sharf. Will I get it right next time? Who knows? To get it right, I merely have to substitute one letter h for c. His name is Sharf, not Scarf.

That concludes the nuts and bolts of memory lite. In the next chapter, we will explore the territory of memory heavy. Make sure your tray tables are stowed, and your seat is in the upright position. Seat belt buckled? Ready for take-off? Let's go.

CHAPTER FIVE
MEMORY HEAVY

CHAPTER FIVE: MEMORY HEAVY

◆ ◆ ◆

Advice to Readers

This chapter covers memory heavy—complex and involved methods to memorize gigantic amounts of material. If you wish to have a super memory capable of memorizing a Shakespeare play, the Manhattan telephone directory, 50-digit numbers, all the presidents of the United States in or out of order, pi to 67,000 digits, the names of the 157 characters in *War and Peace,* the plot structure of *Pride and Prejudice,* the 52 cards in a deck in or out of the order presented (known in casinos as card counting)—if you wish to card count, or anything like such, read on. If having a super memory doesn't interest you, skip the chapter and go on to chapter six about mental math. Most people do not need a super memory, just a better memory than normal and a better memory for what interests them. How about you?

If you can't decide whether to continue with this chapter or not, then read the summary that follows and make a decision on that basis. If you still can't decide, flip a coin.

Summary of This Chapter

Ancient humans, lacking devices to store information, invented and developed systems of mnemonics, which evolved and passed on to modern times. These systems, known as the Ancient Art of Memory, were discovered in 447 BC by a Greek lyric poet named Simonides and were adequately discussed and described by Cicero, Quintilian, and Pliny. After Alaric sacked Rome in 410 AD, the memory arts, just as most other learned disciplines, fell into neglect for about 800 years, a period of time known to us as the Dark Ages.

In 1323, Saint Thomas Aquinas revived memory arts and transferred them from a division of rhetoric (rhetoric is the art of selecting from available resources the arguments most likely to be effective) to ethics (the art of doing the right thing at the right time in the right way for the right reason), using memory skills to recall Catholic doctrines and versions of biblical history.

In 1540, Saint Ignatius Loyola used mnemonic images to affirm the faith with members of his newly formed Society of Jesus, and he and his Jesuits used the memory arts to try to convert the Ming Dynasty in China by teaching these memory skills to Chinese nobles and to the candidates for office who were required to take the imperial examinations in Mandarin.

Today, ancient memory arts have applications in the rehabilitation of brain-damaged patients, pilot training, gambling, mentalism, mental math, and telepathy demonstrations. Objective testing confirms that with the use of the systems and with the adequate development of memory skills, recall is increased, at least ten-fold (1,000%), and the memory deficits of proactive and retroactive inhibition do not exist.

This chapter divides itself into three parts: Part I deals with ancient memory traditions. Part II deals with medieval memory traditions. Part III displays aspects of the modern practical applications of memory heavy techniques. Malcolm Conway, a retired TWA pilot, adapted memory heavy techniques for pilot training and licensed the techniques to airlines for millions of dollars. According to Conway, with the use of the systems, pilot training time is remarkably reduced, and pilot accuracy is remarkably increased. According to Conway, the North American Air Command purchased, for four million dollars, his system to manage training of the people who operate America's nuclear arsenal.

The chapter's purpose: Designed to show concepts, ideas, and techniques that may prove useful to you and help you develop your own memory skills. The chapter is merely an overview of a vast subject, the serious investigation of which has only just begun. Commercial schools of memory, including those run by Harry Lorayne, Bruno Fürst (and wife, Lotte Fürst), and Roy Montsauvage, were the primary sources of some of the techniques used to illustrate the basic memory principles of memory heavy, but those mnemonists were using and copying very ancient traditions and merely adapting those traditions to modern times.

A serious student of memory techniques should enroll in one of the commercial schools of memory for a six-week course (yes, it will take at least that long for you to become a memory superstar) run by these men or similar experts. Alternatively, take an advanced college-level course in memory techniques or a course run in a university's continuing education program. The codes discussed here to convert numbers to letters, letters to words, words to pictures are mainly Doctor Patten's simplified version of the more complex systems used by Harry Lorayne. The simplified codes are easier to apply but just as effective. The memory peg lists (based on numbers), used to hang complex memories or massive amounts of data, are copied from those of our ancient ancestors and are actually over 2,000 years old. Modify and adapt the systems to your individual needs. Take and use what you like. Leave what you don't like or what doesn't work well for you. Memory heavy is a fine art. It is an art in the sense it is an immediate, personal, creative, and imaginative craft requiring adroitness and cunning for successful performance.

For better or worse, to look like a memory genius, you must be a memory artist and work at your craft. The chapter ends with some tips on how to develop a good memory for images, a skill crucial to reaching the goals of memory heavy. Ancient memory arts were an important feature of the educational curriculum for over a millennium and a major medieval tradition for a similar length of time. The pursuit of this subject will open vistas of some of the greatest manifestations of our culture and touch vital points in the history of religion, ethics, music, painting, and literature.

Ready?

If so, let's renew our contact with this important heritage and review some of the highlights of its fascinating history.

BERNARD MICHAEL PATTEN, M.D.

Part I—Ancient Traditions

Prehistory: Somewhere and somehow, in a time out of mind—in a time older than the time of chronometers—an unknown human or several humans learned that making mental images of items in places facilitates recall, and he or she or he and she realized that two items, once linked in the consciousness, forever tend to help each recall the other and in the order originally presented. Aristotle knew this quite well, as discussed in the chapter on memory lite.

The physiological reasons for this natural phenomenon are now known and involve neuronal networks firing together and in sequence. Those interested should consult the editorial in *Science,* March 2020, vol 367, issue 6,482, page 1,087, entitled *Human Brain Activity During Memory.* The detailed scientific article on which the editorial was based appears on page 1,131 of the same issue.

It turns out episodic memory relies on the replay of past experiences, and those experiences are temporally organized during episodic memory encoding and retrieval. Ripple oscillations in the brain cortex reflect underlying bursts of single-unit spiking activity that are organized into memory-specific sequences. This spiking activity occurs repeatedly during memory formation and is replayed and repeated during successful memory recall. The main place of activity is, as expected, the temporal lobes of the brain, but many other modules of the brain may play a role depending on the type of material or task to be remembered and the modalities (vision, sound, touch, smell, taste, kinesthetic) involved.

Back to Ancient Times

This unknown ancient ancestor, or more probably, ancestors, also discovered that the images that worked best were those encoded in a vivid visual way. Make this principle part of you, if you have not yet done so, by memorizing this:

The basic principle of human memory and thought is: Two items once associated in the consciousness forever tend to recall each other.

The items that work best in helping to recall each other for most people are visual images or a combination of visual images with sounds and movements. The use of multiple modalities to encode memory is known as enhanced encoding when you can aim for enhanced encoding.

Ancient Memory Arts

The above-mentioned principle is a basic human mental mechanism and is the "discovery" that is the fundamental basis of the ancient art of memory. This discovery, we can speculate, might have facilitated the finding of the berry patches (mental image of fruits in a particular landscape) or the hunting grounds (animals mentally pictured in a forest or on the plain or in a tree or where ever). This idea of linking images with food may sound trivial to modern humans but finding food, since the dawn of our species, was basic to human survival. In fact, food is needed for the survival of individuals of any species. There is no doubt other animals make clear and persistent images and ideas in their heads concerning food and where to get it. Don't believe me? Watch your cat stalk a rat or a bird. Watch your cat sniff the air when a steak is cooking. Visit the ancient cave paintings of Europe see the paintings that suggest what was on the mind of the artists—animals, lots of them, and most of them already extinct.

Ancient Greece

Every single source, from Cicero in his *de Oratore* (Cicero MT *De Senectute*. Trans. Falconer WA. New York: Loeb Classical Library, 1936), Quintilian in his *Institutio Oratoria* (Quintilian. *Institutio Oratoria,* vol 4. Trans. Butler HE. New York, Loeb Classical Library, 1936) and even the famous and anonymous *Ad Herennium Libri IV,* attributes the discovery of the ancient art of memory to the Greek poet Simonides of Ceos.

All these sources relate fundamentally the same story that the ancient art of memory was invented in 477 BC by Simonides, who had chanted a lyric poem at a banquet given by Scopas, a nobleman of Thessaly.

About Simonides

Simonides was one of the first poets to require payment or fee for service for his poems, and legend has it during the first half of his poem, he praised Scopas and his wealth. But during the second part of his poem, he praised the two gods, Castor and Pollux. In the old days, there was no TV; poetry was **the entertainment,** and you had to pay for it.

At the end of the poem, Simonides requested payment, but Scopas meanly told the poet he would pay solely for the half during which he was praised and that the poet must look to the two gods, Castor and Pollux for payment for their half of the poem.

Cicero tells us that a little later during the banquet, a message came to Simonides that two young men were waiting for him outside and wished to see him. Simonides left the banquet but could find no one outside. During his absence, the stone roof fell in and crushed all the guests to death. The corpses were so mangled that relatives who came to take them away were unable to identify who was who. But Simonides remembered the places at which each had been seated and had a visual image of what they looked like at table. So, he was able to indicate to relatives which were their dead.

This doesn't sound like much of a discovery, but images in places is the key to ancient memory systems and the key to their modern applications, and your key to a super memory.

The invisible callers, Castor and Pollux, the two gods, had paid handsomely and handsomely paid for their share of the poem by drawing the poet away from the banquet just before the collapse of the building. According to the ancient sources mentioned above, it was this experience that suggested to Simonides the principles of the art of memory: Namely, that orderly arrangement is essential for a good memory and that a visual image of the to-be-remembered item in a specific place or locus makes recall easy.

Get it?

Order and image make for spectacular memory. Order is usually a framework or a pattern. So, look for the pattern or use a preexisting pattern. Then hang memory items, especially images, on the pattern.

Still, lost? Don't fret. Multiple examples will illustrate what we are talking about and how to do it and how to use it.

Proof of Invention

The Parian Chronicle, a marble tablet of about 264 BC, which was found at Paros in the 17th century, records legendary dates for discoveries such as the invention of the flute, the introduction of agriculture, and the recitation of Orpheus' poetry. In historic times, the tablet tells about prizes awarded at festivals, the ancient equivalent, I suppose, of our present Nobel Prize. The entry that confirms Cicero's attestation is as follows:

"From the time when Simonides, son of Leoprepes, the inventor of the system of memory aids, won the chorus prize at Athens, and statues were set up to Harmodius and Aristogeidon, 213 years (i.e., 477 BC)."

Notice Cicero got the year exactly right.

It is known from other sources that Simonides won the chorus prize in his old age.

A fragment known as the *Dialexeis,* which dates to about 400 BC and written in Ancient Greek, contains a section on memory and clearly talks about the rules for mnemonic devices (See Frances A. Yates, *The Art of Memory,* Routledge, 1999). The *Dialexeis* talks about memory for things and memory for words—so here are the technical terms for the two kinds of artificial memory already in use in the fourth century BC. Both kinds of memory use images, one to represent and recall things, and the other to represent and recall words. The orderly arrangement so necessary for accurate recall is based on and is supplied by architectural models in which the image of the to-be-remembered item is placed in a set image of the building. The images in that building can be anything, a picture, a door, a fountain. The items to be remembered are attached to the images in the building by an act of conscious thought. This act of conscious thought that associates two items is known in memory schools as the "original awareness."

To facilitate recall, to develop the memory, one walks through the building and looks (in the mind's eye) at the place where the previous image of the item to be recalled was stored. Usually, the image of the thing or word to be remembered will immediately flash into consciousness. Cicero said the item was suddenly donated to him. Remember?

Cicero (remember?) used the same techniques to recite speeches in the Roman Senate. This is probably the reason orators even today advance to different topics by saying "in the first place" followed by "in the second place" or "in the next place" and so forth. The modern orator is using numbers in place of the system of organization based on architecture, but the concept, execution, and results are fundamentally the same. In the ancient system, places were the pattern to which memory items were attached. In the more modern approach, numbers or letters of the alphabet are the pattern used as the scaffold on which the items to be re-membered are attached.

Orderly Arrangement

The orderly arrangement has to be supplied by something, either a set of numbers, letters of the alphabet, or the rooms in a building or the frescoes or pictures in the building or your body parts, and so forth. This organized pattern set, whatever it may be, gives us the pegs on which the items to be remembered are hung. The set must be known in advance and has to be capable of being recalled at will. All this is necessary for the systems to work well and is the very basis of modern thinking about memory systems. Thus, the *Dialexeis,* a simple manuscript itself, shows us that the patterns of human thinking in ancient times do not differ from patterns of human thinking in modern times. This makes sense because the human brain has not changed size or shape in the last hundred thousand years. The thinking machine in the hollow round of your skull is fundamentally the same thinking machine that Cicero had and Saint Thomas had. The thinking machine you are using at present to understand what you are reading is the same thinking machine that had been used by Galileo and Einstein. And it will be the same thinking ma-chine used by your children and grandchildren and great-grandchildren and on and on until the sun becomes a red giant and burns out the earth and extinguishes humanity.

Note by Ethel Patten

Don't you think the human brain will evolve if the species lasts long enough?

Answer: That is a hope, but probably a slim one.

What do you think? Check your view:

_____ Yes, the human brain will evolve.

_____ No, the human brain will not evolve.

_____ Hard to say. We'll just have to wait a few million years and see.

Sophists

The *Dialexeis* reflects Sophist teaching, and its memory section refers to the mnemonics of the Sophist, Hippias of Elis, who is said in the pseudo-platonic dialogues that satirize him and that bear his name to have possessed a science of memory and to have boasted that he could recite 50 names after hearing them once, and also recite the genealogies of heroes and men, the foundations of cities, and much other material, especially material of an eristic nature.

This is firm evidence that Hippias was a practitioner of the ancient artificial memory arts. He taught these things to aristocratic youths whose parents paid enormous fees for the educations. According to Professor Rufus Fears of the University of Oklahoma, the value of the fees paid yearly matched what the usual American private college charges in tuition per year—about $55,000.

In ancient Greece, memory training was part of the science and art of rhetoric. Rhetoric prepared the youth for important positions in law and government and was therefore very worthwhile to master. Rhetoric selects from available arguments those most likely to be effective and effective arguments led to fame and fortune—they still do.

Aristotle

Aristotle was familiar with the art of memory and wrote a book on the subject. Aristotle also wrote, according to Diogenes Laertius, a book on mnemonics, which, unfortunately, has been lost. According to Aristotle (whose name means "master of they who know"), a person with a trained memory can augment the memory by placing visual items in loci, and then, by recalling the loci, the item to be remembered can be recalled. This is the same method used by Simonides. For Simonides recalled his mental image of the banquet table and the places occupied by each of the guests and therefore was able to identify what corpse belonged to what person by mentally placing the image in that person's place. If this idea is still not clear, please don't worry. It will become clearer as we get to the applications of memory arts.

Mental Gymnastic

Have a friend make a list of six grocery items. Take each item in turn and make a mental image of that item and attach it to a part of your home or apartment. For example: if the first item was bread, you might make a mental image of a giant loaf of Wonder Bread with its white and red wax paper layered over your front door. Continue to make the images and attach them to features in your home as you would walk through your home. Then in your mind's eye, picture yourself entering your home and viewing the areas that you attached the images of the grocery items to. Notice how quickly the to-be-recalled items flash into your consciousness.

Whoa! You say you did this before? So what! Memory tasks have to be refined, repeated, and practiced. If you don't do it, who will?

All memory experts repeat themselves. That is an important component of memory training—just as important as the Indian Position is in yoga, or training in the major and minor scales are in music. Repetition in a memory book comes with the territory. It is natural.

The repetition in this book is small compared to the repetition in Harry Lorayne's book on *Memory Isometrics.* His chapter on card counting, for instance, repeats the same card words and pictures over and over again. And Harry tests and retests the reader with his proctor cover technique. The ace of clubs is CAT as a word and as a picture. That CAT—AC (ace of clubs) is tested at least 35 times in the card counting chapter. That is a lot of repetition and a lot of self-testing. But the results speak for themselves. By the end of Harry's chapter, the reader who did the repetitions will be an expert card counter.

Imaginary Places, Palaces, and Memory Rooms

Not content with the architectural features of their own homes, our ancient ancestors pre-built imaginary places, often called memory palaces, in which they placed the things they wished to recall. Those of you interested in examining this architectural place system of memory in more detail should consult the book *Memory Palaces of Matteo Rickey,* a Jesuit priest who used the systems to train Chinese nobles to memorize enormous amounts of material so that they could pass the imperial examinations and get good government jobs.

Ancient Rome

Pliny in his natural history describes the same memory systems. We have already mentioned the same systems appear in the Latin work on rhetoric called *Ad Herennium,* and we have also mentioned Quintilian, who wrote about memory in his handbooks on oratory. These books gave detailed information on how to construct memory buildings and the images one would place in them. As the author of *Ad Herennium* explains:

"We ought to set up images of a kind that can adhere longest in the memory, and we shall do so if we establish likeness as striking as possible. If we set up images that are not many or vague, but doing something, if we assign to them exceptional beauty or singular ugliness, if we dress some of them with crowns or purple cloaks, for example, so that the likeness may be more distinct to us, or we somehow disfigure them, as by introducing one stained with blood or soiled with mud or smeared with red paint so that its form is more striking, or by assigning certain comic effects to our images, for that too, will ensure our remembering them more readily."

Wow! A better description of the qualities of memory images that work has never ever been offered. What she (the anonymous author) is saying is, "Make the images memorable by making them remarkable or interesting or unusual or notable or different. Make them striking in some way to attract attention and help the brain pay attention to them and remember them."

Quintilian elaborated on the same subject by explaining what sort of places one would use to store the images one had chosen:

"The first thought is placed, as it were, in the forecourt. The second, let us say, in the living room. The remainder are placed in due order all around the impluvium [the water storage tank in the center of a Roman home] and entrusted not merely to bedrooms and parlors but even to the care of statues and the like. This done, as soon as the memory of the facts requires to be revived all the places are visited in turn and the various deposits are demanded from their custodians as the site of each recalls the respective details."

Are you still worried that you don't get it? Don't worry. That is the normal reaction. Despite these attempts at explanation, the system sounds elusive and abstract to most readers today, except to those who are actual practitioners of this ancient art and have studied it or taken courses at the commercial schools of memory. Please be reassured that the descriptions given above by the anonymous author of *Ad Herennium* and by Quintilian clearly show procedures in the mnemonic arts that are extremely effective in increasing recall. For example, Cicero was able to recite his speeches in the Roman Senate for several days without resorting to a single note or other written device, and Quintilian as a teacher of the art of rhetoric was able to do the same. Roman generals had actually memorized the name of each person in their army. Caesar did this, and Henry Wadsworth Longfellow was aware of that fact as this quote from *The Courtship of Miles Standish* proves:

"See how bright they are burnished, as if in an arsenal hanging;

That is because I have done it myself and not left it to others.

Serve yourself, would you be well served, is an excellent adage;

So I take care of my arms, as you of your pens and your inkhorn.

Then, too, there are my soldiers, my great, invincible army,

Twelve men, all equipped, having each his rest and his matchlock,

Eighteen shillings a month, together with diet and pillage,

And, like Caesar, I know the name of each of my soldiers!"

This he said with a smile that danced in his eyes as the sunbeams.

MENTAL MAKING MIGHT

We know from Polybius and Tacitus that Publius Scipio was actually able to recognize and name all of the 32,000 men in his army (other ancient sources say he knew the names of 35,000 men). I wonder how many names American generals know. My guess: less than 100. President Kennedy made it a point to remember all the names of the house staff at the white house. Pierce (President 14, 1853–1857), using this technique, actually delivered his first official address entirely from memory. That historical fact was a $64,000 question on one of the quiz shows Doctor Patten watched as a kid. Who was the first president to give his inaugural address entirely from memory? Answer: Franklin Pierce. What president was Pierce? See an arrow in a tire. Tire translates to tr, translates to 14—all by methods soon to be explained.

Miles Standish looks like a memory midget compared to the ancients. Memorizing the names of the 12 men in his troop is nothing to brag about. No wonder the beautiful Priscilla Mullins, the only single woman of marriageable age in Plymouth Colony, thought he was a bore and married John Alden instead. Do you recall her famous question? "Why don't you speak for yourself, John?"

Kennedy and Pierce had great natural memories, but with the use of the memory systems, they looked super because they were super.

And, dear reader, why is it probably good that Publius Scipio Africanus remembered the names of the men in his army?

Pause here and try to recall the answer. We pause for reply.

Answer: Because if his army had not defeated Hannibal in the great battle of Zama (202 BC), ending the second Punic War, this book would probably have been written in a language based on Punic instead of Latin.

Careful reading is an act of memory. You should have, if you were paying attention, noted the date of the battle of Zama and the fact that that battle ended the second Punic War. And if you were really on the ball, you would have looked up Scipio and the Punic War to solidify your knowledge and to enable you to talk about that phase of Roman history intelligently for at least three minutes at the next dinner party. No one else at the dinner table will know as much as you about the Punic war. So, if you can somehow work it in as a topic of conversation, you will look like a superstar.

Give yourself partial credit if you remembered the general idea. Give yourself an A+ if you recalled the battle of Zama and the date.

If you didn't get the answer, figure out why. Probably you need to be more attentive and more awake as you read. By the way, do you know where Zama is? If not, how come you didn't look it up. How are you going to look ten times smarter than you are if you don't do the work? Zama is also known as Xama. The modern name is Tunis. Where is Tunis? North Africa, where ancient Carthage used to be.

How did Scipio remember 32,000 names? Answer: How he remembered the names is not discussed either by Polybius or Tacitus, but we can conjecture that he did it the same way the modern memory experts do—by application of the ancient arts of memory. This task would have been easy to any practitioner of the ancient memory arts. Every Roman had three names: a family name, a given name, and an acquired name. The acquired name was based on an outstanding feature of that person and usually matched up with something memorable about that person. For instance, Scipio was the family name, Publius was the given name, and after the defeat of Hannibal, Africanus was the acquired name. The Romans called him Africanus because the battle of Zama, which destroyed Carthage, took place in Tunisia, which is in North Africa.

What Was Scipio's Problem

The usual problem, then as now, was that there usually was no logical connection between a person's face and the person's name. So ancient generals had to make a connection, often an illogical connection, by looking at the face, selecting a special feature (something memorable or something likely to trigger a memory) like a big mouth or a scar, and then making a vivid visual image that connects the facial feature with the name.

Example: When I think of Africa, I see a lion and would put the lion in Scipio's mouth, making one vivid ridiculous visual image. If I saw him in person, his mouth would remind me of lion, lion recalls Africa, Africa recalls Africanus, and Africanus would remind me of or link to his other two names Publius and Scipio.

Why Did the Romans and Other Ancients Work So Hard on Their Memories?

There is no doubt that memory was important in Roman times. They had to remember things because they didn't have tape recorders and ready access to filing cabinets. They had no computers. No cell phones. No Alexa to tell them the day, time, and the news. Paper from Egypt was very expensive (actually, it was papyrus from which we get our English word paper), and parchment was even more expensive. Only the most important things were written down. Hence, the very heavy reliance on the memory systems of the meat computer in the hollow round of their skull—their brains.

What, No Paper?

Paper did not exist. To write something down for permanent storage, Romans had what came only from Egypt or from Pergamon. From Egypt came papyrus, which was expensive and strictly controlled by the Egyptian Kings. Because it was expensive, one rarely wrote down anything except the most important items. Important books were written on papyrus and rolled into scrolls which were stored in great libraries and guarded as treasure. Even the Egyptians were stingy about how they used papyrus and wrote most of their letters and other trivia on ceramic pots.

Mental Gymnastic

Where does our English word "paper" come from?

Answer: Our word "paper" comes from the ancient Egyptian word for papyrus.

From Pergamon came parchment made from animal skins (sheep, goats, and calves)—untanned skins on which things were written. These were precious and used only for important items. Vellum, a finer quality parchment, was made from younger animal skins, particularly lambskin. It was even more dear and could be bound into books, which were stored in vast libraries and guarded as treasure.

So, what's the point?

The point: Ancient memory arts were essential to the intellectual life of a community as other means for recording things were not readily available. Out of necessity, memory arts were highly developed, much more highly developed than they are now. Memory arts were part and parcel of the intellectual, scientific, political, cultural, and domestic life then and in use as much as our cell phones and computers are today.

Part II—Middle Ages

Europe

Alaric sacked Rome in 410 AD, and the Vandals invaded North Africa in 429. Saint Augustine died in 430, during the siege of Hippo Regius. Ancient memory arts must have been in use then because Augustine tells us that his friend Simplicius memorized and could recite Virgil's Aeneid backward. This is an amazing feat as most of us can't recite Vigil's Aeneid forward. In fact, most of us would not dare to try to memorize an entire book like the Aeneid. But this activity did interest many ancient Greeks and Romans. The past is a different country. They do things differently there.

Although the time of the capture of Hippo Regius was a time of economic and social collapse in the Roman Empire in the west, Martianus Capella published a little book called de *Nuptiis Philologiae et Mercurii,* which was used in the Middle Ages for education and which outlined the seven liberal arts: Grammar, rhetoric, dialectic (the art of critical examination into the truth of an opinion; originally the art of reasoning by question and answer), arithmetic, geometry, music, and astronomy.

Capella's book discussed the ancient art of memory under rhetoric, which is its classical niche since memory was considered one of the five parts of rhetoric. His book is the foundation for the Middle Ages and Renaissance applications of ancient memory arts to the curriculum of those times. *De Nuptiis Philologiae et Mercurii* details all of the commonly accepted rules of artificial memory, including the principles of making vivid visual images and placing them in vivid visual places to facilitate recall. But for a few centuries, this art, along with much of the world's information and learning, got lost. How or why this happened is not known. But we know it did happen.

For instance, memory arts were unknown to Charlemagne (768–814) and to Alcuin (735–804). Alcuin was considered the "most learned man anywhere to be found." Alcuin was commissioned by Charlemagne to restore the educational system of antiquity to the Carolinian empire. We know these arts were unknown to Charlemagne because, in the dialogues concerning rhetoric and virtue derived for the royal master, they are completely omitted. Alcuin only mentions that "we have no other precepts about it (speaking here of memory enhancement) except exercise in memorizing, practice in writing, application to study, and the avoidance of drunkenness."

In other words, that's it. That is all the great man, the most learned man of that age, knew about memory. So, here is good evidence that knowledge of the artificial memory arts and their applications had faded in the Dark Ages. The rules are gone, replaced by "avoid drunkenness," which is good advice in view of the adverse effect alcohol has on second-stage memory. The exercise in memorizing advice refers to repeating the things to be remembered. That is what we moderns would call memorizing by rote. It is and can be somewhat effective but is tedious and time-consuming. Practice in writing is also somewhat effective as a memory tool. Some people write things to get them into their memory. The physical act of writing helps them cement the memory, and so does the visual image of the writing. If writing things out helps you remember what you want to remember, then, by all means, write.

Most memory schools oppose writing as a memory tool. They say the mind likes to be trusted. Writing things down is a sign of distrust. The key point is that writing things down without trying to remember is going against the rules for a better memory. You are not trusting your memory, you are not showing confidence, and you are not practicing your memory skills. Instead, you are displaying a lack of real interest in memorizing the item. The other problem with writing is you can misplace the notebook or the paper. You can't easily misplace your mind.

Back to Alcuin

Poor Alcuin, a great scholar, probably the greatest of his time and specifically recruited by Charlemagne to get ancient wisdom back into European culture. Poor Alcuin—he had few books at his disposal. He was in charge of the re-education of Europe, and yet he did not have access to the works of Aristotle, Cicero, Quintilian, or *Ad Herennium*. No wonder the ancient art of memory lapsed into disuse. No wonder his advice about how to improve memory was so feeble. Alcuin would have devoured a book like this one or any book by Aristotle, Cicero, Quintilian, or Pliny.

Conclusion: Yes, in the Dark Ages, memory arts were lost. But not forever.

The Rediscovery of the Ancient Arts of Memory

The art was recovered by two very important figures: Albertus Magnus and Thomas Aquinas. Both these men, but especially Thomas, were eager to reconcile the teachings of Aristotle with the evolving philosophy of the Roman Catholic church, and indeed, Thomas wrote a very large work called the *Summae* to provide intellectually the unification of Aristotelian ethics and church doctrine. If Simonides was the inventor of memory systems, then Thomas Aquinas, canonized in 1323, was its patron saint.

Saint Thomas transferred the memory arts from a division of rhetoric to ethics and said that memory could be used to recall the important points and components of ethical behavior. His books provide us with memory rules that are now used for memorizing (guess what?) lists of sins, virtues, and vices. Such long lists as these prompted jests by other church officials, including the famous François Rabelais (c. 1494–1553) in his masterpieces *Gargantua* and *Pantagruel*.

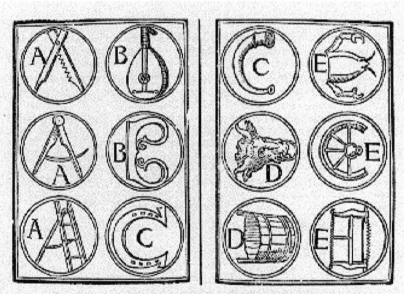

7. Visual alphabet from Johann Host von Romberch's *Congestorium Artificiose Memorie* (No. 46)

Fig5.1 - From Romberch shows some memory pegs based on letters. Note how the objects depicted as the image to be used resemble the form of the letter, especially A, C, and E. This is a simple mnemonic to clue the memory of what image pegs to what letter.

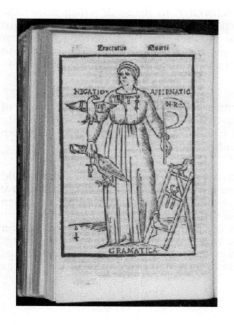

Fig5.2 - Illustrates some of these points with grammar as a memory image, and figure 1B shows the visual alphabet for inscriptions on grammar from Johannes Romberch, Congestorium Artificiose Memorie, Venice (1533), page 170.

Look at Figure 5.2. What do you see? Grammar is a woman! She deals with negation and affirmation. Negation is on our left, her right. This image was used and actually helped students recall the elements of grammar, including usage, sentence structure, and so forth. The tool symbols in her hands and those on her chest and all those birds (one in her right hand and one on her arm) had significance for that era and indicated schemes, synecdoche, litotes, tropes, metaphors, metonymy, onomatopoeia, metalepsis, allegory, irony, hyperbole, and analogy. Exactly what tool means what is not known and will probably never be entirely known. In fact, most modern readers do not have a clear idea of what a trope is, or a metonymy, or an onomatopoeia, or a metalepsis. What do we do when we don't know the meaning of words?

In figure 1B, some of us might have trouble seeing important differences in the images attached to the letters. The key point is that we are seeing these images from the point of view of our own culture, in which they lack significant meaning. A person from the 16th century would have little difficulty distinguishing bird C from K, and after all, C and K in classical Latin are pretty much the same sound. But in church Latin, the C is soft, sounding more like the letter s.

Bird C looks stronger, bigger, and more powerful than bird K. Why? Who knows? Probably bird C reminds them of Coeli, meaning heaven as in the Eastertide anthem chant to the Virgin Mary, Regina Coeli (Queen of Heaven). Yes, admit it. We moderns have trouble with medieval iconography, just as a 16th-century person would have trouble (we imagine) telling the difference between a Rolls-Royce and a Ford. They wouldn't know and probably couldn't guess what those cars were for and what they indicated about the persons who owned them. A 20th-century person wouldn't have a problem with that task because automobiles have an important meaning to us historically and culturally.

The famous Abbey memory system is illustrated in figure 2, which shows the visual images to be attached to numbered places. Looking at figure 2, you might wonder how such a set of numbers and pictures could help anyone remember anything. The explanation is that to a person of those times, each image had immense importance and was a powerful part of the thought process of that era.

Notice the window that is the peg image or locus of the number 1 (figure 2). This window is a church window, and the church was the number one power of those times. In addition, with a little imagination, you can turn that window into something that resembles the number 1 itself. Can you see how the window can be imagined to have a shape like the number one?

When someone wanted to recall an item associated with number 1, they would make a visual image of the item and place it in that window. All they would have to do is see in their mind's eye the image of the item and the window, and then they could forget all about it until recall time. At recall time, they would think of number one, perhaps also recall that the church was the number one power of the time, that and the common shape would remind them that the peg image for one is that window. Usually, as soon as they again imagined the window, the visual image of the item they placed there to be remembered would flash into the consciousness. Don't believe me? Try it.

Image Training—Comment by Doctor Patten

Experience trying to train patients to make visual images taught me that this particular skill is deeply suppressed in modern culture. Children can do it and, in fact, like imagining images. Adults have trouble. Perhaps making a visual image and projecting it onto a wall or onto another image reminds adults of the mentally ill, and that reminder inhibits maintenance of this skill. Multiple ancient texts give convincing evidence, and multiple examples prove that Greek, Roman, and Medieval scholars were well trained to make mental images and did so routinely and without guilt or feelings of mental imbalance.

Your brain is making images all the time. So, we know any normal brain can do it. In fact, everything you see is a reconstructed and highly adjusted image of what is out there in the real world. For instance, color and depth do not exist; they are work products of the brain. The brain gives us the appearance of color and depth to help our orientation to and our interpretation of external reality. In fact, there is no color in the real world. The real world is just various shades of gray due to various wavelengths of light. The brain organizes the various wavelengths into colors as long as we have the functioning elements in our retina to manage various wavelengths. Only three receptors are needed to make millions of colors. For the TV to show all those colors, only red, green, and blue dots are needed.

Some men lack receptors for a certain wavelength and will therefore be "color-blind" for that wavelength. Those men have trouble distinguishing a red light from a green light. In the dark, all humans lack retinal receptors for color so, in a truly dark environment, you will not see color at all. Galileo stated color does not exist, and neither does taste or smell. Those things are products of the brain and do not have an external existence. Some people have trouble understanding all this, but that is their problem, not yours.

Making and Projecting Images

And yes, with practice, you can make a colored image of a giant Coke bottle and project it onto a wall such that it looks as good and as real as any image on TV or in a magazine. In your mind's eye, you can, with application be able to enlarge the image and make it smaller and rotate it, so it is displayed upside down or sideways. A computer with a photoshop program can do that easily, and so can the human brain.

With practice, every normal human can do that as easily as they can say "Coke bottle." However, because of the suppression of such skills in our culture and educational systems, it becomes a terrible uphill battle to train yourself to make and project mental images. In fact, you are probably frightened to even attempt this exercise.

Note from Doctor Patten

In the memory clinic at the Neurological Institute of New York, I gave up trying to teach such skills because the patients complained of being haunted by the images they made, haunted by the Coke bottle appearing and disappearing with every speck of red-brown Coke showing clear. The problem became especially acute just before the patients tried to sleep. They became frightened that they were losing their minds, that the image was out of their control, and so forth. The straw that broke the camel's back was when a 60-year-old patient woke me in the middle of the night complaining about the Coke bottle haunting him and preventing his sleep.

Me: "This is good, George. Practice working with the image. See what you can do. Make it bigger or smaller. Rotate it. Change colors. This is your chance to develop your image-making skills,"

He: "No thanks, Doc. Just make it go away. I need my sleep."

Me: "Relax. The persistent image is like an earworm where a melody you have heard keeps repeating over and over in your head. It's harmless, and you can make it disappear by focusing on something else. Go watch TV, and it will disappear in an instant."

Saints and Images

Some saints had no trouble making images and projecting them. In 1559, Teresa of Avila became firmly convinced that Jesus Christ Himself was visiting her in bodily form. In another vision, a Seraph repeatedly stabbed her in the heart with a golden sword. That vision became the subject of the famous white marble sculpture by Bernini entitled *The Ecstasy of Saint Teresa*. Teresa also had visions of Mary, sometimes with the infant Jesus, and sometimes alone, and Teresa had multiple raptures in which she felt she was being levitated. The levitations frightened her, and she begged her fellow nuns to hold her down so she would not hit the ceiling. Mary Magdalene, according to John 20: 1–10, visited the tomb and found the stone had been rolled back. She saw a man whom she thought at first was the gardener, but the man introduced himself as Jesus, and Mary then recognized him as such. Why did Mary have trouble recognizing Jesus? Your guess is as good as mine. If she believed he was dead, then she might have a kind of brain fog in recognizing he wasn't. On the other hand, maybe she wanted him to be alive and therefore imagined the gardener to be Jesus.

Sacred visions also occurred at Fatima, Lourdes, and outside Mexico City at Guadalupe. Read about them if you wish.

Religious folk are not the only ones who report visions. While Boethius was in prison awaiting execution, a "beautiful majestic woman" repeatedly appeared to him and helped him write a great and noble book, a timeless classic, entitled *"The Consolations of Philosophy."*

In 1951, when I visited my great-uncle John in Ireland, he told me the Virgin Mary had appeared to him in an apple tree and assured him that he would be the richest man in Carrick-ma-Cross, his village. Considering the abject poverty in that place, this isn't much. And it is too bad this miraculous apparition of the Virgin isn't better known. Carrick-ma-Cross could have become a place of pilgrimage like Fatima and Lourdes.

Crazy People Make Images and Project Them

Psychotic patients routinely have auditory and sometimes visual hallucinations. Also, very sick patients report they had visions. Usually, the vision is a special visit from their mother. That mother visit is quite common, especially in patients recovering from surgery who have been placed in a darkened room. The visions also occur in serious infections (and have been reported in the present pandemic), and the visions are common when patients are receiving narcotics for pain control.

She: "My mother appears in this room, and for the life of me, she looks real though she's been dead 15 years."

Me: "Did she say anything, Margaret?"

She: "Words of encouragement. Last time, she said I would recover."

Me: "That's good. Nice to know."

People Can Make Themselves Blind

Illustrations of this type of blindness are discussed in my book *Neurology Rounds with the Maverick*. Depending on circumstances and individual need, the human mind can make images or not make them and can even simulate blindness.

Back to the Abbey System of Artificial Memory

Although much of the meaning of the images and how they relate to the numbers in the Abbey system is lost, we can see that there does seem to be some kind of logical organization afoot: 5, 15, and 25 each have a hand associated with some other stuff. The images for 10, 20, and 30 have a cross associated with other stuff. The 10 has a rosary with 14 beads, suggestive of the stations of the cross. The 20 has a stole with two large circles suggesting 2 x 10 = 20. The 30 has a stool with three legs suggesting 3 x 10 = 30. If the modern equivalents are any model to follow, then it is likely that there were little mnemonics attached to the individual numbers that would help recall the peg image of that number. For instance, in a modern peg system that we might study, we could make a car the image for the number four, and we might remember that a car has four wheels. A hand (say attached to a policeman in the stop position) might be our image for the number five. To remember the peg image of five, we recall a hand has five fingers and that, therefore, the image for five is a hand. Holy cow! Hand associates with fives (5, 15, 25) in all of the images in the Abbey system, probably making as much good sense to our ancestors as it might to us. To us moderns, six might be imaged as a revolver because some revolvers are six-shooters. (Other revolvers have capacity for only five bullets.) The six in the abbey system is a clock. Our ancestors would know nothing about revolvers as they had not yet been invented. For them, six is a weird clock with three counterweights (figure 2.). The clock face reads ten minutes to ten for reasons that we'll probably never understand or know.

Demonstration of Method

Suppose we wanted to use the Abbey system to memorize in order the Roman Emperors. We would start with the first emperor, Octavian, afterward named Augustus (Augustus is his acquired name and means proud or haughty, something like that), and he is the person after whom the month of August is named.

Octavian is a rather abstract word, and we might not have any real idea of what it actually signifies. It might relate to something eight, but it is hard to say how that might relate to the emperor. Perhaps his genes had something to do with eight. No matter. When we can't think of a logical connection, we have to think of an illogical connection, and for someone who loves to play the piano, that connection would be the octave, which is the basic eight notes of the scale of Western music. Hence, let's picture in our mind's eye a note or a scale of notes in the church window. That might work, and it might not. To make sure the image is going to jog the memory, we had better pep things up by adding some blood to the scale or seeing blood drip from the note in the window. Notes dripping blood would remind me of the bloody civil war that Octavian waged against his two friends,

Lepidus and Anthony. The blood is helpful because it is bright red, a color that attracts us, and is associated with violence, which also gets our interest. Now to recall the name of the first Roman emperor, look at the church window, see the bloody notes, which remind us of the Octave, and that reminds us of Octavian. We could do the same with the other emperors, attaching, in turn, their image or something about them to each of the pictures in the Abbey system.

Tiberius is Roman Emperor number two. I don't have to make an image for him because I know he followed Augustus, and if I know Augustus, there will be no trouble with Tiberius. Just to make sure of the connection, I will remind myself (interesting word "remind," meaning bring back to mind) that Tiberius was Augustus's adopted son.

Number three is Caligula which is Latin for little boots, undoubtedly his acquired name from being born in a military camp and carried around on the shoulders of the soldiers. Notice that the more associations you can make, the more you know and can remember, the more you will be able to know and remember. So, knowing about the little boots, we shall hang boots on that tombstone and let the tombstone remind us of death and the fact that Caligula was murdered by the Praetorian Guard. It would have been nice if Caligula had been buried in that nice tomb instead of being fed to the dogs. Ugh! Fed to the dogs. It will be hard to forget that image, especially if we make a mental movie of that event. Dress him in regal clothes and then have the dogs tear him to pieces next to the tombstone.

Wait! Octavian, Tiberius, and Caligula makes OTC or over the counter a part of the less formal international market for stocks. Now, if I can connect OTC with something to remind me of Romans, I will have a neat set of three letters to clue my memory of the first three emperors. Right now, can you think of anything—if not, so what? ONWARD!

Claudius was a nice guy, and that is why he gets the flowers in image four, and Nero's hand worked the fiddle in image five when Rome burned. Try to see in your mind's eye an image of Claudius getting flowers and Nero, number five, watching Rome burn while his five-fingered hand plays the violin. Just think of these associations for a few seconds and dismiss all thought on the subject.

Now look at the pictures and name the Roman emperors, one to five, in order. If you got it right—great. If not, then reread the section and try again. Make your images more vivid, more interesting. in a word—more memorable. Now try remembering without looking at the images. It should be harder to recall the emperors. Images should have helped your recall. Without the images, recall is still possible but more time-consuming and, in some cases, more difficult.

When I did the exercise, window two meant nothing to me, and I then realized I didn't make an image for that window. Instead, I relied on the basic fact that Tiberius followed Octavian and confirmed that fact with my OTC. I missed emperor four probably because the idea of nice associated with flowers wasn't strong enough to suggest Claudius and lazy me did not make a mental image. Now I say to myself Debussy liked flowers, and that reminds me of Claude (Debussy's first name), and Claude reminds me of Claudius. It is not an image, but it is a narrative that can be effective in this setting. From available materials, select what associations work best for you.

Mental Gymnastic

What emperor associates with the hand in image five?

What emperor had little boots?

What emperor is associated with a bloody octave?

What emperor gets the flowers?

What emperor followed Octavian? This last question should prove the most difficult because our associations were least strong for emperor number two. Hint: Think OTC. The T stands for the second emperor.

Hell as an Image about the Nature and Severity of Sin

Figure 3A shows the position of Hell as a memory device for remembering the sins and their relative place in Hell. And also, we are told by Johannes Romberch, the image of hell can be used as a structured place in which to put to-be-remembered items. Note that the very center of hell is occupied by the devil himself surrounded by heretics who in turn are surrounded by the infidels grouped with the Jews, and then the next circle is for idolaters followed by hypocrites. The envious and the irritable and the proud and so forth are in the puteus (dungeon). Purgatory is outside the walls of hell, as is limbo, the place where the just who died before Christ and where infants who were not baptized stay. Limbo derives from the Latin limbus, a prison.

Keeping this image in mind, you should have no problem remembering that being a heretic is more serious a sin than worshiping an idol. By the same token, hypocrisy is a more serious sin than pride or gluttony but less serious than heresy. Get it? Being a Jew was considered a more serious sin than hypocrisy. In that era, the church said only Catholics could enter heaven; everyone else was headed elsewhere.

See how this image was effective in teaching church doctrine and in getting people to remember exactly what was what about sin?

Figure 3B is the memory image for heaven. Notice the angels have a much higher place than prophete, martires, apostoi, and virgines. That's unexpected because I thought the Bible said somewhere that the angels had to bow down to humans.

Dante had a different arrangement. The ninth circle was reserved for the treacherous, those who betrayed a special relation. Brutus and Judas reside with Satan frozen in a lake of ice. Brutus betrayed Caesar and Judas betrayed Jesus. Heretics get off easier in Dante's inferno: They're in circle six. All of Dante's great poem is a memory aide to teach readers about what's what in the world of sin. Later, when the poet approaches purgatory and heaven, we will learn about virtues, works of mercy, and so forth. In this arraignment by Dante, the pious pagans and unbaptized babies are in circle one with Socrates and Virgil. Lovers are in circle two. Knowing that fact, we have to conclude Dante felt fornication was less serious a sin than blasphemy or pride or gluttony. In fact, he tells us that directly in the poem, and he gives a reason: "Lovers are driven by passion that is hard to control. Therefore, lovers are not entirely responsible for their sin."

Now look at figure 4 and try to figure out what the devil that is about. It is a famous painting by Titian showing how the allegory of the three parts of prudence can be presented visually and used as a memory device. Note that the picture is pregnant with symbolism. The wolf, the lion, and the dog below the images of three men are medieval symbols for the past, present, and future. The old man at the left recalls memory, the man in the center looking straight at us represents intelligence, and the young man at the right represents provision for the future. The three parts of prudence are, not incidentally, memoria, intelligentia, and providentia. The whole picture tells us how to be prudent: Remember the past, do an intelligent analysis of the present, and prepare for the future. Pretty good advice, and all of it summarized in a famous painting which is a mnemonic device.

Similar sculptures of the triune god Lugh have been found that depict Lugh as a youth, a young man, and an old man. This was an image to remind pagan Europeans that Lugh had three forms but was one god. Did Titian get the idea for his picture from the ancient Celts?

Late Middle Ages

By the middle of the 15th century, a book consisting of devotions for children circulated in Europe. The children were urged to give characters in the Bible, including Christ himself, the faces of friends and acquaintances so that they could be fixed in their memories. The author of the book told his young audience to place the figures in their own mental Jerusalem, "…taking for this purpose a city that is well known to you." Thereafter, with this scheme, each child could, though alone and solitary, undertake devotions, reliving in his or her mind the story of the Bible by moving slowly from episode to episode—in other words, the recommended spiritual exercises that Saint Thomas Aquinas thought would increase understanding of the events that happened in the Bible. These exercises for children were based on the same scheme of mental images as the ancient art of memory, only this time they were adapted for church use to facilitate the recall of items the church thought important for spiritual salvation.

This vivid restructuring of memory for church things was also a fundamental component of the edifice of discipline and religious training that the converted Spanish soldier Ignatius of Loyola developed for the members of the Society of Jesus, which he founded in 1540. Saint Ignatius wanted his followers to experience more vividly and more personally the biblical narratives in all their force, actually "see" images of Jerusalem, and follow in their minds' eyes the path which Christ traveled toward his passion.

Ignatius of Loyola had been marshaling his arguments in writing in the early drafts of the spiritual exercises, which were to be published in final form eight years later.

The *Spiritual Exercises* (Ignatius of Loyola, Trans: Puhl LJ. Chicago. Loyola University Press, 1952) are the first reference in history of the art of memory in which multiple modalities were used in order to fix the memory in a more vivid way. Ignatius tells his people to smell the indescribable fragrance and taste the boundless sweetness of the divinity, to touch Christ by kissing and clinging, and to use vision to fix the memory. In other words, Ignatius evokes five senses, not just the visual modality, in order to deepen the significance of the memory image and to facilitate recall. No wonder some of the saints to follow him had vivid visual, personal, multisensory, and one might say almost real, experiences of the Blessed Mother and other biblical people appearing to them in the solitude of their rooms. These saints had worked hard to produce such apparitions, and they were rewarded for their work with a very special spiritual experience few modern people will ever know. These saints had vivid mental images, which were the natural extrapolations of the spiritual exercises, projecting an image to the external world that always existed in the internal world of the mind. With training, modern people can do the same. In fact, all that you are seeing—everything in your visual field—at this very moment while you are reading this book is a projection of your brain. You are not seeing the scene itself. Neuroscientists know this for sure. The brain is taking highly coded electrical impulses from multiple relay stations and reconverting those impulses into a projected image you think you see. In the same way, we are sure colors do not exist. Colors are projected images that have been constructed by the brain. Remember: the real world has no color, just various shades of gray.

China

In 1596, a Jesuit missionary, Matteo Ricci, traveled from Goa, a Jesuit outpost in India, to China and taught the Chinese how to build a memory palace (Spence JD. *The Memory Palace of Matteo Ricci*, New York: Elisabeth Sefton Books/Viking Penguin, 1984). He told them that the size of the palace would depend on what and how much they wanted to remember. The most ambitious mental construction would consist of several hundred buildings (yes, that many, believe it or not!), several hundred buildings of all sizes and shapes. "The more there are, the better it will be," said Ricci, although he added that one did not have to build on a grandiose scale right away. Whole imagined villages would be used to place memory items. So instead of walking through an actual building, one could imagine the village and take from it the items previously placed there in various places.

In summarizing the memory system, Ricci explained that the places, pavilions, divans, and so forth were mental structures to be kept in one's head and not solid objects to be literally constructed out of real materials. Here, we recognize the place architectural memory system discussed by Cicero, but instead of using a real home as Cicero did, Matteo is using an unreal, imaginary palace in which to deposit the memory items. Ricci suggested that there are three main options for such memory locations, and he had detailed the whole memory system of his time in a very large book, which was presented to the Chinese emperor. The real purpose of such images and places was to store up the myriad concepts that make up the entire mass of human knowledge. To everything that one wished to remember, an image could be given, and that image could be placed in memory palaces and swiftly recalled by simply returning to the place in which the image was placed. Images and information, previously stored, could now be summoned in an instant using the same meat-tissue computer that we have in our heads.

As useless as all this might seem to us, to the Chinese, it was extremely useful because, at the time that Ricci arrived in China, the Ming Dynasty was sponsoring imperial examinations, and considerable evidence exists that advancement, social standing, and wealth in Chinese society of the time depended, for the most part, only on one's performance during the imperial examinations.

Memory of Chinese art, history, and poetry played a major role in the success of examinees in this setting, and accordingly, the memory systems proposed by Ricci would have been of value to some of the participants in the examination who had been trained to use the systems to recall specific information verbatim.

Because great success in the imperial examinations was the surest route to fame and fortune in the imperial Chinese state, it is probable that Jesuit influence and inroads to China were very much dependent on the use of memory systems as the enticement for interesting the Chinese in European traditions and religion. If you want to know more about the imperial exams and the trials and rewards of the examinees, take a look at Rulin Waishi's novel entitled *"The Secret History of the Forest."* English title: *"The Scholars."* It is considered one of the six classics of Chinese literature.

Ricci also left us a method for learning Chinese.

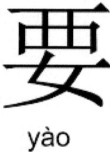

Character: Chinese Simplified
Pronunciation: Hanyu Pinyin
(Mandarin = Standard Chinese)

要

yào

Fig5.3 - The character is yao, which means fundamental, or needed, or want, and several other meanings. Yao said the same way but written as a different character means medicine. Ricci describes this character as a "tribe woman from the West," who we presume he would mentally in some way associate with fundamental and the other meanings.

Only a mind familiar with the art of memory could identify this, the Chinese ideograph yao, as a tribeswoman from the west. The upper part of this image is the symbol for west in Chinese (Xi), and the lower part is the symbol for woman (Nu). It is clear that Ricci mentally divided the entire ideograph into two parts: The upper meaning west and the lower meaning woman. By linking the two—woman and west = fundamental, necessary, want, and so forth, he became able to read and recognize the meaning of yao. Chinese words do not usually have specific meanings. Instead, they have what might be called a word atmosphere. The context in which the symbol appears will often suggest and sometimes actually indicate the meaning. We don't know how Ricci connected woman from the west with yao. But he did. My own modern connection might be an image of a woman dressed in western clothes (a cowgirl) who has a gigantic spoon of medicine (the other yao) and is giving that to some sick man at death's door. My own experience with yao is that the most common use of the word is to indicate medicine taken by mouth. This is no joke. From the medicine idea, I would extrapolate to want and necessary. With this kind of association method, hundreds of Chinese pictographs can be learned. Multiple books are available on Amazon.com that use such mnemonics to teach Chinese characters. Compared to learning spoken Chinese, learning the meaning of the characters is much harder, and mnemonic systems help a great deal, and so does writing the character several thousand times.

Using this method, Ricci was able to learn the Chinese language quite well and quickly. One can see how memory images are well adapted to learning the Chinese language because the Chinese ideographs were in large part in ancient times based on images or are images. Tuttle estimates that about 10% of current characters are based on images, and the others have evolved into an abstract form.

Chinese sources reported that Ricci was able to memorize forward or backward a large number of Chinese characters at first sight. That fact leaves no doubt that Ricci had mastered the ancient art of memory and was a genius in the application of the art of memory.

Mental Gymnastic

Tell the definition of metalepsis.

Did you look this word up? If you did, give yourself a pat on the back. If you did not look it up, think about why you didn't. How do you expect to look ten times smarter than you are if you don't do the work? If you had done the work, you would have opened a world of information and knowledge you previously did not know existed. Words are one of the tools of thought, and the more words you know, the greater will be your range of thought. With that in mind, identify from the list of tropes which ones apply to the sentences that follow:

Listed Tropes: Irony, synecdoche, allegory, litotes, hyperbole, metaphor, metonymy, alliteration, and tautology

1. All the world's a stage, and all the men and women merely players; they have their exits and their entrances, and one man in his time plays many parts. His acts being seven ages.

    Answer: Allegory because of the extended use of metaphor. Hyperbole because of the exaggeration.

2. Sister Suzy's sewing socks for soldiers.

    Answer: Alliteration. Give yourself extra credit if you said sibilance alliteration.

3. That filthy place is really dirty.

    Answer: Tautology. States the same thing twice.

4. I was so nervous I had butterflies in my stomach.

    Answer: Metaphor because of direct statement. Could also be hyperbole.

5. It felt like I had butterflies in my stomach.

    Answer: Simile because of the indirect comparison with butterflies. Simile is often identified by the word "like." Could also be hyperbole as there is exaggeration, a statement that represents something as worse than it really is.

6. Your father and I are not as young as we used to be.

    Answer: Litotes. What she is saying is they are old. She is saying it in an indirect way with the affirmative expressed by the negative of its contrary.

7. The White House said today, "This virus is under complete control and will have little or no effect on the economy."

    Answer: Metonymy. The White House didn't say anything. The dunce in the White House made the statement. He was impeached twice for good reasons.

8. The digital sales over the internet are beating out bricks and mortar.

    Answer: Synecdoche. Parts (bricks and mortar) are used to make up the whole of commercial sales in physical stores.

9. Wow! That is the sixth megachurch within four square miles. That's what we really need around here—another megachurch.

    Answer: Irony. His language signifies he believes the opposite of what is stated. He thinks we don't need any more megachurches.

10. Two cannibals are eating a clown. One says to the other, "Does this taste funny to you?"

    Answer: Humor and Irony. Hyperbole and ambiguous term because funny has two meanings. There is funny "ha, ha," and there is funny "unusual."

Part III—Modern Applications

Although some of the methods of the ancient art of memory were described by Cicero and Quintilian, specific examples of its practical application can only be inferred from our present knowledge of similar systems used by contemporary mnemonists such as Harry Lorayne, who ran a commercial school of memory for over three decades. Harry has written many best-selling books on the subject, but each book is hardly original, and each pretty much restates material present in his other books, all of which claim your memory can be improved enormously.

The extravagant claims that are made by Lorayne and men like him have been tested objectively. The conclusions show that when typical college students are used as subjects, the recall of specific information can be increased enormously by the use of such systems. It has been demonstrated, for instance, that capacity for serial leaning and paired-associate tasks can be increased at least over ten-fold or 1,000% when they use the systems as compared to their performances when they don't use the systems.

Modern Memory Power Demonstrated

In 1972, Harry Lorayne advertised in the New York Times that he could make anyone a memory genius. All you had to do was report to the Hotel Roosevelt that night at 7:30 PM to see a memory demonstration and sign up for a six-week training course in memory augmentation.

That evening, about 50 men were lined up outside a second-floor conference room at the hotel. Each of them wanted a better memory. Most of them were salesmen who wanted to remember customers' names and details about the customers as well as the products they were selling, including catalog numbers and specifications.

Soon Harry arrived, introduced himself, and told the men to shake his hand, tell him their name and occupation and go into the conference room and sit down. When my turn came, I told Harry that I was a physician and that my name was Bernard Michael Patten. And then I went in and sat in the first-row center, waiting for Harry and the rest.

Harry came in and welcomed everyone. He promised he could make us memory geniuses. Harry asked each of us to stand, and he said he was going to tell us our name and our occupation. Harry said that if he got both the name and the occupation correct, we should sit down. If he got either the name or the occupation wrong, we should remain standing.

About the others, I don't know, but Harry got my name and occupations correct. At the end of the naming, no one in the room remained standing.

Harry then pointed to the Manhattan telephone directory on the desk and stated that as a demonstration, he had memorized the Manhattan telephone directory. He then said he was going to prove that he had memorized it by passing the book around and by asking each of us in turn to thumb through the directory, give him a name, and see if he (Harry) could recite the number correctly. If Harry got that number correct, the person who asked was to say so. If Harry got the number wrong, the person involved was to say it was wrong. After about 22 correct answers, my turn arrived. At this point, I firmly believed everyone but myself in the room was a shill and that Harry would get my number wrong. But then, in a sudden act of perversity, I gave Harry a number that I had just looked up and asked him for the name attached to that number. Harry smiled and gave the name Vianney Gonzales, which was correct. The directory continued to circulate, and it was clear the evidence indicated that Harry Lorayne had probably memorized the Manhattan Telephone Directory, which in those days was about two inches thick and contained over a million names and numbers.

Harry then introduced Roy, a boy about 12 years old.

"Roy has just finished the Harry Lorayne six-week course in memory isometrics and is here to demonstrate his memory skills," announced Harry.

Then Harry put a blindfold around Roy and had Roy face the audience and face away from the blackboard. Harry told us Roy was about to memorize a 50-digit number made on the spot by the people in the room. He then asked people in the room to call out digits, and as they were called out, Harry wrote those digits on the blackboard in the order that they were called. When 50 digits were there, we stopped shouting numbers, and Harry asked Roy to tell us the number.

Wow! Roy read off all 50 digits as if he had eyes in the back of his head and had seen through the blindfold. Then Harry asked Roy to read the 50-digit number backward. Roy did. Then Harry asked Roy to divide the number in half and read the number from the middle left and then from the middle right. Roy did. Then Harry asked Roy to add the numbers. Roy started at the left and said 6 plus 5 is 11 plus 3 is 14 plus 7 is 21 and so forth until Roy had said and added all the digits correctly. Then Harry took the blindfold off Roy and thanked Roy for that "wonderful demonstration."

Harry smiled, looking around the room, and said, "Those of you who would like a memory like Roy's, step up here and pay $125 for six weeks of memory training."

Doctor Patten was first in line with the money. The systems that we learn from Harry and several other mnemonists, including Lottie and Bruno Fürst, will be discussed soon. Meanwhile, before we get to the nitty-gritty of the systems themselves, let's be familiar with and review the basic ideas and facts about human memory.

Serial Position

When a list of items is memorized, the items from the beginning and the end of the list are more often correctly recalled than the items in the middle of the list. This peculiar finding that the probability of recall relates to the position of the item in the list is well known to psychologists and is called the serial position effect. Remember?

Unlike the usual results in list learning, serial position effects are completely absent when the ancient mnemonic systems are used. In fact, if a peg system is used or an architectural system is used to encode the items, the items can be recalled in or out of order at will, and all items in the list have the same probability of recall.

Proactive and Retroactive Inhibition

When two lists are memorized one after another, the first tends to interfere with the recall of the second, and the second tends to interfere with the recall of the first. The adverse effect of the first list on the second is called proactive interference, and the adverse effect of the second list on the first is called retroactive interference. These peculiar phenomena, proactive and retroactive interference, are also well known to psychologists. When the ancient art of memory is used to encode one list after another, proactive and retroactive inhibition is notably absent. Why this is true is not clear, but with encoding of items as images in arranged order, each list seems to have an independent existence in the memory and is available for recall without significant trouble.

Concrete Items Are Easier to Encode and Recall than Abstract Items

In general, in memorizing emotionally neutral material (that is, material that has no special personal relationship to the person doing the memorization), the more concrete the item, the easier it will be to recall the item. Conversely, the more abstract the item, the longer it will take to encode the item and the harder it will be to recall the item. This is just a fact of human memory, and there is nothing about it that can be changed. The human brain works better on the concrete than on the abstract, probably because in ancient times, survival was more dependent on concrete thinking.

How do we get around this disability? Often, converting an abstract item to a concrete symbol is needed before the item can be successfully encoded using the memory systems. Concrete items need not be converted into symbols but can be imaged directly. For instance, to remember love, one might have to convert to a red heart with an arrow through it as the image to recall love. Looking at the image in the mind's eye, one would not say that is a heart with an arrow. Instead, it would be immediately apparent that the symbol stood for love. All our numbers are abstract, so we often have to convert numbers to images or something else that is more concrete. On the other hand, remembering our nearest star, the sun, a common concrete experience, would not require any symbols, just the glaring, baking image of our sun on the horizon at daybreak or on the horizon at dusk.

Peg Lists Organized In Some Way and Composed of Images Facilitate Recall

Prior memorization of a peg list and images attached thereto is not necessary, for the peg lists can be written down and used that way to jog the memory. However, pre-memory of the peg list can enormously increase the facility and the dramatic demonstrations of a person's memory. For instance, using peg lists, you will soon be able to memorize almost anything you wish, and recall will be easy, fast, and accurate. The problem is that memorizing the peg list can be a pain, and much work is needed to get the pegs right and attach effective images to the pegs. One hour a day for six weeks should be sufficient. What is six weeks if you wish to be a memory genius? People spend 10,000 hours of study to get to be expert pianists or competent neurosurgeons. With sources of information literally at our fingertips, even those ten thousand hours, supposedly required to become expert on a given topic, according to Malcolm Gladwell (though this has been disputed by the authors of the original study), can be shortened through more efficient learning techniques and memory practices.

Pegs and Their Use

Peg lists were used by the great Russian mnemonist Shereskevskii along with bizarre, crazy images to recall information even when he had no idea what the information was about—such as atomic theory or advanced statistical mechanics of the hydrogen atom. You, like Shereskevskii, given the proper application, will discover that your memory has no defined limits. You will need to practice making visual images, and you will need to memorize peg lists. Little mnemonic tricks to help you will be supplied along the way, but still, you will need to put in some time and effort. Less visual items and more abstract items will need to be converted to something else, usually something more visual. More time will be needed to do the conversions. Sometimes, the conversions will seem impossible if the item to be recalled is a 50-digit number. In that case, a special phonetic system must be applied to convert the number to sounds, sounds to letters, the letters to words, and the words to images so that the number is stored as a group of images and not as a number. Roy, in the demonstration, did not remember any number. He mentally converted the digits as they were called out into images, and he placed each image next to a peg image he had memorized previously.

A number is stored as a linked series of interconnecting images. Without this method, there is no way Roy could have remembered the 50-digit number in the time he was given. The secret was that he did not memorize the number at all. He converted the digits to sounds, then converted the sounds to letters, then converted the letters to words, the words to pictures and memorized the list of pictures probably as a narrative tale interconnecting the images or he attached each new image to the prearranged list of images on a peg list. When Harry asked Roy to recall the number, Roy worked backward. He recalled the image that gave the word. The word gave the number. He saw a shell which was a mike. That translated to 6537 because sh = 6; l = 5; m = 3; k = 7. Therefore, the first four digits were 6537.

Numbers Are Abstract

Just about the most abstract items we deal with in memory are letters and numbers. A number, particularly a pure number not attached to anything concrete, is so abstract that it doesn't give us much memory traction. Take a walk in the woods. Turn over the rocks. Look at the tree bark. You will never ever find an actual number in nature. Numbers exist in the abstract void of human imagination. The way we give numbers some memory traction is by conversion to letters, as mentioned above. Some people do try to twist numbers into something the way 2 can be rotated left to look like an n or a 3 can be rotated left to look like a m. Some people make an 8 a cursive f, and some people make 7 into K because with a little imagination, they "see" a 7 in the K.

Here's How to Convert Numbers into Something More Easily Memorized

Use consonant sounds to represent numbers. In the system below, most of the useful consonant sounds are included. To recall what sound connects with what number, use simple mnemonics. The best results will occur when you have memorized the sounds connected with each digit and can use the sounds to make words. Practice converting numbers to words and words to numbers as the first step to memory heavy.

Example: In the scheme, use number 1 because it has a single vertical line, and that reminds us of the letter t. So, t represents 1 and vice versa. The letter d also has a single vertical line so let d also represent the number 1. Having two letters to represent a number will give some flexibility in making words from the letters. Another association that will link t with d is that tee and dee rhyme.

Stop here and fix in your mind the relation of number 1 (one) to t and d.

1 = t or d

t or d = 1

What number do you think that we will work on next?

If you guessed 2, you are right. The reason the number two seems next is that is the way we learned the order of numbers. First comes 1, and then comes 2.

The number 2 looks like the letter n if you rotate the 2 to the left 90 degrees. By this association, we will always recall 2 is n and n is 2. Pause now and fix in your mind the relation of 2 to n and n to 2. If the flip mnemonic doesn't work for you, think of an association between 2 and n that does work. Multiple associations do not confuse the brain. They, in fact, increase the chance of recall. You might say n has two vertical lines, and those two lines will remind me that n is 2. Whatever you do, do not go to the next number until you have, for one brief instance, fixed in your mind that 2 is n and n is 2. What you are doing is mentally attaching a character tag to the number 2, and you are also attaching a character tag to the letter n. Stop now and actually consciously connect in your mind n with 2 and vice versa 2 with n.

2 = n

n = 2

The letter m is 3. Rotate 3 to the left 90 degrees. It does look like an m. This is usually enough to recall the connection between m and 3. If you need more associations, make them for yourself. Note that m has three vertical lines. That might help firm up the association of m with 3. Now connect the two items m and 3 in your consciousness and go on to the next number.

3 = m

m = 3

The letter r is four. Some people remember this because the last letter in the word four is r. Another idea might be that the word four has 4 letters. Again, the associations you make for yourself will work better for you than the associations others make for you. He is well served who serves himself. Make the association: Some picture a car, which reminds them of four wheels. Remember, the brain doesn't care if your association is logical or not. The brain doesn't know anything. It is just a meat machine for recording coincidences that occur in the consciousness. The more the item or item appears, the greater the chance of encoding.

4 = r

r = 4

The letter L (l) is five. This is somewhat harder to associate. For me, the Roman numeral L means 50, so that reminds me that L (el) is five. Think of an association that might work for you. Don't try to memorize the association of letter L with 5 cold. That will work for a while, but there is going to be lots of things to recall, and you are safer relying on the system rather than on your natural memory for something like this. By now, you know the drill: Some people hold up their left hand with the thumb pointing right and the four fingers together. That does look like an L.

5 = l (small case) or L

L or l = 5

Whew! That was work. But do not despair; we are halfway there. The number 6 presents some problems because the sounds sh, ch, j, and dg are unusual to understand. The sounds sh and ch are easier. Most systems will make j as in the word judge as 6. Sometimes a negative association will work just as well as a positive. In this case, I might ask myself what is the hardest number-letter combination to connect with each other. Oh yea, that's j and 6. A six-shooter serves as the image for six and makes the connection of sh with 6. From that association may follow the ch and the j and maybe the dg. Make your own association, if you can, but don't spend much time on it. For me, it has been sufficient to forget about dg = 6 and just stick to j = 6, sh = 6, and ch = 6. A six-shooter has 6 shots, which reminds me of 6 = sh, and the sh sound itself reminds me of its close neighbor ch. Hence, 6. = j or sh or ch. By the way, sh and ch seem to me to be one sound, although they are represented in English by two letters. In some other languages, Egyptian hieroglyphs, for instance, these sounds are one letter. Or how about this? Shoe and six both start with s, and the sh in shoe reminds us that 6 = sh.

6 = j or sh or ch
J or sh or ch = 6

The letters for 7 are hard c and k. These can be recalled because they both have that hard k sound as in the word kick. There are elaborate ways to connect 7 with hard c and k. Some people take the 7 and add lines so that it looks like a K. What works for you is what you need to do. Say over and over to yourself 7 is K.

7 = (hard c) and k
(Hard c) and k = 7

The letters for 8 are f and v. A handwritten f in cursive does look like an 8, and f and v are closely related consonant sounds, as you can prove by saying fur and vur. Notice the position of the tongue to make these two sounds is only slightly different—one is voiced, and one is not.

8 = f or v
f or v = 8

The letters p and b are 9. Rotate 9 180 degrees right, and it looks like a b (sort of). Rotate the 9 out of the page and put it flat down again, and it looks sort of like a p. Make other associations if you need them. These two consonants are close to each other in the mouth. If that idea helps you remember the association—good. If it doesn't—forget it.

9 = p or b
p or b = 9

And last but not least is the digit zero. The letters soft c, s, and z are the number 0. I usually remember this by the fact that the word zero has a soft s-like sound, and that soft s-like sound reminds me of soft c.

0 = (soft c) or s or z
(Soft c) or s or z = 0

Review the items and the associations to be sure that you know them cold. Then quiz yourself on a piece of paper and check your work. These digits are the only digits you will need to make any number from zero to infinity.

Summary:

1. is t or d
2. is n

3. is m
4. is r
5. is l
6. is j or sh or ch or dg
7. is hard c or k
8. is f or v
9. is p or b
10. is soft c, s, or z

OK?

Mental Gymnastic

What's m? What's 7? What's 3? What's z? What's v? What's j? What's choo-choo? What's wet? What's bat? What's wet bat? Remember, vowels don't count, only consonants.

Answers: m = 3; 7 = k; 3 = m; z = 0; v = 8; j = 6, Choo = 6, choo-choo = 66; wet = 1; bat = 91; wet bat = 191. Choo-choo wet bat = 66,191

With this conversion system, you will now be able to convert any number into letters and any of these consonants into a number.

Mental Gymnastic

Translate into numbers: Bernard M. Patten

Answer: Disregard the vowel sounds or letters for which we assigned no numbers. B is 9, r is 4, n is 2, r is 4, d is 1, M is 3, P is 9, t is 1, t again is 1, and n is 2. Hence, this name is in numbers: 9424139112. What's your name in numbers? Note some memory books disregard double consonants and count them as a single. So, the tt in Patten would be simply 1 instead of 11. To Harry Lorayne, Patten would translate to 912, not 9112. Make up your own mind on how to handle this, and when you have decided, stick to that rule.

Practice with Phonetics

Take the 94241 and, knowing the sounds associated with the digits, try to pronounce the word that those numbers represent. You should come out with something that sounds somewhat like Bernard. 9112 should come out as bttn or pttn. Fill in the spaces with vowels as you wish to make words. In this case, 9112 would come out as battan or pattan or betten or petten or bittin or pittin or botton or potton or buttun or puttun or any combination. The best results would be the ones that make the most sense or have some associative property or those that are easily visualized, but note that each of these nonsense words does decode to the correct number. The word that best connects for me would be button which translates as 9112 and can be made into a nice visual image. Ye gods! What am I talking about? The word that best translates here in this context is *Patten*.

Application of the System to Remember a Number

Suppose you wanted to recall the telephone extension of W. King Engel at the National Institutes of Health circa 1973. My bet would be that King doesn't even know what his extension was at the time since he left that job decades ago. And I don't recall the number either except that I did make a mental image of King riding a train (choo-choo) and swinging a wet bat. That [choo-choo wet bat] would translate to 66191, which had to be King's extension.

Note: King has read this manuscript and says 66191 was, in fact, his extension.

That is how Harry Lorayne memorized the Manhattan Telephone Directory. He didn't memorize the numbers per se but converted them into an image and worked with that image in its association with the name. The more you know about things, the easier it will be to connect items with each other even if the connection is not logical. Time gone by has lost the actual association that Harry made to recall the number of Vianney Gonzales. But perhaps he knew the Hispanic singer who died young of a broken heart named Vianney (I am making this up, but no matter. What matters is does it work for me). What could be more common than a Hispanic named Gonzales? But how would I connect, or how would Harry connect her telephone number with her name? By association, of course. Her number is 370 9410.

The problem is now how to convert that number into a word. Let's try. 3 is m, 7 is k or hard c, and 0 is s or soft c or z. Hence MKS. That would be easy for me because that is the type of Lincoln. But MKS sounded out sounds like the word "makes." Makes, a verb of action, might work, and it might not work.

Let's look at 9410. That could be PRTS = parts. Makes parts would be Vianney's number. But is that good enough? Probably not too memorable, so I will scout around for something else. Looking at 9410, I could fall back on my prepared peg images for 94 and 10, which are pear and toes. Makes pear toes. Sounds sufficiently weird that it might work. But how would that connect with Vianney, the Hispanic singer? I could make a picture of Vianney up there on the platform looking around puzzled. She then announces that she is not a singer, but instead, she makes pear toes (whatever they might be—looking at my feet, I see my toes are not toes, they are pears!).

Whoa! 9410 is also BRDS. So, she makes breads. Or she makes birds. That would work too. And so would bards. Which is it? Birds or breads or Bards? You decide.

When Harry expected to hear the name Vianney Gonzales he would see a picture of a confused Hispanic singer who would announce that she doesn't sing. She makes breads instead. Makes breads would then be read out by Harry as 370 9410, and everyone would be amazed.

But, of course, that is not what happened. I read out the number 370 9410, not realizing that was even an easier trick for Harry. He would take the number, get "makes breads" from the sounds of the consonants, and then picture the singer as Vianney. Once he got her first name, the Gonzales would follow as the two names were linked in his consciousness when he originally sat down to memorize the Manhattan telephone directory.

This was the same system that I used when I was on the Dave Kennedy TV show coming out of Chicago. Dave announced that people should call in and talk with me and tell me their phone numbers. The numbers were written down where I couldn't see them, but the audience could. After I talked with ten Chicago house-wives who were wasting their lives watching this crap, Dave then gave me the name of the caller and asked the number. Having practiced working the systems, I got them correct. For example:

"Hi. My name is Allegra, and my number is 300 2944."

Allegra is an unusual name, so I don't think I would forget it, especially since it's my daughter's name. I made a narrative. She is the first to call but could have been number 300. Allegra had better watch out and not nap (on) the railroad. Nap RR will be her number after the 300. I didn't need anything more because I knew test time, when I would be asked the answer, was close by, and there was no need to make firmer associations for such a short-term test. The recency effect would be on my side. When Dave said Allegra, I think Allegra could have been 300, so her number is 300 something. Then it occurs to me that Allegra shouldn't nap on the railroad, nap is 29, and the abbreviation for railroad is RR: "Dave, Allegra's num-ber is 300 2944." It took some time for you to read this, but the thinking time to get the memory occurs very fast, almost instantaneously.

Hi this is Sally, and my number is 291 9232.

Stop and work on this number yourself. See what you can come up with.

This looks difficult, and I didn't have time to think of suitable translations, so I fell back on my predetermined peg list of double-digit peg names and images. In this case, I saw a big sign with a pit crossed out in red. The kind of sign you see around that indicates no smoking. Only, in this case, it is no pit. No pit is, of course, 291. 9232 is easy: 92 is pan, and 32 is man. Pan and man rhyme, and I could construct a story: Sally chews on an olive, thinking there is no pit, but she is surprised by the fact that instead of a pit, she bites into a pan which jumps out of her mouth and assumes the form of a man. Nopit-panman = Sally. To complete the associa-tion, though, I would need a way to connect Sally (the name) with the narrative mnemonic. Something about Sally, something intrinsic to Sally's name that will trigger an association. In this case, I used sallied as in sallied forth out of the fort. So Sally reminds me of sally forth, which will give me a picture of her coming out of the fort chewing an olive with no pit and so forth. How long did it take to actually construct all this narrative scheme to recall Sally's number? Answer: Not long at all. When you train your mind to work the systems, the brain works at the speed of thought, which is not as fast as the speed of light but is actually very fast and pretty close to the speed of light.

What are the colors in the American flag? See how fast you can say the answer. Any well-encoded memory can be brought to consciousness that quickly.

Such associations have to be practiced so that they come quickly, almost at the speed of light. Otherwise, the demonstration of super memory, especially on a TV show, may fall flat.

Although I hate TV, I did enjoy being on TV. For this bit of hypocrisy, I beg pardon. My time on the show was paid for at the rate of $300 per hour camera time, and I had a dressing room with a big yellow star on it, and a young woman did my make-up so that I looked four times better on TV than I did in real life. My sister-in-law, Emily, who lived near Chicago, watched the show and was impressed. With her, I now had status.

TV has been attacked many times. It has been called "the wasteland," the "boob tube," and many other undesirable names by people who want to make it something other than what it is and has been. Major networks understood from the start TV is entertainment. Most people watch it to be amused. My approach to the Dave Kennedy show was that I was there for one purpose only, and that was to entertain. Try to make something else out of TV, and you're fighting a losing battle. And that, the entertainment thing, friends, is the reason TV has to move fast. Most stories last for about twenty seconds; even big news stories run less than a minute. The scene, even in the documentaries, changes every few seconds, and that may be the reason TV watching has been associated with decreased attention span. The commercials are a problem also. It was not unusual for Dave Kennedy to be interrupted in mid-sentence for a commercial break. Of interest was the fact that Dave shut off the commercial, so we in the studio were not subject to seeing it or hearing it. Dave didn't want to be bothered by the sponsor, and neither did the crew.

Mental Gymnastic

What's Allegra's number?

What's Sally's number?

Success? Failure? Part success and part failure?

Didn't try? Shame on you

Mental Gymnastic

What number makes breads? How about birds? Why are bards, birds, and breads the same number?

Mental Gymnastic

Let's work out on memorizing a serial number. Here's the number of a hundred dollar bill that I just took out of my wallet. It is a beautiful 2009 series with a big picture of Franklin. It is colored bluish-green, and the number in the upper left-hand corner and the number in the lower right-hand corner are the same, namely: LB 94537432 S.

Go to work on this number and test yourself before you look at the work product below.

Ready? Need more time? OK. Let's wait. Your processing time at this stage in your memory development is probably pretty slow. That is normal and OK. Slow and steady wins the race.

Answer: Divide and conquer. LB is easy. For me, it is Franklin on the bill, but I will bet LBJ would have liked the privilege. Now let's attack the number. Probably better to break it down to smaller parts.

How about making two numbers four digits each. Four and four? That would give us 9453 and 7432. There are only eight digits in the serial number, so these two four-digit numbers in combination will do the trick.

Let's start with 9453, which translates to p or b, r, l, and m. PRL could be PARL. Whoa! That's too good. Some of you out there in reader land will now be thinking I deliberately selected an easy number. That's not true. That I am forbidden by law to photograph, I would have attached a picture of this bill. Anyway, do you see what I am driving at? PARL could easily be Pearl! That is a nice concrete thing for which a ready image is available. But, that means the m (the 3 at the end of 9453) will have to attach to something down the line. Wow! 374 nicely translates to maker, and 32 is man. So, the serial number is pearl maker man or 94537432.

Try this exercise with some dollar bills in your wallet. Here are two more hundreds in case you don't have a wallet handy: KC 07172966 A (from series A 2006) and KC 07172915 A (series A 2006). Isn't that interesting? Two hundred-dollar bills drawn from my wallet today (May 14, 2020) have similar numbers.

Ugh! Since I am a memory junkie, I can't resist attacking these two numbers.

Since I see 66 (choo-choo) at the end, I will work on three digits at a time from the beginning. Then number KC one will end with a 66 (choo-choo), and bill number two will end with a tile 15. Except for the two last digits on each bill, the serial numbers are identical, e.g., 071729.

Consider 071. That could be s or c or z with k and t or d.

SKT looks great to me because it can spell skate, which would make a nice image. 729 has to be KN with P or B. KNP looks good to me as it could spell KNAP, which is the old English spelling of nap, or a small hill like a knoll but smaller. KNIP would also do and eight other combinations. Hence, this serial number translates to *skate knap a choo-choo*.

Sounds absurd. Right? But it does get us where we want to go. We memorized an eight-digit number easily. How many of your friends can do that?

Add KC in front by telling yourself the bill could have come from Kansas City. Bill two would then be *skate knap a tile*. As an exercise, translate that phrase back to a number.

This Is a Nice Party Trick

You are entitled to your own opinion. But as for me, I think this is pretty cool that I have memorized two serial numbers in less than a minute. You need more practice, so you probably took longer. This trick may help you when you pay with a hundred-dollar bill. It will also work just as well with a twenty or a ten or a five or a one as every dollar bill has a serial number. For some reason, serial numbers are not on coins.

Succorance for the Faint of Heart

Don't worry. All this is easy when you know the system and have worked it a few hundred times and can apply it with finesse. The way to learn it is to do it while thinking about what you are doing. And remember to study the problem before jumping to it. Analysis will save time and energy. Before you act, think! Seeing the similarities and differences in the last two hundred-dollar bills saved me the trouble of independently memorizing the skatknap twice.

Mental Gymnastic

Time yourself on this. You should finish in less than five minutes. To do the gymnastic, you will need a blank sheet of paper and a pen or pencil. Follow the directions exactly. I repeat: Follow the directions exactly.

1. Read everything *before you do anything*.
2. Write your name in the upper right corner of the paper.
3. Print NAME under your name.
4. Draw a circle on the upper left side of the paper.
5. Draw a triangle in the circle.

6. In the middle of the page, calculate 43 times 956.

7. Make a large Q with a question mark in the right lower corner of the paper.

8. Draw a rectangle around your answer in item 6.

9. If you have carefully followed the instructions write "I have followed the instructions" at the bottom and sign your name.

10. Now that you have finished reading everything do only as directed in the first sentence (item 1) and place the blank sheet of paper back where it came from.

Ha ha ha.

At Rice, where Doctor Patten's clone taught the course, most of the students set right to work and did not read everything before starting. The demonstration proved to them and perhaps proved to you that there is a tendency not to follow directions. There is a tendency to just plunge in. Telling students that fact would not have been as effective as showing them. More than that: People see things more clearly when it is directly applied to them.

Assemble Your Peg List from 1 to 100

You can't have prearranged peg lists unless you prearrange them. Let's work on a few so that you get the main idea on how to do the pegs and the images. Starting with the number 1, we know that that is a t and t reminds me of tea, and to make the idea more concrete, picture a teacup, and to make the teacup more memorable, coat the inside of the cup with fur, the red fur of a red fox. Now when you want to remember something attached to number 1, picture that item with the teacup or, even better, picture the item in the red-fox-fur-coated teacup.

Suppose you wanted to recall the name of the first Roman emperor. Instead of picturing the bloody notes in the church window, you would picture the bloody notes in the furry teacup. Just make the image once in your mind's eye, and it will work.

Number 2 is n, and n reminds me of Noah (whose name translates to 2 because oah doesn't count). See him not in the ark but as the pilot of a 747. His long gray-white beard is hanging out the window of the jet plane. Hope the white beard doesn't get caught in the jet engine. Now when you want to associate something with 2, attach an image of that something to the peg image of Noah. Did you remember the second Roman emperor? Attach Tiberius to the Noah image. That's not Noah. It's Tiberius. What the hell is Tiberius doing piloting an airplane? Any such nonsense associations or narrations will do if you deliberately make the association in your mind.

Number 3 is m, and m reminds me of my mother. M is for the many things she gave me. I see her, but to make the image more memorable, I see she has a light bulb in her mouth, and it is blinking on and off. When I need to remember something associated with three, I will place an image of that thing with the image of my mother. Now my mother has little boots on her. Can you tell why?

Stop! Think about the boots. Hint: we are still on the Roman Emperor list.

Make your own personal image of what you associate with m or mother or anything you like that will connect that image with 3 and 3 with m.

Number 4 is r so see a car because it has four wheels.

Number 5 is L, so see your hand or a policeman's left hand, which has five fingers. See the left hand in the "stop" position but with thumb extended to the right and the other fingers held together. That looks like the L, which is number 5.

Number 6 is a six-shooter, so see one of those old revolvers, the kind that stole the west from the Indians. Six-shooter will remind you of sh, and that will recall ch and j. Some people are more comfortable with the 6 image as a shoe. What works best for you?

Number 7 is k, so see a cow kicking someone. The kicking reminds us of 7 and vice-versa. Key also works for 7. You could visualize a big golden key sticking into the thing you are trying to remember. Add some blood to the key to make it more memorable, make the key larger than life, so it is more memorable.

Number 8 is f, and the written cursive f looks like some ice skater was there showing off, so the image for 8 will be a pair of skates. No, wait—I've got a better idea: 8 will be ivy, so see the ivy on the wall of your favorite college or high school. This will make ivy personal and relate to you. No ivy on your school? So what! Put it there in your mind's eye.

Number 9 is a pea. The pea is a giant—the biggest pea in the world, bigger than the giant green giant on the can of Green Giant peas.

Number 10 is toes. Notice how we combined the t and the s sound to produce a word that has the potential to make an image. 1 + 0 = toes because t is 1 and s is 0. Toes is better than does because it is a definite and concrete image. Does does not do well because it is hard to make an image as good as toes.

Don't continue reading until you are familiar with these 10 digits and the sounds and images associated with them. Practice converting sounds (not letters) to numbers. The phonetic alphabet should become part of you, part of your nature. When you hear an r sound, you should think of 4. If you hear or see a 3, you should think m.

Memorize the Rules

A few rules: all vowels have no number value. W, H, Y have no number value. Th = 1, the same as t or d. Q is the same as k. X is 70 because it is the sound of Ks = 70, except when X is sounded as Xsh, as in complexion. In that case, X becomes 76.

Enough Review. Now on to New Territory

Number 11 is tt, so see a tot, a baby. Make this image memorable for you.

Number 12 is tn, so see a tin can.

Number 13 is tm, so see a tomb.

Number 14 is tr, so see a tire.

Number 15 is tl, so see a towel or a tile or a tail or a… You choose.

Number 16 is tsh or dsh or tch or dch or dj. I like DJ running a record shop, but dish could work well too if it was jazzed up as a memorable image. Dish would work, and so would touch.

Number 17 is tk, so see a tack pinning an insect to the wall.

Number 18 is TV, so see a TV. Probably should have some effective image on the TV to make 18 more memorable. Grant was president 18, so whenever I think of 18, the image of Grant flashes across consciousness. He is drinking whiskey, of course.

Number 19 is tp, so see a tap.

Number 20 is nose, so see a giant nose. It wouldn't hurt to have some blood coming out of it or sticky green snot.

The Rest Is up to You

And so on. If you want to construct images for the numbers 1–100, go ahead and do it. The idea is to use the numbers to make letters and from the letters make a word that can convert to a visual image. Once you have your peg numbers and images in place, you can use them to recall vast amounts of specific information. For instance, can you tell me the names of the first 20 presidents of the United States? This might seem to be a daunting and dauntless task, but it isn't. Everyone knows Washington was first, so we don't need to do anything special to recall number one. Or do we?

At the course in Mental Gymnastic at Rice University, I asked for a volunteer to recite all of the presidents of the United States in order.

Here's how the volunteer started: "One—I see a teacup. But it is full of red fox hair and needs to be washed. A great deal of wash is needed. In fact, a ton. Therefore, Washington was the first President."

Ho ho ho. The class had a big laugh at that.

Me: "Excuse me, Sir. Where were you born?"

He: "Romania."

Me: "Please continue."

And he did—getting them all right except his English had a Romanian accent.

George Washington Was the First President

Most people know Washington was the first president, but this man from Romania had to use a mnemonic narration to recall that fact. John Adams is two, but if you didn't know that, you would have had to associate an image of Adam and Eve with Noah in the 747 or some such ridiculous image. Jefferson is three, and for some reason, most Americans know that Jefferson is the third president. But now we come to four, and most people draw a blank. Most people have a problem with four, and probably so do you.

Who was the fourth president? It's hard to know because there is no logical connection between the number four and the fourth president of the United States. It is just an accident of history that that person, whoever he was, was president in slot number four. There is no logical connection between the number and the name.

So, what do we do when we don't know something? What should you do when you don't know something?

Answer: Look it up. And after we look it up and know the fourth president was Madison, we will imagine a narrative and an image that connects, however illogically, the number four with Madison. How about four is a car so see a car driving down a street. The street is Madison Avenue? Got it? Four associates with car because a car has four wheels, and now that car is driving down Madison Avenue, a very famous street in New York City, and therefore, president four is Madison.

Number five, you see a hand on a policeman; he is signaling stop! The stop position. What the devil does that mean? It could be some mind relic from childhood when we were taught the fifth president was Monroe, who stopped further European influence in the western hemisphere with his famous Monroe Doctrine.

MENTAL MAKING MIGHT

Review Time

OK, let's take a break and then review presidents four and five.

Madison was four, and Monroe was five. So how will we remember those facts? Four wheels has a car. See the car going down a street. Recall Madison Avenue in New York City. Then five—see a policeman with the hand held in a stop sign. That should remind us of Monroe and the famous Monroe Doctrine.

Onward!

President 6 was John Q. Adams. I recall this fact because it was the first time a presidential name repeated. President 7 might be more difficult. I see a cow kicking a man. The man is unhappy. The cow kicked him because he was trying to jack up the cow with one of those carjacks. Therefore, president 7 is Jackson. President 8 is easy for me because I see the ivy on my High School, which was named (believe it or not) after Martin Van Buren. President 9: I see a giant pea pod. Opening the pod shows the peas are not normal and smooth. They are hairy. That reminds me of Harrison, our 9th president. Ten is toes. Remember, 10 is ts, which can make the word toes. These toes are attached to a foot, attached to a leg, attached to a man in a canoe. Tipper Canoe and Tyler too. (Actually, Tippecanoe and Tyler too.) That was a famous campaign slogan for William Henry Harrison and his running mate, Tyler. Tippecanoe was the name of the Battle of Tippecanoe, November 7, 1811, wherein Gov. Harrison of the Indiana Territory defeated a Native American (Indian) army led by Tecumseh.

Harrison was lucky in that battle because the Indians, supplied by the British, ran out of ammunition. Guns become ordinary clubs when there is no ammo. And what's a club against real guns that are firing at you?

Yes, Harrison was lucky at that battle, but Harrison was unlucky as President because he died of typhoid fever after only 31 days in office. Thus, Harrison was the first president to die in office, and Tyler was the first vice president to become president.

Notice how you should pile on the information. The more associations you have and make, the easier it will be to recall information from third-stage brain storage.

Tippecanoe and Tyler Too: TCTT

This was a campaign song of the Whig Party during the Log Cabin Campaign (1840). But most people remember slogan TCTT better than the song. Why? Because it is euphonious. It uses devices to promote memory that we discussed in memory lite. There are 3Ts—a triple alliteration. There is an internal rhyme—canoe and too, and there is (nearly) a nice iambic tetrameter. TCTT is memorable because it is poetry, poetry lite, but poetry nevertheless.

BERNARD MICHAEL PATTEN, M.D.

On with the Presidents

Wow! Now we know the presidents to ten. Check to see that you do know them. Start your initial check by going through the numbers. If you draw a blank or make a mistake, try to figure out what went wrong and correct the defect if you can. The usual mistake is to try to jump ahead and not do the sequence: Number, image, association, name of president. Unfortunately, most Americans don't know much history and these presidents for them are names only and not associated with images, personalities, or the events that would facilitate recall.

Mental Gymnastic

Memorize the next ten presidents using the peg system and your images. My examples are good for me. But the best images for you are the ones you make for yourself. President 11 is tt or tot. I see a baby in a cradle. Someone lifts the veil and sees that is not a baby! It is a pig, a pig in a poke.

President 12 is tn, tin. I see a tin can well-dressed, and, therefore, it had a Taylor. President 13 is tm. I see myself driving up to a filling station in a tombstone car, and I tell the attendant to fill her up, which reminds me that president 13 is Fillmore.

President 14 is tr or tire. I see a tire with an arrow in it. The arrow has pierced the tire, and that means president 14 is Pierce.

What image will you use for 15? Poor James Buchanan. He knew the Civil War was coming and was eager to leave office before it started. Seven states had already left the union, and Buchanan didn't know what to do about them. My memory clue for Buchanan is simply that he was the president before Lincoln. But how about Cannon towels? Towel is 15, so Cannon towel might suggest Buchanan.

The 16th president everyone knows is Lincoln, so there is no need for any images. The 17th is easy because Johnson was the first president to be impeached but was acquitted. For 18, see U.S. Grant watching TV and drinking whiskey. The 19th is a little difficult: Tp. See a tap. Water should be coming out, but instead, there is hay, and that reminds us of Hays. As an exercise, you may wish to work through all the presidents. Using the images and pegs, you should be able to memorize and correctly recite all the presidents in or out of order. It may take about an hour to do this. No kidding! Try it and see. You already know the first 19. It may take less time for some people and more for others. But in relatively short order, you will know more presidents than any other kid on your block.

What president was nose? Who is nose? Hint: A garfish has a big nose.

Mental Gymnastic

Who was president 22?

Answer: Cleveland.

How do I know?

22 = nn = nun—see a nun cleaving the land.

How about those serial numbers on those 100-dollar bills?

It is now two days since I memorized those numbers. Correction—since I memorized the words and images. The actual numbers were not memorized.

LB was one and came out to pearl maker man, which translates to 94537432. The two LC bills were skate knap choo-choo and skate knap tile, which translates to 07172166 and 07172115.

How did you do? If you did the exercise, then you and I are probably the only two people in the whole world who have memorized the serial numbers of three bills. Tell you what. If you didn't memorize the serial numbers, you deprived yourself of the experience of knowing you could.

Mental Gymnastic—Memorizing a Big Number

By now, you probably get the idea behind how to store vast amounts of information and recall that information exactly. As an exercise, let's practice memorizing an 11-digit number. Any number will do, but for this exercise, it is better to have a number that is randomly generated and that has no special significance for you. Use your own number. But if you must, work out on this one, which I just generated by flipping a pack of cards from which the pictures were removed:

11185796620

Method: Don't just plunge in. Most people will plunge in, and that is wrong. Study the number for a pattern. If this is a party trick demonstration, it might be more effective to make sure you get the last few digits correct because that is what will count more. In this case, the last digits are easy. 20 means the number is going to end with a nose. And 966 is going to be a pea choo-choo. So we have already mastered five of the digits or about 45%. I also like that 857, which would spell flick. So flick pea choo-choo nose gives me eight digits, and I will just recall that before the flick, there are three 1s. So now I know 111 flick pea choo-choo nose = 11185796620. Encoding those 11 digits took me less than 20 seconds. It might have taken more time or less depending on your insight, skill, attention, and imagination. OK, I admit dealing three aces (111) from the pack did make it easier for me to get the 111 part. Arthur T. Benjamin, a famous math-professor, taught me the trick of using cards to generate random numbers for memory practice.

My thoughts are in parentheses; the words I say to myself are in quotes.

"The number is"

"111"

(flick) "857"

(pea choo-choo nose) "96620"

Telepathy Demonstrations

All telepathy demonstrations are memory tricks. The usual method is to have an actor pretending he is psychic. He might even be dressed as a swami. The assistant will put a blindfold on the psychic and will then pass through the audience and stop at a table, collect an item, preferably an item selected by a person at the table, and not selected by the assistant. The assistant will then ask the swami to identify the item. Let's say that the item is an American Express credit card. The assistant will then ask the swami a question such as, "Oh swami, are you ready?" The form of the question will tell the swami what list they are working on. The assistant and the swami will have three peg lists memorized, each with 100 peg items and images, just as we have discussed above. The form of the question might indicate that they are working with list two. Then the swami may put on a show on how hard it is for him to get on the same wavelength as the assistant. Or there may be some patter about how it is so difficult to mobilize psychic power late at night after drinking all that Wild Turkey 101 whiskey, and when you have a headache and are not in the mood, and so forth. Somewhere along the line, the assistant will give a word that has the number of the peg item. The assistant might even say something absurd that is actually the number of the item on list two. "Come on, swami, get with the program. Since you seem to be having trouble, I will give you a hint. I will give you a big hint. What I am holding in my hand is not a choo-choo train." Lots of laughs, of course, but item 66 (choo-choo) on list two is none other than the green American Express card, and now the swami knows what the item is and will soon get it right, just as he will get right all the other items that night. Naturally, the assistant will never select an item that has not been pre-encoded. To give a more effective demonstration, the assistant will then ask the audience members to hold up items that they want identified. It is unlikely that anyone in the audience will have on their person an item not on one of the three lists. The assistant will select the items from the audience members, making sure the items are on one of the three lists, and send the code number to the swami. The show people may even pretend that some members of the audience have the psychic powers by asking them to think of the item and send it telepathically to the swami. Every show benefits from having the audience participate in some way. Old-time magicians knew that for sure and frequently asked for a volunteer to come up to the stage and help. And so it goes.

Don't believe this? Doctor Bonomo, a fellow physician, and friend, and Doctor Patten had no trouble doing this demonstration. They even did it at neurology grand rounds at the Neurological Institute of New York before an audience of neurologists and medical students, not a one of whom figured it out. Of course, Doctor Bonomo and Doctor Patten memorized three lists of 100 items each and, by the way, choo-choo was item 66 on list two, and that was (you guessed it) a green American Express Card.

Pilot Training

The application of the ancient memory arts to pilot training has shortened training time and increased accuracy. These systems for training mainly rely on visual imaging, and they have been patented by a former TWA pilot, Malcolm Conway. Because of the patent and copyrights owned by Conway's heirs, the systems and their application cannot be explained here. Sorry. When demonstrated, the systems allowed a pilot to glance at all the instruments on the panel and be aware of and be able to recall the exact readings.

Do you remember how much Conway got when he sold the use of the systems to the North American Air Command (the people who run America's nuclear arsenal)?

Answer: Four million dollars. When large amounts of money are mentioned, most people pay attention and remember.

Conway also said he sold the systems to Sabena Airlines for two million dollars. Pilot training shortened according to Conway by 18%, but pilot accuracy improved over 400%. At the time of these sales, a million dollars was a lot of money. Still is, but not as much.

By agreement, Conway gave up the patent rights when the systems are used for education or for the rehabilitation of brain-damaged people. Which is the reason such systems or similar systems are used worldwide for those purposes and were discussed here.

Gambling

Using systems, it is possible to keep track of what cards have been played and to calculate the changing probabilities as the game continues. Betting when the odds are favorable and not betting when they are not will work better than relying on pure luck. Consult Harry Lorayne for details. But watch out! The technical term for memorizing cards and calculating probabilities is "card counting."

Most casinos have watchers who are trained to spot the card counters. Card counters—that's what they call them. But the gamblers who do this are not card counters; they are card memorizers, and they have a preset image for each card and apply the images as the cards are played much the way Cicero progressed through his villa and used the villa as a memory palace with multiple memory pegs. The card counters are not gamblers either. They are just working a system such that the odds, which usually are in favor of the house, instead tend to work in their favor. Over the long haul, when odds are in your favor, you will win.

Card Counting

Fürst's system is complicated, and so is Lorayne's. Dominic O'Brien's system is more or less similar to theirs. Doctor Patten's is easier to work and easier to work fast. Each card has an image. There are four suits, and each suit can be made into the image. Clubs is a club, probably black and bigger than life. Hearts is hearts or a red heart with an arrow in it. Spades is a .... (guess). Diamonds is a diamond, made big and beautiful and sparking and scintillating, perhaps even radioactive.

We can attach the given image to the number in the suit and make a picture. So 2 of clubs becomes C2 or CN = can. Ace of hearts would be H1 = HT = HAT. Aces are 1. The picture cards supply pictures. Make all jacks themselves. So, the jack of clubs is a club. The jack of hearts is the heart image. The jack of spades is a spade. The jack of diamonds is ...... (guess). Make the king of clubs a real king and the queen of hearts a real queen. With the others you have to be creative. Use a mnemonic based on a kind of rhyme or a clue based on a first letter. Queen of clubs is cream because clubs starts with the letter c, and so does cream. King of hearts is a hinge for the same reason, hearts and hinge start with the same h. Queen of spades is steam. King of spades is sing. That leaves only queen of diamonds—dream and king of diamonds—drink.

If you are interested in card counting, make up your own images and test yourself repeatedly to make sure you are fast and accurate. Attach the card image to your peg list images to keep track of what cards are played. Adjust the odds accordingly. If you don't understand how to adjust the odds, do not gamble. If you can't memorize cards as fast as you can recite the pledge of allegiance or the Hail Mary, you are not yet ready to hit the blackjack table or the shoe of chemin-de-fer.

Poker

A memory of what's been played is helpful in most games. Good players know the poker odds cold. Do you know the chance of drawing to an inside straight? And the odds change according to cards played. In an open or stud poker game, it would be foolish to keep betting if you are waiting for a 10 card when you know two 10s have already been dealt to others. A good player will note the cards dropped as a player turns cards down and play accordingly. In five-card draw, where you see none of the other cards, memory systems help you remember the odds for bettering your hand. Example: you have three spades, and you want to know whether or not it pays to stay in and draw two more cards of the same suit to get a flush or should you drop out. The odds are about 23 to 1 against drawing the flush. The mnemonic for this is flush = flame-name. Fl for flush and flame to name gives you the 23 (n = 2; m = 3; 2A3E). Flame = fl = flush; m = 3, designating the 3 card flush idea. The odds of drawing one card (you have four) to flush is about 5 to 1. This is the flare-law flush mnemonic. Fl = flush and r = 4, meaning the four cards in your hand. Flare-law makes flush 4 with 5:1 because 5 is law. Some players may stay in the game holding a pair and a "kicker," then drawing two cards. In that situation, the odds of making a three of a kind are 12 to 1. The odds of making two-pair under this situation are 5 to 1. Exact odds under varying conditions are available. If you really want to work at this game, study combinatorial mathematics. How many kinds of five-card hands are there? 52 choose 5 equals 2,598,960.

What is the chance of getting a full house right off the bat? First, select the card that will be three of a kind. There are 13 choices. Then select the card that will be part of the pair. There are now 12 cards left, so the pair has to come from one of those 12. OK, now we have 13 x 12 and need to choose the three cards for the three of a kind. There would be four chose three or four ways. The pair is similar and would be four chose two, which is six ways. Therefore, the number of possible subsets of five cards that can make a full house is 13 x 12 x 4 x 6 = 3,744. Pretty cool, right? This is exactly the ways a full house can be made from a deck of 52 cards.

3,744/2,598,960 equals 1/694.17, about 1/700. How about a flush, where each of the five cards is the same suit. There are four suits to choose from, so four choices. Now we have the suit consisting of 13 cards. So the next choice is 13, choose five, which is 13!/5!. 8! is 5,148 possible ways of making a flush.

How about a pair? Probability of one pair is 0.42. Straight is 10 x 4 to the 5th power equals 10,240, about 1/254. The chance of being dealt a garbage hand, a hand of no value, is 0.501.

See why a flush is more valuable than a straight? A flush is less probable. See why a full house beats a flush? Four of a kind is even rarer and beats a full house.

Mental Gymnastic

Calculate the probability of getting a straight flush in the first five-card deal of poker.

Answer: There are four choices for the suit, and there are ten ways of making a straight because the Ace can be a one at the bottom, or it can be at the top of a 10, J, Q, K, A. Hence, the number of possible straight flushes is 4 x 10 = 40. As there are 2,598,960 possible poker hands, the probability is 40/2,598,960 or 1/64,974 or 0.0000154.

How about calculating a hand of four of a kind?

Answer: There are 13 choices for the first card, and that leaves 48 choices for the card that does not match because 52 − 4 = 48. Hence, the probability of 4 cards of the same denomination is 13 x 48 = 624. As there are 2,598,960 possible poker hands, the probability of getting four of a kind is 624/2,598,960 or 0.000240.

When doing calculations like this, always step back and see if the answer is reasonable. I call this the sanity test. Recently, I made a purchase of several items worth $233, but the two clerks said I only owed $2.33! They insisted they were right because they had done the calculation on a calculator. Their failure to apply the sanity test cost Office Depot over $200.

Probability calculus is discussed in the logic book *Truth, Knowledge, or Just Plain Bull: How to Tell the Difference*. In many games, like craps and poker, you can calculate the exact odds, ditto in bridge, in canasta, in roulette with one zero or two zeros, and so forth. The study of probability was initially stimulated by the needs of gamblers. Remember? Can you name them? Who were the two mathematicians? Who was the gambler? If you forgot, go back and get it right. Specific information is much more impressive at dinner parties. Show off with facts!

Games of chance are still used to provide interesting and instructive examples of probability methods. Probability now finds applications in a large and growing list of areas besides games of chance. It forms the basis of Mendelian genetics. Modern theories in physics concerning subatomic particles make use of probability models. Cancer treatment results are often stated in probabilities derived from experience. The spread of infections is studied in the Theory of Epidemics. Queueing theory uses probability models to investigate customer waiting times under the provision of various levels of service like numbers of checkout counters, telephone operators, computer terminals, etc.

The bottom line here is that it is not enough to know what cards have been played, what numbers have been rolled in craps (the point), and whatnot in your real-life situation. You have to also know how to determine the real odds. Real odds are the chance of an event versus the chance of its complement. If you can't do that, you are guessing and just gambling, and you will probably lose to another player who is more in the know, another player with a fiendish computational ability, a phenomenal memory, and seemly limitless energy who will belly up to the green baize table and take you to the cleaners.

"To every man upon this earth, death cometh soon or late. And what a better way to die than facing fearful odds for the honor of our fathers and the temples of our gods," said Horatius Cocles in heroically defending a Roman bridge in 509 BC.

Facing fearful odds may be a good way to die, but I can't think of a worse way to gamble. Ian Fleming, in his James Bond books, tells us James never makes a bet unless the odds are pretty close to even. What's right for Bond is probably right for the rest of us.

The Card Counting Champ

Dominic O'Brien, eight-time world memory champion, got into the *Guinness Book of Records* because, in May 2002, he memorized a random sequence of 2,808 playing cards (54 packs) after looking at each card once.

Yes! Amazing! But he did it and without much apparent effort.

O'Brien correctly recited the sequence making only eight errors, four of which he corrected right away. O'Brien said the inspiration to become a memory genius came when in 1987. He saw Creighton Carvello on BBC TV memorize a pack of 52 cards in three minutes. Carvello holds the record for memorizing pi to 20,013 digits, beating Hans Eberstark's 11,944.

Take a Break to Memorize Pi to Eight Digits—3.1415926

You can easily memorize pi to eight digits by recalling, "May I have a large container of coffee." The number of letters is the digit: May = 3, I = 1, Have = 4, A = 1, Large = 5, Container = 9, Of = 2, Coffee = 6. See how easy hard memory tasks become if you have a framework to hang the memory items on. The problem then devolves to memorizing the connection of pi and the framework. In this case, you might picture a large container of coffee poured onto a big pie. That might clue the memory of the sentence, and then you can read the digits from the number of letters in each word. Most people have trouble with the container, which is 9. Review the sentence and then write the first eight digits of pi and check your work. Correct? Great! Not correct? Great! That gives you a chance to learn it again and this time (we hope) correctly.

Or convert 3.1415926 into letters, then words, then an image or images. That is much harder. This illustrates the importance of flexibility in approaching a memory task. From the available tricks, choose what works best for you under the circumstances you are dealing with in real-time.

Back to Counting Cards

A nice party trick is to have an audience member take five cards from a shuffled deck. She doesn't look at the cards, nor do you. Have those cards put aside face down on the table. Then have someone shout out each and every card remaining in the deck. As they shout out the card, make a mental image of that card and then mentally set it on fire. When all the cards have been shouted, mentally go through the deck and see what cards are not burned. Those are the five that were removed from the deck at the start of the demonstration. Announce what cards are face down and have them uncovered to prove you are right.

Some performers prefer to put an imaginary black line through the cards as they are shouted, but burning the cards is more vivid and therefore more effective as a memory tool.

What Happens If the Casino Catches You Card Counting?

Don't worry. Nothing much happens (or can happen) if they catch you. They merely ask you to leave. When I ask why I am being escorted to the door, they usually say something like, "We don't allow people to play that way." My next question is usually, "May I cash in my chips?"

"Of course."

One time in Las Vegas, I was told directly, "Card counting is not permitted." Modern casinos get around the problem by using multiple decks, particularly in blackjack, and not dealing the last ten cards from the bottom of the deck. One deck is easy to work with, and so are two, but once you get above two, you would need to be an expert mnemonist to keep track of things. Chemin-de-fer, same problem. In Europe, the shoe has six shuffled decks. Las Vegas usually three. Atlantic City only two, which may explain Ivey's multimillion-dollar wins.

Advanced training in probability theory helps. Probability theory is a major advantage in playing craps. Don't play dice without knowledge and understanding of what's what. The chance of rolling a two, for instance, is 1/36. If you don't understand why this is true, stay away from the crap tables. The chance of rolling a crap is 1/9; a seven or eleven, 2/9. Your chance of making your point depends on the number. If you don't get this, don't gamble. Initial odds always favor the shooter on the first roll by exactly 2 to 1. When a point has to be made because the first roll is not a crap or a seven or eleven, then the odds are against the shooter because the chance of rolling a seven is greater than that of making the point. A smart way to play might be to bet light on the first roll if you are not the shooter and then bet heavily that the shooter doesn't make her point.

Achieving Optimal Memory for Music

This is a complex, technical subject, detailed, very long, and particular. It, therefore, doesn't have a place in this book, which is intended for a general audience about the general principles of making mental might. Music memory will be a separate book entitled: *How to Memorize Your Music Pieces in Less Time with Fewer Tears.* **Look for it on Amazon.com**

Absentmindedness

As soon as you notice you are not concentrating on the task, stop and take a break. When you don't know if you locked the door, you don't remember if you locked it or didn't, that is absentmindedness—basically a memory problem and one of the most common minor annoyances because you have to go back and check the door. Is the stove on? Did I take my medicine? Where did I leave my iPhone? How come I looked high and low for my reading glasses, and they were perched on my forehead all the time? How come I just finished this page in this novel, and for the life of me, I don't know what I read?

To solve these common problems, you have to think of what you are doing at the time you are doing it. You simply say to yourself, "I am locking the front door and testing it to be sure it is locked." "This is where I parked my car: Level 3, row L, and column 8." All this is easier said than done, so you must train yourself to pay attention to these minor things when you are doing them in order to save yourself time in the future.

How Do You Know You Are Absentminded?

You are absentminded when your mind is absent, when you do a task unconsciously, without thinking. We see with our eyes, but we observe with our minds in full gear. We hear with our ears, but we understand what we hear with our minds.

There is a mismatch between our modern lives and ancient brains that is most evident in the problems of working memory and attention in complex tasks like memorizing music, memorizing poetry, learning a foreign language, etc.

But there is another culprit.

Our Brains Overvalue the New and the Now

We are easily distracted because we overvalue what happens to us now compared to what comes in the future. This attention to now was, of course, a major survival technique when the saber tooth tiger was at the cave. You addressed that problem now, or you got eaten (and if you got eaten, you weren't around to worry about anything else—end of story).

Furthermore, as discussed, the human brain likes and pays attention to novelty. Thus, interruptions take advantage of the brain's natural bias toward paying attention to something different and new. The biases of attention to now and the attention to new served well in our species' evolutionary past when the future was uncertain, and the new could well be a threat that deserved immediate attention. Nowadays, the new is more often trivial than essential, and sacrificing immediate rewards can yield greater rewards in the future.

Seniors, Do Not Hide behind Your Age

Some contests, festivals, and recitals allow adult students to play from notes or read their poem or speech, whereas the younger students must work from memory. I have been to poetry slams where some senior poets actually read their poems from a sheet of paper. That is wrong and always flops.

Every student, every contestant, should be on an equal footing, and every student should be judged equally. No exceptions. The memory power of (some not all) young people is pretty good. Even little children can repeat long poems and whole pages of books and (worse) the advertisements on radio and TV. But so can adults. This pall parrot memory is in all of us. Adults just tend to think they don't have it. And in a certain sense, they don't have it as much as they used to have it. Young people have highly impressionable minds, and even small children like my granddaughter, Miranova (age 2), can repeat by heart whole pages of a book of which she may have grasped the sense but dimly. She was also pretty good at imitating Italian when we were in Italy.

Because pall parrot memory tends to diminish with age, many people (including some well-known psychologists) convince themselves that after 35 (at the latest 40), it is useless to learn anything new. This belief in the decay of memory with age is highly convenient to the average mind, which is probably the author of it. Taking the line of least resistance, most people prefer to relax with the idea: "I am getting too old to memorize anything." Wrong! Old dogs are learning new tricks all the time.

Frankly, you are much better off carrying out the better idea: "Every day I am going to learn something new."

Those who pride themselves in their physique know that exercise is needed to maintain muscle tone, bulk, and power. Ditto for memory: Exercise is needed to maintain memory skills and memory power. Make sure you get it. Most Americans have not memorized anything in several years. They are way out of practice and are suffering and will suffer for it.

The (probably false) belief in the significant decay of memory with aging permits some adults to convince themselves that it is useless to try to memorize anything new. As mentioned, this attitude is self-defeating. If you think you can't do a thing, it is for sure that you will not be able to do it. Such thinking gets adult students to take the line of least resistance, most of them relaxing with the thought that "I am getting too old to learn." A better attitude is "Each new piece is a new adventure that must be learned anew. My mind, like my muscles, needs daily exercise, and music or poetry or counting cards or _____ (fill in the blank) is an ideal exercise for both mind and muscle. Boy, am I lucky!"

Adult memory is a power that is useful and reliable. Let's give it a special dignity by giving it a special name: the selective memory of maturity.

If I can, at age 79, joyfully undertake memorizing a sonata, so can others. Cato started learning Greek at age 80. Rumor has it that George W. Bush read a book after he left office. Trump—not yet.

The power of a great memory depends upon habits of learning much more than is supposed, and in memory's growing obedience to the will is to be found the compensation for the passing years. Vladimir de Pachmann (Odessa 1848–Rome 1933), at age 70, said he was only beginning to learn how to practice on the piano. Senior students like maestro de Pachmann need to find a sense of renewal, a sense of adventure, a sense of progress, and a sense of wonder, by finding new methods, new pieces, new ways, new habits, new things.

You Have to Try New Things

Seniors need to hold fast to the spirit of youth, for that spirit will serve them best. Studies of adult Americans (sadly) prove most adults are not interested in anything new with one exception—information about health and how they can live longer. That is pitiable. Don't be that way. Resolve here, and now you will try new things.

Hold Fast to the Spirit of Youth

Kids are not afraid to make mistakes. Ever watch a child working on how to feed itself? The kid pushes the food on the face, lips and makes a big mess. Eventually, by trial and error, they figure out where their mouth is and how to place the food there where it belongs. Children of that age haven't yet learned that mistakes are supposed to be bad. They are gung-ho learners, fearless, really. Watch a one-year-old learning to walk. It is all gusto, trial, and lots of errors, but fun. Look at that big smile on the child's face after they master how to stand and walk on two feet. That kind of personal satisfaction can be yours if you work for it.

Children, by and Large, Are Not Afraid of Failure

Adults, on the other hand, many of them, are afraid of failure. Hence, they are reluctant to learn or try to learn new things. For decades, Doctor Patten has been teaching social dance to seniors. Usually, the first thing he hears as the one-on-one lesson starts is "I don't know how to do waltz." or "Excuse me, I am such a poor dancer." or "So sorry, I have two left feet."

What they need is an injection of courage. Grown-ups want to appear competent. They feel making mistakes is a sign of incompetence. This attitude is wrong from the start. Get over it. This phobia is bad and will interfere with your learning anything new and different. To the new dance student, say, "So what! That's normal. You are here to learn. If you knew how to dance, you wouldn't have signed up for lessons. Just relax. Mistakes will be made, and we will learn from them. Think of what it was like when you first tried to drive that stick shift car. You learn by doing and by making mistakes, and now driving is automatic and second nature. The same will happen if you stick (pun intended) to the dance lessons."

As with many types of learning, in social dance, we need to perform the dance repeatedly. The more practice and repetition, the better you get. And you already know the drill: The more that practice is spaced over time with rest intervals in between, the better your retention. But unlike touch typing and target shooting, results are hard to quantify or judge. That is why feedback from a teacher or friend is needed. Your feedback sources will shift in time as you develop more skill within a given area. In social dance, the initial experiences of learning motor movements are verbal because you are told what to do and cognitive because you are shown what is needed. Gains at this stage are rapid and large because you are starting from almost no skill. Later, progress will be slower. Of course, there is lots of variation in how fast dances are learned. Unfortunately, some people do have two left feet, and some are truly hopeless. One man, a retired physician, was discovered at the Clear Lake Senior Center to be truly rhythm deaf. No matter how hard he tried, he couldn't hear or get the beat. This problem was solved by having his partner tap out the beats on his shoulder while they danced.

Bottom Line

Old people, do not hide behind those grey hairs. Stop being self-conscious. Try new things. Expect to look bad, make mistakes, and feel awkward. All that is normal and is the usual road to learning how to make a chocolate cake, roller skate, or fly an airplane. It took Doctor Patten 91 hours of instruction before he passed the flight test for his pilot's license. Other students got their licenses in half the time. So what!

Final Advice If You Are Old, That Is, over 30

It may be useful to try to learn something truly new every so often—something that is radically different from the usual things you do, something outside your comfort level, but that is still meaningful and enjoyable. Try a new dance class or sculpture course, or learn a new language. Try something!

Know the Usual Sources of Misinformation

"Facts" are usually not facts from people who have a personal stake in the matter. Statements from people who have little knowledge or training in the experience in that field—take with a grain of salt. Hastily prepared data that has lots of errors—ignore. Simple and superficial reports from biased sources—forget them and it.

Beware any sources that don't go thoroughly into details. There are too many simple and simplistic people out there. Watch out for preconceived notions that were never right in the first place. In considering any important matter, the first thing you should do is gather and consider the evidence and the facts. Evidence is anything that leads to the truth. Facts are truth itself. What facts are indisputable? What facts might be questioned? What important information is missing? Ask pointed questions. Establish your own network of reliable information. If you wish to have a reputation for reliable information and opinions that count, you must pay particular attention to your sources. Never send out black thoughts. They live on like sound waves and get into the stream of consciousness in which we all swim.

Maps

How would you recall the planets in our solar system? If you have a map in your head of how they line up starting from the sun and working out, you will do better than most people. Visualize Mercury, Venus, Earth, Mars, asteroids, etc. Then see in your mind's eye the outer planets: Jupiter, Saturn, Uranus, Neptune (JSUN). Pluto. Serious questions have been raised about Pluto because in all the time we have known about it, it has not orbited around the sun. It is also pretty small for a planet—about the size of the United States. Those facts should help you look pretty smart at the next dinner party if the topic of Pluto comes up. Because Neptune's orbit is irregular, there is probably another planet out there.

That planet is now known in scientific circles as planet nine. No one has seen it, but we know it is there.

The same is true of your mental map of your memory task. Be patient when first learning. No impression is lost. Your second view will take more readily, the third still more readily. If rightly spaced, your mind will learn with each repetition and review. But repetition, though needed, cannot take the place of conscious thought; and here you must not make the mistake that most students make. In order to memorize a map, to look at it frequently may not be enough. You must study it! You must think about it. You must associate what you know with what new information is there depicted. We see with our eyes, but we observe with our minds. The ancient saying goes, "None are so blind as they who won't see." Review the maps of your subdivision and your city. Get a general orientation to where things are. This will serve you well, and you will be better positioned to give and receive directions. Not a week goes by here in Texas when we don't get a report of some senior getting lost in their car. The usual problem is forgetting the way home and eventually panicking. I have a nice video of some poor woman who was confused about what side the gas port was on her car. She kept driving up to the pumps, getting out of her car, shaking her head when she discovered the gas port was on the other side. The problem was solved when a woman pointed out the port was on the driver's side and explained the driver's side had to be close to the pumps. The confused woman needed a mental map of the size, shape, and position of things on her car. On the other hand, maybe she needed a neurologist more than a map. Confusion of that magnitude may be due to a brain tumor in the right hemisphere. Some patients with strokes do have difficulty figuring out which way (right or left) to turn into their driveway from the street. Another senior lost his license to drive because he kept confusing the gas peddle with the brake and vice versa. One neurology resident diagnosed his own brain tumor when he discovered he didn't know whether to turn left or right to get from the street into his driveway. Many people learn they have had a stroke when they discover in the morning that they have forgotten how to dress themselves. This is called dressing apraxia and is due to a stroke in the region of the brain in the right hemisphere that remembers how to dress.

Shapes

To recall shapes exactly, you have to think about them, comparing one feature with another. If the courses of two rivers are somewhat alike, you must notice the differences, and the conscious understanding of the differences will help you remember the map. So, this is the only way to easily remember with certainty— to analyze it, making conscious associations and making a mental scheme of the material to facilitate recall. Here are two passages or roads that begin the same but end differently. Here is route to the theater; here the path to the park. You recall at will only what you notice and nothing else. Train yourself to notice as much as you can, especially the similarities and differences, repetitions and sequences, and the distances, preferably in exact numbers.

Parts of Speech

Knowing there are eight parts of speech gives you a head's up on remembering them. If you count off only six on your fingers, you know you missed two. Attaching some letter code would also help. NVAAPPCI. Nouns, verbs, adjectives, adverbs, pronouns, prepositions, conjunctions, and interjections. Nouns name a person, place, or thing. The noun can be concrete like mountain. Or abstract like faith, hope, charity. Verbs give action or state of being. Adjectives qualify nouns. Adverbs qualify verbs, adjectives, or nouns. Pronouns stand for nouns. Prepositions govern nouns. Conjunctions link items, and interjections express emotion. Notice by staying organized, you can sound very authoritative about the parts of speech. The secret is having some kind of mental structure on which you hang what you know. Once you know the structure, your chance of reproducing it goes way up.

The next chapter is easier and lots of fun. Read and learn from it if you want to look like a mathematics genius.

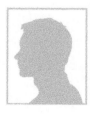

CHAPTER SIX
MENTAL MATH

CHAPTER SIX: MENTAL MATH

◆ ◆ ◆

Attention! Mental math requires brainwork. Take it easy on this chapter, and take frequent rests. A little bit every day, say 10–15 minutes, should eventually make you look like a math genius. If you find your brain is getting bored or fatigued, stop and do something else or just take a rest or a walkabout. You can play with the problems or read some of the other chapters or just relax and do nothing. But whatever you do, don't watch TV! TV is junk food for the mind.

Summary of Chapter

Mental math helps build mental might in one realm and one realm only: Mental math. But the study methods needed for success in mental math will help you develop your memory skills and make your reviews, studies, work, and adventures in Memory Lite and Memory Heavy less taxing.

Mental math provides you with a fun, interesting, and effective way to memorize important math vocabulary, ideas, symbols, and operations. Properly applied mental math can make people with little or no interest in mathematics look like a Fields Medal recipient.

Interested? Read on. This stuff is complicated and will be explained in detail later on. Please don't get scared. Just skim through this review to get a general idea of what is ahead.

In some cases, mental math will serve a practical purpose, even save you money. All four math operations are better performed mentally if you first study the problem, think of a way of making the problem easier, and then do the operations in small steps. As with everything else, you have to take things one step at a time. Alas, we have to learn how to walk before we can enter a decathlon.

Stepwise—that's the ticket. Addition estimates are easier if you add the left-hand column first as that is the most important column. Any digit in the left-hand column is actually worth more than what the digit in the column on the right next to it is worth. Look for complementary digits (also known as compatible numbers) that add to 10 or some number like 10 that is an easy number to recall and easy to work with, and easier to keep in mind. Try to take several digits at a time, not just two. When you see 3 + 2, you should immediately think 5 and not think 3 plus 2 equals 5.

Fair estimates can be made by taking the number of numbers and assuming each is close to 5. Thus, if there are eight numbers, each with four digits each, assume that the average of each number is about 5,000 and that the total of the eight numbers would be about 8 x 5,000, 40,000. Better estimates can be made by summing the left column and then taking the number of other numbers to the right, multiplying and adding the result to the sum of the left column.

Subtraction is made easier by converting the subtrahend to a multiple of ten by adding a number to it and then doing the subtraction. After that, add the same number to the result. Fractions are subtracted by converting the subtrahend to an even number by adding a fraction to it or subtracting a fraction from it and then adding or subtracting the same from the minuend and then doing the operation. If you continue reading, you get examples and some practice in doing this. It sounds difficult, and it is unless you have mastered the simple techniques.

For example: In most change problems, it is easier to think of what number, when added to the cost, will make the change. Let's say you bought gas for $16.23 and gave a $20 bill. How much change is due? Instead of subtracting 16.23 from 20, which would be a monumental task to do mentally and a pain to do on paper, think of what number you can add to $16.23 to make $20. Thus 23 plus 7 would make 30 cents, and from there, it is an easy 70 cents to make a dollar. To get to $17, we need 77 cents. After that, it is another easy $3 to get from $17 to $20. So, the correct change would be $3.77. Try doing this on a calculator. Which was faster? Your mind or the calculator?

Multiplication requires a fundamental rote knowledge of the times tables from 1 to 10. A rote knowledge of times tables from 1 to 20 is even better. When you are stuck, the times tables from 10 to 20 are easy to recall by using the teen rule: Add the last digit of the second teen number to the first teen number, multiply by 10, and then add the product of the two-unit digits. For example: $17 \times 18 = ?$ Procedure: Add 8 to 17 to get 25. Tack on a zero to indicate that you times by ten to get 250. Then add the product of $8 \times 7 = 56$. Then add the 56 to 250 to get the answer. Thus, $17 \times 18 = 306$. But stepwise, in our minds, the operation would be better thought of as $250 + 56 = 250 + 50 + 6 = 300 + 6 = 306$. The teen rule is a special case of the general distribution rule for multiplication:

$$(ab) \times (cd) = ac + ad + bc + bd.$$

Example: $23 \times 45 = (20 + 3) \times (40 + 5) = 800 + 100 + 120 + 15 = 1,035$. Stepwise, this would be: $20 \times 40 = 2 \times 4 = 8$, tack on two zeros $= 800$, add $5 \times 20 = 100$ makes 9,00; add $3 \times 40 = 120$. $900 + 100 = 1,000 + 20 = 1,020$; add $3 \times 5 = 15$ makes 1035. With a little practice you will be able to do this with ease and confidence in the result. Example: $12 \times 13 = ?$ Adding the 3 to 12, gives 15, put the zero to indicate you times by 10, gives 150 and then add the product of $2 \times 3 = 6$ to get the answer 156.

The same distributive system can be used to multiply numbers with three digits or, for that matter, any number of digits.

Division is done breaking the number down to easy parts and doing the division on each of the parts. Here multiplication comes in handy. Example: What is 14 divided into 105? 15 into 90 is 6, and into 105 would be 7. But 14 is one less than 15, so the result, the quotient, must be larger than 7. Multiplying 7×14 is $7 (10 + 4) = 70 + 28 = 98$. Subtracting 98 from 105 gives 7. 14 divided into 7 is .5! Therefore, 14 divided into 105 must be 7.5! Another trick is to reduce the size of the numbers you are dealing with so that they are easier to handle mentally. Divide 14 and 105 by 2 to get 7 and 52.5. Now divide 7 into 50 to get 7 (because 7 x 7 = 49) with leftover. Then divide 7 into 1 + 2.5 = 3.5 to get .5 because .5 x 7 = 3.5! Answer is the same: 7.5. No matter what path you use in mental math, the correct answer will always be the same if you have calculated correctly. Therefore, you can use different paths on the same problem to check your work.

Why Study Mental Math?

Good question. Here are some reasons:

1. Mental math is practical. The majority of our daily calculations are simple enough to do mentally, without the aid of a calculator or even a pencil and paper. And even if they were not, most of the more complicated calculations can still be handled mentally because, as you'll see, approximate answers are all we usually need. This week I bought gas. The credit card reader at the pump was not working. After I filled, I went inside to pay. The counter young lady, looking at my white hair, explained that the cash register was out too. "I can't make change," she said. "But I know you can. If you tell me the change, I'll give it to you." My gas cost $17.68. I gave her a 20, and she looked at me expectantly. "The change is $2 dollars and 32 cents," said I.

   Here's how I did it: I didn't subtract 68 from 100. That's too much work. I simply thought what number added to 68 makes 100. Two added to 68 makes 70, and 30 added to 70 makes 100, so 32 cents would get me to $18. $20 – $18 makes $2. Therefore, my change was $2 + 32 cents or $2.32. Early in my mental math career, I might check my answer by adding it to the $17.68. $2 + $17 = $29 (just kidding to see if you were awake). 2 + 17 = 19 and .68 +.32 = 1. 19 + 1 = 20—check.

2. Mental math can be faster than written math. Although it took 47 seconds to explain how I calculated the change for my gas bill, it actually took less than 3 seconds to do the calculations in my head. Later, I will show you how to make estimations in less than 13 seconds that are accurate to 1%, whereas punching the same numbers in the calculator would take several minutes with the added risk and danger that you might miss-enter, double enter, or omit an entry. Many types of everyday computation problems like this must be solved mentally. In fact, at the supermarket and airport, you probably will need to do the math mentally because you won't have a calculator or pencil and paper handy.

   When I buy something at a store, I don't have pencil and paper handy. Do you? When I shop, I don't have a calculator handy to discover if I am being treated fairly. Believe it or not, some people still think that it is necessary to have pen and paper to calculate 10,000 x 945. They will do this operation by multiplying 5 x 10,000 to get 50,000, then multiply 4 x 10,000 to get 40,000, and then multiply 9 x 10,000 to get 90,000. They will line up the 50,000, the 40,000, and the 90,000 as they were taught in grade school to get the answer. Mental math would just tack the zeros of 10,000 on to the 945 to get the correct answer, 9,450,000.

Because of neglect of mental math in elementary school, most people are not proficient mental calculators. Studies have shown that a large majority of children and young adults cannot do even the simplest mental calculation. The third National Assessment of Educational Progress in mathematics found that less than half of the 13-year-olds in the sample correctly calculated the product of 60 and 70 (6 x 7 = 42, then tack on 00 to get 4,200.) According to the survey, most of the children were not aware that a mental calculation is often the most convenient method of calculation. Only 38% of the 13-year-olds thought that the above-mentioned problem of 945 x 10,000 could be done mentally. None of those prescient teenagers, though, actually knew how it could be done or could actually do it. They just gave it for their opinion that someone somewhere somehow could do the calculation mentally. The majority, 62%, claimed either paper and pencil or a calculator would be needed. How do you feel about that? In my view it is sad.

3. Mental math is a good mental exercise. In the beginning, your head may ache, especially with the big multiplications. But after your brain gets accustomed to the task and has grown the appropriate synapses, you will find mental math quite satisfying. And, believe it or not, much later, after you can do these calculations with facility, you will find that mental math is fun. Yes, fun!

4. Part of the fun is that mental math will help you show off. Think of what a pleasure it will be for you to impress your friends and grandchildren with your ability to do 17 x 18 in your head almost instantaneously or square the 75-mile-an-hour speed limit in your head while the grandchildren struggle with the calculator on their iPhone to check to see if you are right or wrong. The answer for 17 x 18 is 306. And was arrived at mentally in less than three seconds. The square of 75 is 5,625 and was arrived at mentally in less than three seconds. What is 110 x 106? 11,660! Done in four seconds. Later, you will be shown how to do this fast and accurately.

5. This book guarantees that with due application, you will be able to do the same calculation (multiply any two teen numbers) in three seconds and square the speed limits in the same amount of time.

6. Mental math gives a better understanding of place value, mathematical operations, symbols, and other math properties, an awareness that will put you way ahead of all the other people on your block and light years ahead of the average American who is (unfortunately) steeped in innumeracy. Innumeracy is a condition analogous to illiteracy. Innumeracy is illiteracy for the significance and proper use of numbers.

Mental Gymnastic

Evaluate this statement from a local newspaper: "Scientists report in a recent study that drinking two cups of coffee a day will double your risk of stroke within a year."

Answer: Yes, the study did show that. Doubling your risk of stroke does sound serious. But in order to appraise the significance of the risk, we need to know the incidence of stroke. It was one chance in 3 million. Therefore, drinking two cups of coffee would increase your risk to two chances in 3 million. The odds **against** having a stroke from drinking those two cups are, therefore, quite good. A subsequent study failed to show any association of drinking coffee with causing strokes. The Harvard nurses' study showed coffee helps prevent cardiovascular disease, and colon cancer, and depression, and suicide, and gall stones.

Key point: Do not confuse percentages with absolute risk. The percent might go up 100%, but the absolute risk might be quite small.

Points about Mental Math

a.   In mental math, thinking is critical. And thinking in shortcuts can be critical. You can't do mental math without thinking. Don't even try. In mental math, the best thinking is visual and verbal. If at all possible, try to train your mind to think of the numbers in images as if they were written on your mind and also talk to yourself to get the auditory input. Talking to yourself encourages cross-modal thinking (image and sound), a quality that helps clearer thoughts.

Whenever possible, simplify the problem (by breaking it up) so that you have a better chance of doing it in your head. At least in the beginning, before you become a pro, follow the rules and the methods and advice given in this book. Keep all operations organized, stepwise, and as simple as possible. That is what you should do. What you shouldn't do is approach a math problem laboriously on a digit-by-digit basis, methodically plodding along in certain rote patterns. Example: Faced with the following addition.

$4 + 6 + 7 + 2$

You should not have to think 4 plus 6 is 10, plus 7 is 17, plus 2 is 19, or some such gibberish. Instead, you should be able to look at the number and read off the sum: 19. You will eventually see the $4 + 6$ as a ten and the $7 + 2$ as 9, and you will therefore know the answer is 19.

Try this one:

$24 + 36 + 17 + 52 = ?$

$24 + 36 = 60 + 69 = 129$. Mentally you should look at $24 + 36$ and say $4 + 6$ is 10 and $20 + 30$ is 50. Therefore, $24 + 36$ is 60. Or even better, borrow the 6 from 36, tack it on to 24, and you now have $30 + 30 = 60$. But what about $17 + 52$? Look at the numbers and try to break them into easy-to-digest component parts. The bite-size of $17 + 52$ is $10 + 50 = 60$ and $7 + 2 = 9$. So now, looking at the original problem $24 + 36 + 17 + 52$, I have $60 + 60 + 9 = 129$.

b.   Later, when you are on your own, you can branch out and innovate. If you discover a trick or two, let me know so I can use it myself, and I can let others know. For the moment, practice the strategies of the pros as illustrated herein. Oh yes, pay attention to place values. It's a shame to see someone arrive at the exact right sequence of numbers but be off by several thousand because of missing the place values. Recall that in the number 7,625, the 7 is more than ten times more important than the 600 because it represents 7,000 versus 600. The 7 is more than 100 times more important than the 2 because it is 7,000 versus 20, and the

7 is more than 1,000 times more important than the 6. Give every number its due, no more and no less. The 7 should receive more attention in our mind's eye, and we must in our mental calculations give the thousands more care, attention, and respect than the hundreds and the hundreds more respect than the tens, and so forth. In numbers, size counts. Pun intended.

c.   Get a feel for the nature of numbers. The number 649 is actually a coded way of indicating 600 + 40 + 9, and that is the way you should think of numbers, and that is the way you should think of breaking apart numbers as it suits your convenience for mental calculations. That is also the way you say 649—six hundred forty-nine. In addition to knowing the nature of numbers, you need to know the vocabulary of calculations:

addend + addend = sum, e.g., 2 + 3 = 5.

minuend—subtrahend = difference, e.g., 10 – 7 = 3.

factor x factor = product, e.g., 6 x 5 = 30.

dividend / divisor = quotient, e.g., 12 / 3 = 4.

d.   Compatibles—numbers are compatible when they together make it easier to do a mental calculation. Example: 8 + 2 are compatibles because together they make 10, which is a number easier to work with and easier to remember. In 65 + 25, just add the tens digits to get 80 (60 + 20 = 80) and then add 5 + 5 = 90. Or send one of the unit digits to the other side to get 60 + 30 or 70 + 20. In a like manner: 35 + 48 = 35 + 45 + 3 = 83. Look at that 35 + 45 and see a transfer of one of the 5s to the other number, so you get either 30 + 50 or, even better, 40 + 40. After the 80, just add on the 3 to get 83. Sometimes you can make your own compatibles: 25 + 79 looks hard until you realize that 25 + 75 = 100 and add 4 to get 104. What happened? The 79 was broken into 75 + 4, and then the 75 was added to 25 to get 100, and then the 4 was added to get the final sum. Another way of doing this problem would be to add 1 to the 79 (because 79 is harder to work with than a number that ends in a zero, and then do the calculation. 25 + 80 = 105. Then take away the 1 you added to get the correct answer: 104. Bottom line: Compatibles are important. Always search for them, and when you can't find them make them up.

e.   The number 10 is always your friend. So is anything with a zero after it, as that is a multiple of 10 and easier for the human mind to think about. To multiply by 10, just add a 0 to the number. Example: 20 x 10 = 200. Why we think easier about 10 is not known but may have something to do with the fact that most of us (who have not been working with chain saws) have ten fingers and ten toes. Therefore, when you can, make a 10 or a factor of 10. Example: 38 + 45 is easier if you make the 38 a factor of 10 by adding 2 to get 40. Then add 40 to 45 to get 85 and subtract 2 to get the answer, which is 93. Just kidding—to see if you are still awake. Staying awake is very important for success in mental math. For instance, 35 + 45 = 40 + 40 = 80, then add the 3 you took off of the 38 to get 83. Thus, 38 + 45 = 83, now and forever. Can you think of another way of doing 38 + 45? How about 70 + 13?

f.   Thinking about 5 is easier too, perhaps because we have five fingers. And five can help us almost as much as a 10. In fact, working with 5 or numbers ending in 5 can be as easy to work with as working with numbers that end in 0. 5 is your friend and almost as much fun as 10, and 0. How come? Well, the number 5 is your friend because the number 5 can be thought of as 10 divided by 2. Thus, if we had to multiply by 5, we could just multiply by 10 and divide by 2 or divide by 2 and then multiply by 10. Example: 26 x 5 = ? 26 x 10 = 260 / 2 = 130 or even better 26 / 2 = 13 x 10 = 130. Five is also a friend because it is 3 + 2 and 10 is a big friend because we can break down 10 to: 9 + 1, 8 + 2, 7 + 3, 6 + 4, 5 + 5 to suit our convenience in solving specific problems. It is important to get yourself into the habit of looking at numbers in their many different forms. 3 + 2 is actually 5 stated in a different way.

g.　　　Yes, in mental math, it is helpful to look at a number in its multiple different forms because several of those forms might be easier to work with than the number itself. Example: Look at 12 as a combination of 2 x 2 x 3 or 2 x 6 or 4 x 3. This is because breaking 12 up into components can make a mental calculation easier. Example: 268 / 12 = ? 268 / 2 = 134 / 2 = 67 / 3 = 22.333. Instead of trying to divide 268 by 12 directly, it is easier to divide by the components of 12 in steps. In general, the smaller you can make the components, the easier will be the steps, and the easier will be the mental math. Get used to breaking up numbers into components. For instance, when you look at 9, you should also see 3 x 3. When you look at 20, you should see 2 x 10, or 4 x 5, or 5 x 4, or 2 x 2 x 5.

h.　　　Here is a suggestion how to study mental math at home: Set aside a time. Do a little each day. Ten minutes is enough. Think about what you want to accomplish. Set reasonable goals. Example: "Today, I will spend ten minutes on the times tables 1–10 and try to get to 6 x 6 = 36." After you have set the goals and the time, do what you set out to do. And then, if you meet your goal, reward yourself.

Mental Math—Lesson One—Making Quick and Dirty Estimates

Look at the array of numbers below and by inspection, tell what the sum might be:

65,738
49,851
72,579
84,281
36,295
24,851
54,592
94,567

Analysis: There are eight numbers, and they all are in the ten thousands. Since there are eight of them, if the numbers were randomly distributed, we would expect that they would each average out to about 50,000. If that were true, then a fast and easy estimate of the total would be 50,000 x 8 or take away the 0s and do 5 x 8 = 40. Then add the four zeros back to get 400,000 = 400,000. That estimate took less than three seconds. And by the way, (remember?) a fast way of multiplying numbers with zeros is to take all the zeros away and just multiply the numbers, then add the zeros back. Hence, 500 x 6 = 3,000, because 5 x 6 = 30, and adding the two zeros makes 3,000. My wife is always harping on the fact that I am a zero. My usual reply is, "So what: I know I am a zero. But sometimes zeros make all the difference, especially when they follow a number."

Ugh! Now for the hard work—checking the answer with the calculator. To use a calculator, you must have one. That can be a problem if you are out in the field and you just don't have a calculator. Fortunately, in the field or not, you will (almost) always have your mind.

A Word of Caution

When using the magic of mental math for parlor or dinner table tricks, make sure the volunteer who is to verify your mental answer with a calculator knows what they are doing. Try to keep the number of digits you deal with to no more than five or six. The longer the numbers, the longer it will take the volunteer to do the calculation and the greater the chance that he or she will make a mistake.

Calculators

OK. Let's assume you have a calculator. Then you have to turn it on and hope that it is working. Next, punch in the numbers: Presto! By mysterious means, the calculator shows 432,903. The process took one minute and 13 seconds, not including the several minutes it took me to find my calculator and figure out how to turn it on. But alas, alack—I forgot to note the number down and turned off the calculator by mistake. Turning it on again and redoing took the same amount of time and produced (what looks like) a different result: 482,754. Ugh! That looks different from the first result. Both can't be right, so to it again. This time I am timing exactly. Ugh! Again, a different number! This time 406,901. That took three minutes and six seconds, not counting time to turn the calculator on. But which calculator result is correct?

The quick and dirty estimate (400,000) was off by 82,754. Not so good. That might be OK for government work, but for the rest of us, it's a little too inaccurate. So, let's try actually adding a column and then estimating the remaining numbers. Which column should we add?

Keep in mind that the numbers on the left are much more powerful than the ones on the right—ten times more powerful. Thus, the best bet is to add the extreme left column, that is the column that starts with the 6 in the number 6,5738. This is the first rule of mental addition: Always add from left to right; that is, add the left column first. Don't add from right to left the way you were taught in grade school. Right to left is wrong; left to right is right.

Sorry about that. It is shocking to learn that you haven't been going about it in the right way all these years. The schools have taught you inefficient methods. These are easy to teach but result in a lot of wasted time in the years that follow.

In truth, the school-taught methods make it nearly impossible to do even the simplest calculations in your head, thus making the kids even dumber than they would have been. The practice of adding from right to left, for example, makes paper and pencil practically a must. Look at these two numbers:

5,894

7,136

The usual practice in grade school would be to add the 4 and 6 to get 10, write the 0 and carry the 1 to the column on the left. Then your teacher probably taught you to add the 9 and 3 and the carried 1 to get 13, write the 3 and carry the one, followed by the 8 and 1 and carry, and finally the 7 and 5. If you tried to do this in your head, you might arrive at the right numbers, but you would have them in reverse order. Down the road in this book, you are going to learn how to add more quickly from left to right, and you'll pick up a bunch of other techniques that will give you a lifetime of benefits using Quick Math. Before we do that, let's concentrate on the quick and dirty estimates.

In the quick and dirty estimates, we pay attention to the important numbers and don't worry so much about the unimportant ones. Let's return to 5,894 + 7,136 = ? The most important numbers are on the left. So just add the 7 and 5 to get 12,000. Then add the next left column, the 8 and 1, to get 9, and that gives an approximate answer of 12,900, which is pretty close to the exact answer, 13,030. In fact, our estimate is only about 1% off. Not bad. Actually, a trained mental mathematician would have looked at the problem and said 12 + 1 would be about 13,000, which is real close to the 13,030.

65,738

49,851

72,579

84,281

36,295

24,851

54,592

94,567

Next rule: Never add one number at a time. That is not necessary and takes twice as long as adding two numbers at a time. Thus, that first column in our original eight numbers example should be added (in your head) as 10 (6 & 4) plus 15 (7 & 8) makes 25 plus 10 (3 & 2 & 5) makes 35 plus 9 makes 44. The first column should not be added, repeat should not be added, as single numbers: You should not say 6 plus 4 is 10 plus 7 is 17 plus 8 is 25 plus 3 is 28 plus 2 is 30 plus 5 is 35 plus 9 is 44.

Notice also, it's nice to look around for compatibles—numbers that lend themselves to ready mental assimilation. Such numbers usually result in an easy-to-hold number that has a zero or a five in it. Numbers that are related to 10 or 5 are easier for us to think about because our number system is based on the number

10. This fact probably relates directly to the fact that we have ten fingers, five on each hand, or at least most of us who have not been playing around with chain saws have ten fingers. Note that I repeat on purpose. Repetition is good. It helps seal the learning. Is there anyone out there now who doesn't believe the normal hand has ten fingers? This is a solid fact that you can rely on.

This means that in a column of figures, pictured below, instead of adding 6 & 3 makes 9 & 4 makes 13 & 2 makes 15, we should say 9 & 6 is 15 right off the bat. But even better would be to find by inspection that we are dealing with some nice compatibles—the 6 & 4, for instance, makes a nice 10, and the 3 & 2 makes a nice 5. How much easier to say 10 + 5 = 15. This is a startling illustration of the benefits you get when you inspect the problem and plan an approach before you tackle it. The inspection will often reveal a nice easy path to take to the correct result. The easier you make the problem, the less likely that you will flub.

In Mental Math, Think First and Study the Problem. Don't Just Plunge In.

$$
\begin{array}{ll}
 & 6 \\
10 & 3 \\
 & 4 \qquad 5 \\
 & 2 \\
\end{array}
$$

10 + 5 = 15

What you are aiming at is to immediately see the 10 and the 5 arrangement to make 15. You do this by inspecting past the 3 to find the 4 that goes with the 6 and then recognize the 5 that goes with the 10 to make 15.

65,738
49,851
72,579
84,281
36,295
24,851
54,592
94,567

Back to the example: OK, so that first column adds up to 44. What about the second column from the left, the column headed by the number 5 in the top number 65,728? We could add that too. Just the way we added the first column on the left and carry the answer to the 44, or we could just estimate again the average value of the numbers in the thousands place would be about 5,000, and that would make the sum of the second column from the left about 40. Carrying that 4 to the 44 gives the estimate of 480,000, less than 1% off, and pretty good considering that it took less than 13 seconds to mentally add the first column and estimate the second.

Later, as was told, we will learn how to add such numbers exactly. But now we are just interested in estimates. To examine your skill and understanding, work out on the following set of numbers arriving at an estimate in 3 seconds or less:

934,756
377,454
246,793
594,324
975,362
026,548
193,563
918,579

Four million. Right?

There are eight numbers, each in the hundreds of thousands except for number six, which is 26,548. As there are three numbers with 900,000, the average number probably is about 500,000, and therefore the quick and dirty three-second estimate would be 8 x 500,000 = (cast out five zeros and do 8 x 5) 40. Adding the five 0s back makes a 4 with six 0s: 4,000,000.

Now do a 15-second estimate by adding the first column. Remember to pair numbers looking for compatibles or other shortcuts.

Then add the estimate of column two from the left.

Four million two hundred thousand. Right?

Here's how: Looking at the first column on the left, read out 12 + 7 = 19 + 10 = 29 + 9 = 38. The estimate of column two 5 x 8 = 40 again, so carry the 4 forward to the 38 giving 4.2 million. That's not bad, considering the exact sum is 4,267,379 million. Our 15-second estimate was off by 1.6%. If we had taken the trouble to add the second column, we would have gotten 10 + 13 = 23 + 10 (9 & 1 at the bottom) = 33 + 9 (the remaining digit) = 42. Carrying the 4 to the 38 gives 4.2 million, plus the 40 that is the estimate of the numbers in the third column makes 4.26 million, an answer only 0.16% off—pretty close.

Mental Gymnastic

Work out on adding by looking for compatibles. Remember, a compatible is any number that is easy to use.

25 + 38 + 72 + 75 + 9 + 13 + 27 = ?

Answer: The first number is 25. Looking down the list, see a 75, and that plus 25 makes 100. Next number is 38. Looking down the list, the next number is 72.

Wow! 2 + 38 is 40, plus 70 would be 110, which when added to 100 makes 210. Now we have only three numbers to do. Bingo! 27 + 13 makes 40, which, added to 210, makes 250. Now only the 9 is left. So the answer is 259. Notice that this was done mentally and in less time than it would have taken us to use a calculator. My actual time to get to the 259 answer was 11.9 seconds, and that included going over the numbers to make sure the answer was correct. Another way of doing this would be 25 + 75 = 100 and 13 + 27 = 20 + 20 = 40. Add the 2 from the 72 to the 38 to get 40, so we are now 100 + 40 + 40 = 180 + 70 = 250 + 9 = 259.

The wrong way to do this problem is to take 25 and add it to 38 by doing 5 + 8 = 13, and carry the 1 to get 63. Then 63 + 72 = 3 + 2 = 5 and 6 + 7 = 13. Hence, 135. Now 135 + 75 is 5 + 5 = 10. Carry the 1 to get 1 + 3 + 7 = 11. Carry the one to get 210. 210 + 9 = 209. 209 + 13, 9 + 3 = 12 carry the 1 so 1 + 1 = 2. OK. We are almost there. We have 222 and need to add 27. 2 + 7 = 9. 2 + 2 = 4. So, the answer is 249. Ugh! This doesn't match up with the 259 we got mentally, so one of these answers has to be wrong. This is the frustrating thing about the long method taught to us in grade school. We are likely to fall asleep or get bored or be distracted and, consequently, make an error. With pencil and paper, it is too easy to lose track of the digits. Looking things over, we are ten short, and the error was 210 + 9 = 219 and not 209. Then 219 added to 13 gives 232, and that plus 27 gives 259.

Check with Digit Sums:

259 = 7 because 9 = 0 and 2 + 5 = 7

Therefore, the digit sum must equal 7. Let's see:

25 is 7; 38 is 2; 72 is 9 is 0, 75 is 12 is 3, 9 is 0, 13 is 4, 27 is 9 is 0.

Thus, the digits are 7 + 2 = 9 = 0 and 3 = 4 = 7. Check. Digit sums are both 7.

You may think that the mental gym example was made up to suit my convenience, but if I did do that, I am unaware of it. Try it yourself. Make a list of random numbers that you select from nowhere or from dealing out a shuffled pack of cards. You will find that there are always compatibles, and there is usually a simple stepwise way to do the addition.

Summary Proof of Answer:

The proof is not going over things with the calculator. That is time-consuming and may be inaccurate. Digit sum of the answer is 7, and the digit sum of the numbers added to get the answer is also 7. Therefore, the answer is correct, and we need not go to the calculator to check it. The digit sum method is cool, real cool, and real fast and will be soon explained for those of you who are gung-ho about numbers and mental math.

Checking with Calculator

Oh hell. Let's get the calculator and punch in the numbers. With the calculator, it took me 55.5 seconds, and that time did not include getting up and finding my calculator. And by accident, the answer got erased. Checking by redo mysteriously, 518 turned up as the answer using the calculator. Since I know the answer must be 259 (numbers never lie, and there can only be one correct answer). Redoing the calculation and paying careful attention to punching in the right numbers does indeed give 259. Total time for recheck with calculator: 2 minutes 35 seconds. So, where did the 518 come from? Looks like 259 is 250 + 9, 250 x 2 = 500, and then add the 9 x 2 = 18. Conclusion: Somehow, the calculator or I or the devil doubled the answer. Total time with calculator to get answer and check it: 3 minutes 30 seconds. Therefore, mental math in this example was 17 times faster than the calculator. Test conditions may vary, and you may get a different result from this experiment. My calculator skills are slow and obviously deficient.

Proof of Principle

Solve 40 x 32 mentally, and then check your answer with the calculator. Then solve with pencil and paper.

Me: 4 x 30 = 120 + 4 x 2 = 128, then add back the 0 we took from 40 to get 1,280. Time: Less than 3 seconds.

Calculator: Six keystrokes are needed. Four strokes for the digits, one for the times, and one for the equal.

Pencil and paper: Eight steps are required assuming the problem was already written on the paper.

Mental Gymnastic

Practice with some of these problems. Think of your answer and then look at my suggestion. There is no right or wrong mental math method as long as you get the correct answer. If your approach is different from the suggestion, don't worry. The idea of this is for you to do your own thing and be creative if you can.

1,150 + 250 = ?

Suggestion: Take 50 from the 250 and add it to the 1,150 to make 1,200. Then add 200 to get 1,400. Or, take the 50 from 1,150 to get 1,100, add the 50 to 250 to get 300, and then add the 300 to 1,100 to get 1,400.

115 + 18 = ?

Suggestion: Make the 18 into 10 + 8, then add 10 to 115 to get 125. Break the 8 into 5 + 3. Add the 5 to get 130, and then add the 3 to get 133. Or change the 18 to 15 + 3. Add the 15 to get 130, and then add the 3. Or change the problem to

100 + 15 + 15 + 3 = 133. Here's what I like the best: Add 2 to 18 to get 20. Add 20 to 115 to get 135, and then subtract 2 to get 133. After a while, with practice, you will look at a problem like this and immediately (and almost automatically) know the answer.

3.6 + 1.9 = ?

Suggestion: Make the 1.9 a 2 by adding a .1 and add the 2 to 3.6 to get 5.6, then take away the .1 to get 5.5. Perhaps, you are already at the stage where you can look at this kind of problem and immediately know the answer.

62 + 28 = ?

Suggestion: Put the 2 on the 28 to get 30, then add 60 + 30 to get 90. Think of some other approaches that work and work them.

$1.75 + $1.50 + $1.75 + $1.38 = ?

Suggestion: Imagine the first three as $1.50, which would make 1.5 x 3 = $4.50, add the .50 you took away from the $1.75 and the $1.75 to get $5.00. Then add the $1.38 to get $6.38. Checking this answer with digit sum, we get 638 = 98 = 8. 175 is 4,150 is 6, 175 is 4, 138 is 3. Hence, 4 & 6 is 10 is 1 and 1 + 3 + 4 = 8. Check.

Subtraction

- Work left to right and not right to left.
- Look for compatibles, i.e., 100 − 38 is easier to do if you don't subtract but think 38 + ? = 100.
- Add the same number to the subtrahend and minuend to make things easier.
- Before attacking the problem, think.
- Keep the cumulative totals in your head.
- Make quick estimates when an estimate is all you need.

Practice

    a. 78 − 23 = ?
    b. 54,976,498 − 43,523,171 = ?
    c. 62 − 48 = ?

Solutions:

a.   Add 7 to 23 to get 30. Take 30 from 78 to get 48. Add 7 to the 48 to get 55, which is the answer. What you are doing is adding 7 to both the subtrahend (23) and the minuend (78). Another way of doing the same thing would be to add 7 to 23 to get 30 and add 7 to 78 to get 85, then subtract 30 from 85 to get 55. This is mentally a little more difficult for some people and easier for others. Do what works best for you. But come to think of it, this problem is even easier. Take the 2 from the 7 to get 5, and take the 3 from the 8 to get the other 5. Some subtractions are that easy. For example: 7.45 − 3.34? 8.14 − 6.01? 4.27 − 1.13?

Remember, think before you attack a mental math problem. In this case, inspection shows that each digit in the subtrahend is smaller than the corresponding digit in the minuend above it. Therefore, it is possible to simply read the answer from left to right: 7.45 − 3.34 = 4.11; 814 − 601 = 213, and putting back the decimal makes 2.13. For some reason, working with whole numbers is easier than working with the decimals. 427 − 113 = 314, then 3.14. Some subtraction problems are easy like that. Don't miss the easy ones. Think first before you start to calculate.

62 − 48 should be easy. Think of what you would need to add to 48 to get 62. Add 2 to get 50 and then another 12 to get 62. Hence, the answer is 14. Another way of doing this is to add 2 to the 48 to get 50, and then subtract the 50 from the 62 to get 12, and adding the 2 to the result gives 14, which is the answer. Or add 2 to both the 48 and 62, then subtract (64 − 50) to get 14.

62 + 2 = 64
48 + 2 = 50
64 − 50 = 14

Mental Gymnastic

Work out on tombstone problems:

Born 1865, died 1892
Born 1941, died 1987
Born 1872, died 1932
Born 1532, died 1561

Suggestions follow. Your methods may be the same, better, or worse. The mental exercise is the important thing, not the answer.

Born 1865, died 1892. Forget the 18s. Now the problem is 92 − 65. Add 5 to 65 to get 70. Take 70 from 92 to get 22. Add 5 to 22 to get 27. They died early in the old days.

Born 1941, died 1987. Forget the 19s, as they cancel. As this is one of those easy subtractions, just read off the answer left to right 8 − 4 = 4; 7 − 1 is 6. Therefore, this person lived 46 years.

Born 1872, died 1932. Think what number added to 72 would make 100. Well,

72 plus 8 would give 80, plus 20 makes 100. So from 1872 to 1900 would be a space of 28 years. Now add 28 to 32: 28 + 2 = 30. 30 + 30 = 60. Actually, when I look at 28 + 32, I mentally take 2 from the 32 and transfer the 2 to the 28. Then I have 30 + 30 = 60. Even easier is to look at 1,872 and 1,932 and take the 2 from both those numbers. Then the problem becomes 1870 to 1930, which, by inspection, is 60 years because 1870 to 1900 is 30 and 1900 to 1930 is 30.

Born 1532, died 1561. Adding 1 to the 1561 makes 1532 to 1562 or 30 years. The 2s cancel, leaving 1530 to 1560. Now subtract 1 (because we gave the death date an extra year) to get 29 years.

This is fun, so how about working out on some real death dates:

Elizabeth Bishop 1911–1979

Easy, right. Forget the 19s. 1 from 7 is 6, and 1 from 9 is 8. So, 68. Notice we work left to right.

John Keats 1795–1821

Add 5 to 21 to get 26. Pay attention to the shifts in centuries. Early death was due to TB.

John Donn 1572–1631

Take 2 from 72 to get 70. 1570 to 1600 makes 30. Take 2 from 31 to get 29 and add to 30 to get 59. Or add 1 to 31 to get 32. Take the 2s away to get 1570–1630, which makes an easy 60. Then subtract 1 to get 59.

Emma Lazarus 1849–1887

Make the 49 a 50 by adding a 1. Then subtract 50 from 87 to get 37 and add the 1 to get 38. Or add 1 to both 49 and 87 to get 50 and 88, then subtract to get 38. She wrote The New Colossus in 1883. Emma died of Hodgkin's lymphoma, but her words now inscribed on the Statue of Liberty will live forever.

Robert Burns 1759–1796

Same as Emma. Adding 1 to 59 and 1 to 96 makes 60 and 97, 37 years.

Mental Gymnastic

Help Frank by telling him his age:

"How old are you, Frank?"
"I don't know, Bernie. But I was born in 1919."

Answer: 1919 to 2000 is 81 plus 10 (the question was posed in 2010) is 91. "You are 91, Frank, if you have had your birthday this year. If not, you are 90." Frank seemed to agree. Notice Frank didn't know how old he was, but he did recall the year he was born. Very interesting.

Subtracting Fractions

Same drill. Simplify, where possible, by adding or subtracting from the subtrahend to make the problem easier:

- $12 - 1\frac{3}{4} = 12\frac{1}{4} - 2 = 10\frac{1}{4}$. Here you added ¼ to the subtrahend to get 2. But don't forget to add the ¼ to the minuend also.

- $1 - \frac{3}{8} = 1\frac{5}{8} - 1 = \frac{5}{8}$. Here you added 5/8 to the subtrahend to get 1. But don't forget to add the same to the minuend also. Some people see this answer right away because they know there are eight 8s in 1, and taking three away would leave 5.

- 24 feet − 16 2/3 feet = 24 1/3 − 17 = 7 1/3 feet. Here you added 1/3 foot to the subtrahend to get 17. But don't forget to add the same to the minuend.

- $5\frac{1}{4} - 3\frac{7}{8} = 5\frac{1}{4} + \frac{1}{8} - 4 = 5\frac{3}{8} - 4 = 1\frac{3}{8}$. Here you added 1/8 to make the 3 7/8 a 4. But adding 1/8 to 5 ¼ is a little more difficult because you have to convert ¼ to 2/8 and add the 1/8 to that to get the 3/8.

Which problem would you rather do in your head?

- 3.42 − 1.96 = ?

or

- 3.46 − 2 = ?

- They look different, but they are the same problem. Balance by adding 0.04 to the subtrahend and to the minuend to get the answer the easy way.

Time Problems

- Your flight leaves at 3:35. Your watch says 2:49. How much time do you have?

  Answer: Adding 1 minute to the 49 minutes makes 2:50. Then 10 minutes to get to 3. So that's 11 minutes added to 35. Thus 35 plus 10 (work with 10 whenever you can) is 45 plus 1 is 46 minutes to take off. You have enough time to get a snack and go to the bathroom.

- Concentrate on compatibles when making change

- You buy gas costing $17.17 and give the guy a twenty. How much change?

- You know you get $2 plus something.

- Instead of subtracting 17 from 100, think of the number that, when added to 17, will make 100. Thus, you get 83 cents in change, plus $2 makes $2.83.

Mental Gymnastic

Help me make change. Write your answers and check with calculator. If you get it wrong, find out why.

I hand over $1 for a purchase costing _____.

What is my change for these amounts: $0.25, $0.45, $0.10, $0.78, $0.57, $0.32.

Mental Gymnastic

Same drill:

I hand over $5 for a purchase costing _____.

What is my change for these amounts:

$4.25, $0.98, $2.55, $1.95, $3.65, $3.80

Multiplication

- 10 is your friend, and so is anything with a zero after it
- To multiply by any number that has a zero after it, just take away the zero or zeros and then do the math and add the zeros back
- 9 x 10 = 90
- 20 x 300 = 2 x 3 = 6. Add back 000 to make 6,000.
- 40 x 50 = 4 x 5 = 20. Then add the 00 back. Attention: 20 ends in a zero. That zero must be kept there, and you must add the other zeros that were taken away to that number. Hence, 2,000 is the answer.
- 9 x 100 = 900
- 20 x 14 = 2 x 14 = 28. Add 0 gives the answer 280.

Mental Gymnastic

Always look before you leap into a solution. The main idea is to look for compatible numbers that will simplify the task:

16 x 25 = ?

Answer: As 16 is 4 x 4, this problem can be redrawn as 4 x 4 x 25 = ? But 4 x 25 = 100 and 100 x 4 = 400. Another way to do this one is to consider 25 as actually 100 divided by 4. So 16 x 100 / 4 = 1,600 / 4 = 400. Another: 16 is 4 x 4 and 25 is 5 x 5, so we could do 4 x 5 = 20 and 4 x 5 = 20 and 20 x 20 = 2 x 2 = 4 and then add the 00 = 400. Checking the digit sums gives $7 \times 7 = 49 = 4$ and $400 = 4$. The digit sums show we are correct. Mysterious right! Digit sum will be explained soon.

Attention! Getting brain fatigue? The human brain can take only so much. So why not take a break now. And come back when you are ready.

$3 \times 25 \times 2 \times 4 = ?$ Same thing again. You should be able to read off the answer as 600 because 4×25 is 100, and 2×3 is 6, and 6×100 is 600.

$12 \times 25 = ?$ Same thing again. $12 \times 25 = 3 (4 \times 25) = 300$. Or $12 = 4 + 4 + 4$. Therefore, $12 \times 25 = (4 \times 25) + (4 \times 25) + (4 \times 25) = 100 + 100 + 100 = 300$. Always use what you know to do the calculation. In this case, we know $4 \times 25 = 100$. Or $12 = 10 + 2$, so $10 \times 25 = 250$ and $2 \times 25 = 50$, so $250 + 50 = 300$. Also possible is using the distributive rule. This is nice for bigger problems than this one. But $ab \times cd = ac + ad + bc + bd$.

Once you truly understand the algebra of the distributive rule, a world of easy calculations will open to you. For instance, $(z + a) (z + b) = z \times z + za + zb + ab = z (z + a = b) + ab$

So 110×108 would add 8 to 110. Or the same thing: Add 10 to 8 to get $118 \times 100 = 11,800$ and then add ab, which is $8 \times 10 = 80$ to get the answer 11,880. Try this method on other two-digit x two-digit problems. This can also be a cool way of squaring numbers. For instance, $12 \times 12 = ?$ Answer: $(12 + 2) (12 - 2) = 14 \times 10 = 140 + ab = 140 + 2 \times 2 = 144$.

Work this out for yourself if you wish.

Five Is Almost as Good as a 10 in Multiplication

- Five is a 10 divided by 2
- Therefore, you can multiply by 10 and divide by 2 whenever you need to times by 5
- or divide by 2 and multiply by 10 whenever you need to times by 5

Example: $26 \times 5 = ?$ $26 \times 10 = 260 / 2 = 130$ or better $26 / 2 = 13 \times 10 = 130$

Four Is Your Friend

- Four is 2 x 2
- Therefore, you can multiply by 4 by doubling and doubling again

Example: 23 x 4 = ?

- Twenty-three doubled is 46 and 46 doubled is 90 + 2 = 92. Notice that to double 46, we converted 46 into 45 + 1. Double 45 is 90, and double 1 is 2. 90 + 2 = 92. Work out other ways of doing this if you like.

Eight Is Your Friend Because 8 = 2 x 2 x 2 or 2 x 4

Multiply by 8 by doubling and doubling and doubling. Thus, 8 x 22 = 44 x 2 = 88 x 2 = 160 + 16 = 176. Notice to double 88, convert 88 to (80 + 8), and then do the operation 2 x (80 + 8) to get 160 + 16 = 176. Keeping things simple in mental math helps a lot, and you should try to keep things as simple as possible. For me, it is easier to change the 8 to a 10. Then, 10 x 22 = 220. Then take away 2 x 22 = 44. The problem becomes 220 – 44. 220 – 40 = 180 – 4 = 176! Or 8 x 20 = 160 + (2 x 8) = 176.

Six Is Your Friend

By the same token, 6 can be a friend because it is 2 x 3, and 9 can be a friend because it can be 3 x 3. 12 can be your friend because it is 3 x 2 x 2. Eleven is your friend because of special properties that pertain to 11, which will be illustrated after the next mental gymnastic.

Aren't you lucky that you have so many numbers as friends? You may only have a limited number of friends on Facebook, but you have an infinite number of number friends.

Mental Gymnastic

Use your knowledge of how numbers break down to divide by 12:

56,824 / 12 = ?

Answer: What you do is up to you. Make this problem as simple as possible by dividing first by 2, then by 2 again, and then by 3. So 56,824 / 2 = 28,412 / 2 = 14,206 / 3 = 4,735.333

Now divide the same number, 56,824, by 24.

Answer: 4,735.333 / 2 = 2,367.6667.

Use your knowledge of 8 to divide 682 by 8.

Answer: Make sure you are doing this stuff in your head and not on paper: 682 / 2 = 341 / 2 = 170.5 / 2 = 85.25. Some of you, I am sure, can look at 682 and actually divide by 8, saying 8 into 68 is 8 with 4 carried. 8 into 42 is 5 with 2 / 8 = .25. If you can do this, more power to you. Sometimes the mental math is better and faster and usually less work, and sometimes, it isn't.

Use your knowledge of 12 to multiply. Suppose you expect to get $9,800 per month interest on your Ford Motor Company bonds. How much would that amount to in a year?

Answer: Do this in your head. Take the zeros away and store them to bring them back again later on. Now the problem becomes 12 x 98 (with two zeros held in reserve). Very interesting. You know multiple ways of mentally solving this problem.

Quick and dirty: Well, $9,800 is pretty close to $10,000, so take 12 and times it by 10,000. Do this by taking away the four zeros and then multiplying 12 by 1 to get 12. Then add back the four zeros to get 120,000, which is the estimated answer. But because 9,800 is smaller than 10,000, we know the estimate is too high. Too high, all right. But not by much. In fact, it is over by 200 x 12 = 2,400. We need to subtract 2,400 from 120,000. No problem. 120,000 − 2,000 = 118,000, and then take the 400, which gives 117,600.

Quick and dirty with refinement: We know the estimate is too high and that the correct answer is lower. But how much lower? Some people are pretty good at money problems, so they will simply say $200 x 12 lower. $200 x 12 is 2 x 12 = 24. Add back the two zeros to get 2,400. Now I must subtract 2,400 from 120,000. That is what we did before, but that looks a little hard, so we can add 600 to 2,400 to get 3,000 and then subtract 3,000 from 120,000 to get 117,000 (in my head, I did 120 − 3 = 117, then added back the zeros to get 117,000). But we must add 600 to the result to get the true answer of $117,600.

Other methods:

The problem is 9,800 x 12. Start by taking away those zeros. They are important, but they can clutter the mind. So the problem is 98 x 12. Breaking 12 to (10 + 2), we would get 98 (10 + 2) = 980 + 180 + 16, 98 x 10 = 980 + 98 x 2 = ? (98 x 2 is easier if you do 90 x 2 + 8 x 2). Then, 980 + 196 = 980 + 200 = 1,180, then − 4 = 1,176, and put back the two zeros to get 117,600. OK? Notice whatever method you use will result in the same answer. Mental math is like that—always consistent.

The problem is 9,800 x 12. Take away the zeros to get 98 x 12. Try to make the problem easier. How about 98 = (100 − 2)? Then we have 12 (100 − 2) = 1,200 − 24. Taking 24 from 1,200 in steps gives (−10) = 1,190 (−10) = 1,180 − 4 = 1,176. Add back the two zeros to get 117,600, which again is the correct answer. Notice the great advantage of thinking before doing. Not thinking will often make things harder. And, of course, not knowing what you are doing will kill your performance altogether. In general, 8 and 9 can be your friend if you make them into a 10 and work from there, applying the needed correction later.

Multiplication of Two-Digit Numbers

This trick is hard, but you can do it if you try. The more you do it, the easier it will get. The secret is to break the numbers down and then add what you get. Example: 23 x 35 = (20 + 3) x (30 + 5). Quick and dirty would be 20 x 30 = 2 x 3 = 6, adding back the zeros to get 600. By inspection, see that this answer is too small, probably by about 200. (3 x 30 = 90 + 5 x 20 = 100). The correct answer would be the sum of 20 x 30 + 100 + 90 + 15 = 600 +100 = 700 + 90 = 790 + 15 = 805.

Working with outliers sometimes makes the problem easier to see;

23   20 (3)
35   30 (5)

Hence: 20 x 30 + 3 x 30 + 5 x 20 + 15 = 600 + 190 + 15 = 805.

Still awake? Still with me? Here's something real cool:

Teen Trick

Any multiplication problem involving teens can be done mentally by following this rule: Take the single digit from one number and add it to the other number, multiply by 10 and then add the multiple of the single digits. Example: 13 x 17 = ? Method: 13 + 7 = 20 x 10 = 200 + 3 x 7 = 200 + 21 = 221.

Example: 18 x 18 = ? Method: 18 + 8 = 26 x 10 = 260 + 64 = 260 + 40 = 300 + 24 = 324.

Example: 13 x 19 = ? Method: 13 + 9 = 22 x 10 = 220 + 27 = 247. Ans yes, you could do it many other ways. Like 13 x 20 = 260 – 13 = 250 – 3 = 247.

Squaring Speed Limits

Here's a good way to impress people while you are driving. Have them ready with their calculators while you square the speed limits in your head. If the speed limit ends in a zero, just take away the zeros, do the math, and add the zeros back. Example: 70 x 70 = 7 x 7 = 49. Adding two zeros = 4,900. If the speed limit ends in a five, apply the special case of the distributive rule: Take the tens digit and add one to it. Now you have two tens digits, the original and the one you just made. Multiply these two digits and tack on 25 to the result. Example: Speed limit is 55, so 55 x 55 = ? 5+1 = 6. 6 x 5 = 30, tack on 25 (tack on, do not add to) = 3,025. Example: 45 squared = 5 x 4 = 20. Tack on 25 to get 2,025. Example: 65 squared is? Do this mentally to get 4,225.

Try squaring 75. Then check your answer with the calculator.
Mental method: 7 + 1 = 8 x 7 = 56, then tack on 25 to get 5,625!

This trick also works with space-age speed limits. For example: 115. Take the tens and add one to get 12. Multiply 12 x 11 to get 132. Tack on 25, and the answer is 13,225. 12 x 11 should be easy by now. You can use the teen rule or the special properties of 11. With 11, just double any single digit. So 11 x 5 = 55; 11 x 8 = 88; 11 x 9 = 99. With a two-digit number like 12, just add the two digits and stick the result in the middle. 12 x 11; 2 + 1 = 3, so 132 is the answer. Larger numbers do the same: 75 x 11 = ? 7 + 5 = 12; 7 (12) 5 = 825.

Mental Gymnastic

25 x 25 = ?

Answer: 625. Knowing that 25 x 25 = 625 helps you mentally calculate products that hover around that number. Example: 24 x 25 = 625 – 25 = 600, 25 x 26 = 650, 25 x 27 = 675, 25 x 28 = 700, 25 x 23 = 575, and so forth. What you are doing is building on what you already know, 25 x 25 = 625, and working from there by adjusting the problem to suit your needs. So, 25 x 28 becomes 625 + (3 x 25) = 700.

Of course, you can do 25 x 100 / 4 = 2,500 / 4 = 1,250 / 2 = 625. Do this if you forget 25 x 25 = 625.

By the same token, knowing that 50 x 50 = 2,500 helps you mentally calculate 49 x 50, 50 x 51, 48 x 50, 50 x 52, and so forth. The more you know, the better, and the more you know, the more you can know.

Estimates from the Speed Limit Tricks

Use the speed limit trick to make quick and dirty estimates. Example: 34 x 45 = ? We know 35 x 35 is 1,225, and we know 45 x 45 = 2,025, and so the answer is probably halfway in between these two numbers. But how do we calculate halfway? Method: 2,025 – 1,225 = 800 / 2 = 400. Add 400 to 1,225 to get 1,625 as the estimate. Another estimate could involve moving the 34 up to 40 and the 45 down to 40 and then do 40 x 40 = 16. Adding the zeros back makes 1,600. Using the distribution rule, we could get (30 + 4) x (40 + 5) = 1,200 + 150 + 160 + 20 = 1,530.

Mental Gymnastic Review of the 11 Trick

- 8 x 11 = 88
- 23 x 11 = 253
- 12 x 11 = 132
- 13 x 11 = 143
- 14 x 11 = 154

- 15 x 11 = 165
- 19 x 11 = 1 (10) 9 = 209

Do you see the relationship? You can times by 11 by doubling the digit if it is a single digit. If it is a double-digit, simply add the tens digit to the unit digit and put the result in the middle. Example: 34 x 11 = (3 + 4 = 7), so the answer is 374. Example: 90 x 11 = 990.

- The 11 trick works for larger numbers also:
- 234 x 11 = ?
- First working left to right is 2
- Second digit is 2 + 3 = 5
- Third digit is 3 + 4 = 7
- Last digit is 4
- Answer is 2,574

Mental Gymnastic

- 2,341 x 11 = ?

Answer:

- First working right to left digit is 2
- Second digit is 2 + 3 = 5
- Third digit is 3 + 4 = 7
- Next to last digit is 4 + 1 = 5
- Last digit is 1
- Answer is 25,751

Review the 11 Trick

If the digits add to a number greater than 9, carry the extra digit to the left. Hence, 11 x 97 = (9 + 7 = 16) Answer: 9 (16) 7 gives 1,067.

848 x 11 = ? This is easy if you stick to principles and keep the digits in your head. 8 is the first digit. Digit two is 8 + 4 = 12, so add 1 to the 8 to get 9. Now we have 92. The next digit is 8 + 4 = 12. So add the 1 to the 92 to get 93. Digit 3 is a 2, and of course, the last digit is 8. Therefore, 848 x 11 should be 9,328. Why check the answer with the computer when we can check the digit sums? 848 is 128 is 38 is 11 is 2. 11 is 2, and 2 x 2 should equal the digit sum of 9,328. Let's see if it does. 9 + 3 = 12 is 3, 3 + 2 is 5, and 5 + 8 is 13, which is 4! Check and perfect!

More Tricks

Pattern detection helps with mental math. The mental math expert Arthur Benjamin came up with this pattern. See if you get it:

10 x 10 = 100
9 x 11 = 99
8 x 12 = 96
7 x 13 = 91
6 x 14 = 84
5 x 15 = 75
4 x 16 = 64
3 x 17 = 51
2 x 18 = 36
1 x 19 = 19

Did you get it? If so, great. If not, so what. The answers are not what makes mental might. What makes mental might is the mental struggle to get the answer. If you did not study the list for at least 10 minutes before giving up, you missed the chance to develop your mental might. Here's the same pattern with some help:

10 x 10 = 100 (10 x 10 – 0)
9 x 11 = 99 (10 x 10 – 1)
8 x 12 = 96 (10 x 10 – 4)
7 x 13 = 91 (10 x 10 – 9)
6 x 14 = 84 (10 x 10 – 16)
5 x 15 = 75 (100 – 25)
4 x 16 = 64 (100 – 36)
3 x 17 = 51 (100 – 49)
2 x 18 = 36 (100 – 64)
1 x 19 = 19 (100 – 81)

Here's the general rule: if you want to find the product of two numbers that add up to 20, take the unit digit from the larger number, square it and subtract it from 100. Example: 14 x 6 = ? First test: Do 14 and 6 add to 20? Answer: Yes. Conclusion: The rule will apply. Take the 4 and square it to get 16. Subtract 16 from 100 (100 – 10 = 90 – 6 = 84) to get 84.

Mental Gymnastic

Examine the pattern and see if you can make head or tail of it:

20 x 20 = 400
19 x 21 = 399
18 x 22 = 396
17 x 23 = 391
16 x 24 = 384
15 x 25 = 375
14 x 26 = 364
13 x 27 = 351
12 x 28 = 336
11 x 29 = 319

Answer: This is the same thing again, only applied when the sum of two numbers makes 40. Make sure the numbers add to 40. If they do, take the unit digit of the larger number and square it. Subtract the square from 400 to get the answer. Example: 28 x 12 = ? 8 x 8 = 64. 400 – 64 = (340 – 4) = 336.

Generalize the rule and practice:

Mental Gymnastic

65 x 75 = ?

Answer: the numbers add to 140. 70 x 70 = 4,900. Therefore, 65 x 75 will be 4,900 – 25 = 4,875.

Using the outliers would give 60 x 70 + 300 + 350 + 25 = 4875.

If this stuff pleases you, work out other patterns that might amuse you also. For instance:

What is the sum of all the numbers from 1 – 20? Do you know? What do you do if you want to know? Answer: Think!

Answer: line up the numbers in two rows:

1 2 3 4 5 6 7 8 9 10
20 19 18 17 16 15 14 13 12 11

This shows the profound advantage of thinking in patterns rather than plunging in and doing the math the hard way. Notice all the numbers add to 21, and as there are ten columns of them, the sum must be 210. I am too lazy to do this by calculator, but feel free to check the result.

Mental Gymnastic

What is the sum of all the numbers from 1 to 100?

Answer: Here, it pays to visualize the situation. See a top row of numbers from 1 to 50 and a second row of (left to right) 100 to 51. All columns add to 101, and as there are 50 columns, the answer must be 50 x 101. Now the problem is to do 50 x 101. That looks a little hard, so use the trick that 50 is 100 / 2. Hence, multiply 101 by 100 to get 10,100 and then divide by 2 to get 5,000 + 50 = 5,050. Another way would be 50 x (100 + 1) = 5,000 + 50 = 5,050.

That must be the sum of the numbers from 1 to 100. Again, I am too lazy to check it on a calculator. But please feel free to check the result yourself. It may take quite a while by calculator, and you might, you just might get the wrong answer. Another way of doing 101 x 50 would be 101 x 5 x 10 = 505 x 10 = 5,050.

Using this form of alignment, you can do any series in your head. If you wanted to show off, you can. Have someone select a series of consecutive numbers for you to add up. Have them work out the same problem with their calculators while you do the problem in your head. Example: What is the sum of the numbers from 1 – 10? Just divide the big number in 2 and add the big number to the small number and multiply. Here, the big number is 10. Divided by 2 is 5. Add 10 and the small number to get 11. 11 x 5 = 55. just for grins, I will check this answer by adding digits in my head:

1 + 2 + 3 + 4 + 5 + 6 + 7 + 8 + 9 + 10

Looking at compatibles, see 5 tens = 50 and a 5 (in the middle) = 55. Did you see the compatibles? Compatibles start with the 9. See 9 and 1 is 10, then 8 and 2 is 10 (notice how orderly we are in approaching the problem and how in sequence) 7 and 3 is 10, and 6 and 4 is 10. That's four 10s, and the 10 on the end makes five 10s makes 50. Only one number is left, and that is 5, so the answer is 50 + 5 = 55. Notice we get the exact same answer we got with the alignment analysis, except it took ten times longer.

If they ask for a sequence that has an odd number, just hold the big fellow over and add it to the result that you get from alignment.

If they want you to add a sequence of just odd numbers or just even numbers, you should have no trouble doing that. Example: What is the sum of odd numbers from 1–20? And how does it differ from the sum of even numbers?

OK, get out your calculators and take 15 minutes to do this. Chances are you will get distracted or bored or flub in some way. Or do it the easy way:

Odd numbers 1–20:

1 3 5 7 9
19 17 15 13 11

Notice the pattern? All add to 20, and there are five columns, so the answer is 100 (5 x 20).

How about even numbers?

2 4 6 8 10

20 18 16 14 12

Notice the pattern? All add to 22, and there are five columns, so the answer is 22 x 5 = 220 / 2 = 110

So the sum of even numbers from 1–20 is exactly 10 larger than the sum of odd numbers. Does that make sense? Yes, it does, because each even number is one unit larger than the odd number that came before it, and there are 10 numbers and 10 x 1 = 10.

If the reasoning is right, the sum of all numbers from 1–20 should equal 100 (the sum of the odd numbers) + 110 (the sum of even numbers) = 210.

Mental Gymnastic

Prove the sum of all numbers from 1–20 = 210.

Answer: The last number is 20, and the first is 1. Therefore the sum of the ten columns will always be 21. 21 x 10 = 210. Check this with your calculator if you like.

Division

Division and multiplication are operations that are to each other in the same relation as subtraction and addition. They are obverse. So just as it is possible to use addition in a subtraction problem, as in making change, it is possible to use knowledge of multiplication to do divisions. For instance, 64 / 8 = ? To do this operation, you could just think of a number which when multiplied by 8, would equal 64 or something less than 64. As we know 8 x 8 = 64, it is obvious that 64 / 8 = 8. In fact, you were probably taught to check your division by multiplication. Apply all that you learned already about mental math to division problems. Think about the problem before you rush in, try to simplify the problem, and proceed stepwise, preferably in small bite-sized steps that are easy to keep in your mind.

Divide the Larger Part of a Number First

36,540 / 9 = ? Make the 36,540 two numbers: 36,000 and 540. 9 into 36,000 is 4,000 and 9 into 540 is 60. Therefore, the answer is 4,060.

Usually, there is more than one way to divide a number. You need to choose the way that serves you best. Consider 126 / 3 = ? You could break the 126 into 100 + 26, but how much good would that do you? Neither the 100 nor the 26 are evenly divided by 3. So forget them. Breaking into 120 + 6 looks more workable as both numbers are easily divided by 3. Hence, 126 / 3 = 120 / 3 = 40 + 6 / 3 = 2; therefore, 126 / 3 = 42. Of course, by now, just looking at 126 / 3, the 42 would pop into your mind.

Magic Number Tricks with 11

Sometimes 11 can help you divide. Take advantage of the fact 11 x 91 = 1,001.

34 / 91 = ? Method: Times top and bottom by 11 = 374 / 1,001 = .374. Calculator gives .3736.

Also 9 x 11 = 99. So times top and bottom by 11. Example: 34 / 9 = ? Method 374 / 99 = 3.74.

Plus a one percent correction because we divided by 100 when we should have divided by 99. Add 1% to 0.374 (0.0374) to get 3.7774. By calculator 34 / 9 = 3.7777...8. Take advantage of 909 x 11 = 9,999. So, 3,724 / 909 = 3 (10) 964 / 9,999 = 4.0964. Calculator gives 4.0968.

Division by 10

To divide by 10, just drop a zero off the number you are dividing or move the decimal point to the left one place. Thus, 350 / 10 = 35; 23 / 10 = 2.3. Division by multiples of 10, such as 100 and 1,000 are just as easy. Example: 35,000 / 10,000 = 3.5. The three 0s cancel each other, and then you divide by 10, pushing the decimal point to the left.

Five Is Your Friend in Division Also

Remember how we could multiply by 5 by remembering that 5 is really 10 / 2? So to multiply by 5, we just divided by 2 and multiplied by 10. Division by 5 is the obverse because 1 / 5 is equal to 2 / 10. So to divide by 5, first divide by 10 and then multiply by 2. Example: 586 / 5 = ? Method: 586 / 10 = 58.6 x 2 = 100 + 16 + 1.2 = 117.2. By now, some of you will be able to just look at 586 / 5 and reel off the answer.

MENTAL MAKING MIGHT

Twelve Is Your Friend In Division Also

Recall 12 is 2 x 2 x 3, so to divide by 12, just divide by 2 and 2 again and then 3. If the number looks like it is easily divisible by 3, you might want to divide by 3 first and then 2 and 2. Example: 636 / 12 = ? Method: 636 / 3 = 212 / 2 = 106 / 2 = 53.

Mental Gymnastic

Divide 486 by 16 using your knowledge of how 8 is your friend.

Answer: 16 is 8 x 2 and 8 is 2 x 2 x 2. So 486 / 2 = 243 / 2 = 121.5 / 2 = 60.75 / 2 = 30.375. That would be the exact answer, but sometimes an estimation is enough. So if you are bothered by the decimals, just adjust the problem to make it easier. Example: 486 / 2 = 243. That was no sweat. But the next division is going to make a decimal, so just change the 3 on the end to a 2 and make the number 242 / 2 = 121. Dividing again by 2 gives a decimal, so make that 1 on the end a 2. Last time we lowered the number by one unit, so this time, how about we raise it by one unit. Now the problem is 122 / 2 = 61. Same deal—make 61 a 60 for easy figuring, and we arrive at 30, not far off and good enough for government work. The easy way: 486 / 16 = 243 / 8 = 30 3/8 or 30.375.

The 11 Trick Helps in Division Also

Here the problem is imagining what number times 11 would come close to the number we are dividing by 11. For instance, 236 / 11 = ? Method: We know that given a three-digit number as the result of multiplication by 11, the middle number is the sum of the two numbers on the ends. Here we know the left number has to be a 2, so the middle number 3 probably came from the addition of 2 and 1. Therefore the product we are looking for is 21 x 11 = 231. So 236 / 11 = 21 plus 5 leftover would make 5 / 11. But what would 5 / 11 be in decimals? It looks pretty close to .5 or a little less, say 10% less, because 11 is 10% greater than 10. So, a quick and dirty estimate would be 236 / 11 = 21.45. But suppose we are building a submarine, and we must know exactly what 5 / 11 equals. In that case, multiply the 5 by 10 to get 50, so we won't have to work with decimals until later. Then figure what number times 11 comes closest to 50 on the downside. That number would be 44 as 4 x 11 = 44. Taking 44 from 50 gives 6, and that makes us think of 55 because 5 x 11 = 55. Now we have 4.5, and as there is a 5 leftover from the 60 − 5, we see that we are going to have an infinite progression of 4.545454545... So dividing by 10 to correct for our multiplying by 10 at the start to make the problem easier (remember?), we get 5/11=.45454545... No calculator could do better. Therefore, 236 / 11 = 21.45454545...

Special Nines

9 18 27 36 45 54 63 72 81 90

See any pattern?

If the digit sum is equal to 9 or 9s, then the number is easily and evenly divided by nine. If the digit sum is different from 9, the digit sum is the remainder after division by 9.

Example: 268 / 9 = ?

Digit sum is 2 + 6 + 8 = 16 is 7. Subtract 7 from 268 to get 261 which should be an evenly divided number by 9 because the digit sum is 9. If it is evenly divided by 9, it should be evenly divided by 3 and 3 again. Is it? Do this in your head. You should get 261 / 3 = 87 / 3 = 29. Then the answer is 29 remainder 7 or 29 and 7/9 = 29.777777....

Squares

Squares are your friend. The squares are 4, 9, 16, 25, 36, 49, 64, 81, 100. You can also develop squares for 10–20. Use the teen rule and after practice memorize the results. Example: 12 x 12 = ? 14 x 10 + 2 x 2 = 144; 13 x 13 = 160 + 9 = 169. 14 x 14 = (do this in your head) = 196 and so forth.

Squares help some people who have trouble keeping track of the times tables. For instance: What's 7 x 8? If you know 7 x 7 = 49, all you need do is add another 7 to get 56. This is taking advantage of the fact that 7 x 8 = 7 (7 + 1). Of course, there are other ways of jogging your memory and it might be helpful to review them. 7 x 8 can be 7 (2 + 6) = 14 + 42 = 56. Or how about 7 x 8 = 7 (3 + 5) = 21 + 35 = 56. Or 7 x 8 = 7 (4 + 4) = 28 + 28 = 56. Or 7 x 8 = 7 (2 + 6) = 14 + 42 = 56. Or 7 x 8 = 7 (2 + 2 + 2 + 2) = 14 x 4 = 40 + 16 = 56. Or how about, 7 x 8 = (1 + 6) 8 = 8 + 48 = 56. And 7 x 8 = (3 + 4) 8 = 24 + 32 = 56. But why bother with the rigamarole when you can use the squares? 49 + 7 = 56 or 8 x 8 = 64 – 8 = 56. No matter what path you take, the answer is always the same. That is the beauty of math. It is nice to know that in this uncertain world, some things are certain.

Probability

The mathematics of probability was worked out in the 17th century by the collaboration of a gambler, Chevalier de Méré, and two mathematicians, Blaise Pascal and Pierre de Fermat. But you knew that already. Probabilities are important in investments, medicine, nuclear physics, elections, gambling, insurance, and in many aspects of personal life. Some probabilities are completely accurate, especially in a gambling situation (provided the cards, coins, and dice are fair), and some have to be based on estimates. Before you can handle probabilities, you have to understand conjunctive and disjunctive statements. Recall: A statement is a sentence that makes a definite claim.

Conjunctive Statements

The probability of two events occurring is the product of their probabilities: Pr (P&Q) = Pr (P) x Pr (Q). Example: A single die has six surfaces, each with the number of dots from 1 to 6. When the die is rolled, by chance alone, one of those numbers will come face up. As there are six surfaces, the chance of any one number coming up is 1/6. A coin has two surfaces, heads or tails. The chance of a head is ½, and the chance of a tail is 1/2.

Question: What is the chance of two heads coming up one after another in the toss of a fair coin? Pr(H&H) = Pr(H) x Pr(H) = 1/2 x 1/2 = 1/4. One chance in four. What is the probability of having three boys in a row? 1/2 x 1/2 x 1/2 = 1/8. What is the chance of rolling a two when a pair of dice are rolled? 1/6 x 1/6 = 1/36.

Disjunctive Statements

The probability of a disjunctive statement is the sum of the probabilities. Pr(PVQ) = Pr(P) + Pr(Q). What is the probability of a head or a tail coming up in the toss of a fair coin. Pr(HVT) = Pr(H) + Pr(T) = 1/2 + 1/2 = 1. Get it? You will always get a head or a tail when you toss a coin. You can prove this to yourself by tossing a penny a hundred times. There will always be either a head or a tail.

Sidebar by Doctor Patten

When I was studying for my master's in philosophy, there was much discussion about the possibility of the coin landing on its edge and staying there. In that case, the probability of a head or a tail would be less than one but not much less. You can bet on that. In class, during a demonstration of probability with coins, a penny did actually land on its edge and stay there! An amazingly improbable event—who knows—one in a million or less. That is one of the difficulties with probability calculus—the unreasonable and unexpected and unexpectable does occasionally happen.

Practical Applications

What is the probability that he loves me and will marry me? Here we have to estimate probabilities. Let's say the Pr(Love) is 8/10 and marriage Pr(M) is less, say ½. Therefore, the Pr(L&M) = Pr(L) x Pr(M) = 8/10 x 1/2 = 8/20 = 4/10 = 40%.

"We can fix your toilet today if I finish my current job and my assistant gets over his bad cold."
"What's the chance of your finishing?"
"Pretty even, 50%."

"What's the chance of your assistant getting over his bad cold?"

"Not good. I would estimate no more than one chance in ten."

"I guess I won't be seeing you today as 1/2 x 1/10 = 1/20. One chance in 20 is slim odds."

Calculation of Possible Value of an Investment

What might be the future value of my Gilead stock?

Whew! That requires some research and some sophisticated guessing. But we can do some estimating. Let's guess there is an 80% chance that GILD will go up 20 points ($20 a share) in the next year, and let's guess there is a 20% chance that it will go down 5 points in the next year.

To do the probability calculation math, we must first make a statement. Future value equals either up 20 or down 5.

Pr(Future value) = Pr (.8 x 20) VPr (.2 x –5) = 16 – 1 = 15. Add this to the closing price on December 24, 2020, which was $57.07 + 15 = 72.07. Hence the prediction is next year, GILD will be $72.07, giving a return on investment (not including dividends) of 26.4%. Add the current yearly dividend, $2.72, which makes a return of 31%. Not bad! But is it true? We won't know until next year. Life has to be lived forward but can only be examined and (hopefully) understood in retrospect. A year from now, we will know if we were right or wrong and by how much. That knowledge may or may not help us make future predictions about the stock price. That's the trouble with the future. The future is contingent and not entirely predictable. Note: GILD closed on February 12, 2021, at $66.89, and the dividend was raised to $2.84 a year. Bulletin: February 14, 2021 Analyst SVB Leerink adjusts Gilead Sciences Stock Price target to $72 from $73. Keeps outperform rating. Nice to know someone got the same result we did.

Digit Sum

In the beginning of your mental math adventures, it is a good idea to check your answers with a calculator. If the result on the calculator is the same as what was in your head, then it is likely you did things right. If the result differs, then find out why. The problem could be your calculator in your head or the calculator in your hand, or both. Always review what happened and see if you can find the problem or problems and correct them. The most common problem with mental math is mental laziness, especially in keeping intermediate step numbers in your mind. That is why it is best to do all mental math in a set sequence such that you need to keep a minimal number of digits in your mind.

In the old days, you were probably taught how to check your work by redoing the sum in reverse order. That doubled your time on the problem. If the problem was division, you multiplied the answer by the divisor. In multiplication, you put the bottom number on the top and the top number on the bottom and started multiplying all over again with your pencil and paper and work. Whew!

A shorter way of checking is to use the digit sum method. After decades of doing mental math, you won't need to check your work because it will be a waste of time. You will be that good and that sure of your calculations. But when starting out, it helps to check calculations to discover mistakes. Try using the digit sums because calculators are too clumsy, and sometimes when a large number of numbers is entered, too slow.

Digit sums allow you to check calculations in about one-tenth the time you would spend with the calculator. And digit sum will allow you to check calculator work in one-tenth the time or less. If you do use a calculator routinely, it is a good idea to check the work because lots of errors occur with calculators.

Digit Sum Is So Accurate Some Accountants Use It to Check Their Calculators

It is easy to make a mistake with a calculator by punching in the wrong numbers or punching the right numbers twice or pressing the wrong function key, and so forth.

Definition: The digit sum is the sum of all the digits in a number.

The digit sum of 13 would be 4 because $1 + 3 = 4$. The digit sum of 12 is 3 because $1 + 2 = 3$. Anytime the number has more than one digit, the digit sum is the sum of the digits. Thus, 343,214 adds up to 17 ($343 = 10 + 7$). Therefore, the digit sum is $1 + 7 = 8$. Another way of doing this would be the hard way: 3 + 4 is 7; 7 + 3 is 10; 1 + 0 is 1; 1 + 2 is 3; 3 + 1 is 4; and 4 + 4 is 8, which is the same digit sum number answer we got the easy way.

Important Advice about Digit Sums

Ignore 9's. Count them as a 0. There is a simple way to prove 9's are zeros, but we will leave this to you to figure out. For instance, 925 is $9 + 2 = 11$; $1 + 1 = 2$ and $2 + 5$ is 7, the same result we would have gotten if we had ignored the 9. What is the digit sum of 94? $9 + 4 = 13$; $1 + 3 = 4$! How about 457? Answer: 7 because $4 + 5 = 9$, and we have learned to forget 9 or treat it as a zero. How about when the digit sum is a 9? Just treat it as a zero. 387 would make 15 and 3 or 18. Therefore, the digit sum of 387 is 0 because it is a 9.

Stop! Take some time to master digit sums. Write some numbers and do the digit sums. When you feel fairly competent, then tackle the next sections, which cover how to use the digit sums as a check.

Mental Gymnastic: Add These Three Numbers and Check with Digit Sum

437

285

164

Add these in your head or, if you must, add them on paper or with a calculator.

886, right? Digit sum of 886 is 8 + 8 = 16 = 7 + 6 = 13 = 4. The digit sum of 886 is 4.

Now you have to decide whether it is easier to do the digit sum of the numbers or the columns. Numbers look easier. Hence, 437 is 5; 285 is 6; 164 is 2. 562 is 112 is 4. Check.

The digit sum of our answer is the same as the digit sum of the numbers we added. Check.

Yes, you could have done all the digit sums on paper. But it is faster to do them in your head.

Subtraction

537 – 241 = 296 Add the digit sum of the answer to the digit sum of the number that was subtracted and get the digit sum of the number that was subtracted from. Example: 296 is 8 (remember 9 is a 0). 241 is 7. 7 + 8 is 15 is 6. Now let's see if 537 is a 6. Bingo!

It is because 8 + 7 is 15 is 6.

Multiplication

437 x 24 = 10,488 Do 10,488 in your head to get digit sum 3. 1 & 4 is 5; 8 & 8 is 16; 5 & 7 is 12 is 3. But does digit sums of the 437 x 24 come out to 3? 437 sums as 14 = 5; 24 is 6 of course and 6 x 5 = 30 whose digit sum is 3. Check.

Division

324 / 4 = 81 So 4 x 9 is 0, and 5 + 4 is also 0. Check. If, in division, there is a remainder, add the digit score of the number you divided, and it should equal the remainder. Example" 325 / 4 = 81 remainder 1. The digit sum of 325 then should be 1, and it is 5 + 5 is 10 is 1!

Think about This

If during the first reading of this chapter, you were lazy and did not practice each of the quick math tricks, you can still learn them any time you wish. This chapter will be here waiting for you anytime you wish to use it. The point the chapter really wanted to get across is that there are quick and easy mental ways to do calculations. For some people, these math tricks are interesting and fun. When you are ready for them, they are here and ready for you. The best results will come with time. Spread the tasks over time, doing a little each day and reviewing and practicing what you have mastered. Don't binge! Be easy on yourself. It took 20 million years to make a masterpiece like the Grand Canyon. Surely you can wait several weeks for a great math brain.

Closing Statement from Doctor Patten

As a neurologist, I state with a reasonable degree of medical certainty that mental math and mental work will do good for your brain. It certainly will be better for your brain than watching TV. So, ditch the remote. Start thinking!

Closing Statement from Doctor Patten

Full disclosure; Doctor Patten had nothing whatever to do with the above statement or with this book. Doctor Patten would not waste his precious time on such things. Instead, he set me, his clone, to do the work. Years ago, Doctor Patten was reading his favorite magazine, *Soldier of Fortune,* and he ran across an ad that promised if you send $50 and a hair sample, they would make your clone. Patten thought it was a scam. But when he saw the same ad in the *Magazine of the Veterans of Foreign Wars,* he decided, for $50, what the hell. Six weeks later, I (his clone) arrived, and ever since, he has been using me to do the work. For instance, it is a universally acknowledged fact that he never showed at that course in Mental Gymnastics at Rice. While he tended his garden or relaxed in his pool or read pulp fiction or tap-danced with his friends, I taught the course and continuingly complained bitterly, and to no avail, that he was pocketing all the money.

Uhm! Talking about Mental Gymnastics course and that class reminds me. The last class would find me saying the same thing I now say to you, dear reader—the same thing what I said to the students at Rice—namely:

"As always, thanks for joining me. I hope to see you all again soon."

Review Time

Square the speed limit 65.

4,225! Good!

6 + 1 = 7. 7 x 6 = 36 + 6 = 42. Then tack on (remember do not add) 25 to get 4,225.

What is the digit sum of 4,225?

4! Good!

4 & 2 is 6; 2 & 5 is 7; 7 & 6 is 13 is 4.

Is that the digital sum of 65 x 65? Yes, 65 is 11 = 2, so 2 x 2 = 4. Check.

Multiply in your head: 5 x 7 x 5 x 8 x 2 x 2

Answer: 5,600. You should have rearranged the problem to 10 x 10 x 56 by noting the two 2 x 5. Another: 4 x 25 = 100 x 56 = 5,600.

150 x 4 x 2 x 30?

Answer: 36,000. Take off the 0s: 15 x 4 = 60 x 2 = 120 x 3 = 360; add 0s back to get 36,000.

260 / 13?

Answer: 20

56 x 25?

Answer: 1,400. Remember 100 / 4 is 25. 56 / 4 = 14 x 100 = 1,400.

Double 29?

Answer: 58 (60 – 2)

11 x 5 x 2 x 9?

Answer: 990. 10 x 9 = 90 x 11 = 990. Or 10 x 99 = 990.

Double 535?

Answer: 1,070. 500 x 2 = 1,000 + 70 = 1,070.

16 x 15?

Answer: 240. 16 + 5 = 21 x 10 = 210 + 30 = 240.

5 x 48?

Answer: 240. (10 / 2 x 48)

35 x 12?

Answer: 420. 350 + 70 = 420.

369 / 9?

Answer: 41. 369 / 3 = 123 / 3 = 41. Most people at this stage will see this answer directly.

Vale

Here ends the book on *Making Mental Might*. The next appendix is optional if you wish to exercise your thinking powers.

Working on the problems and writing this book has increased my mental power quite a bit. Good for me. I hope you gained mental horsepower also. If so, good for you!

As always, thanks for joining me. I hope to see you again sometime soon. Meanwhile, stay well.

And -
Goodbye and good luck.

Your friend,
Mickey

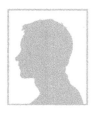

APPENDIX: CHAPTER SEVEN
PROBLEMS

AFRICAN CONTEMPORARY
PROBLEMS

APPENDIX: CHAPTER SEVEN—PROBLEMS

◆ ◆ ◆

Increase your mental might by working on problems. Think long and hard about the problem and write down the answer, so you don't deceive yourself into thinking you got it when you didn't.

Self-Testing is Important

One of the most important principles of mental might is self-testing to see if you really know something or you don't. It is better for you to know you don't know something before someone else (your professor or teacher) finds out. Socrates famously said he knew nothing, and everyone else knew nothing but thought they knew something. Therefore, Socrates said he was ahead of the crowd. Always review your answer and the given answer. Pay particular attention to the method used to solve the problem so that you can apply that method to other problems. Always try to explain your answer so that you know after the smoke clears where you went right or wrong.

Problem One

A notorious robber has made a lucrative living by robbing travelers in the forest. Three suspects are identified. Their statements follow. One makes two true statements; one makes one true and one false statement; one makes two false statements. Which one is the robber?

A.   1. I am not the robber.

         2. C is the robber.

B.   1. C is innocent.

         2. A is the robber.

C.   1. I am not the robber.

         2. B is innocent.

Stop! Pause and think. Work on the problem yourself. That is the way to grow your mental powers. Even failing to solve the problem will benefit you because even your failure required you to stay alert and concentrate and use your brain.

Solution

Assume A is the robber, then do an analysis of the statements

A.   1. F 2. F

B.   1. T 2. T

303

C.   1. T 2. T.

Therefore, if A were the robber, B and C both make two true statements. As this violates the premises given, A is innocent.

Assume B is the robber. Then

A.   1. T 2. F
B.   1. T 2. F
C.   1. T 2. F

As all have one T and one F, this violates the premise, and B is innocent

No need to worry who is guilty because A and B are innocent, but it wouldn't hurt to prove the point. So, if C is the robber, then:

A.   1. T 2. T
B.   1. F 2. F.
C.   1. F 2. T

So if C is the robber, we get two true statements from A, two false statements from B, and one statement true and one false from C. This is exactly as specified in the facts, so we have proven the answer. C is the robber.

Note that to solve this problem, you had to completely understand the given facts. It wouldn't hurt to recite the facts several times because they are the premises of the problem that the solution must satisfy. If your solution didn't have two true statements, two false statements, and one true and one false statement, you did not solve the problem. Try your hand on the next problem, which should come easier.

Problem Two

Your company is to undergo an RIF (reduction in force). Try to get the contract, and try not get the pink slip.

You get two envelopes, A and B. You are told the envelopes may have a contract or not. You ask a question and are told: "Both envelopes may have a contract. Both may have a pink slip. Either one may have a pink slip or a contract. But what envelope A says is false if and only if it has the contract, and what envelope B says is true if and only if it has the contract. Otherwise, the reverse is true.

Summary: Two envelopes, each with a pink slip or a contract. If A has the contract, what it says is false. If B has the contract, what it says is true. So what's written on the envelopes?

304

Here's what is written on the outside of the envelopes:

Envelope A: "B has the contract."

Envelope B: "It doesn't matter what envelope you pick."

Pause. Think. Formulate and answer. It will help for you to write your answer and the reasoning you used to get the answer. Only then should you look at my answer.

Answer: Usually, it is best to start with the truth. So, B says it doesn't matter, and if B has the contract, then that statement is true. If it doesn't matter what envelope you pick, then A must have a contract also. So now let's look at envelope A. If B has a contract, then A must have one also. But if A has the contract, what it says is false. It says B has the contract. Therefore, B cannot have the contract and not have a contract. That is a contradiction. A contradiction can't be entirely true. Therefore, B cannot have the contract. If B can't have the contract, it has the pink slip. Therefore, what it says is false, and it does make a difference which envelope you open. Therefore, A had the contract.

Let's check this reasoning. A has the contract, so what it says has to be false. It says B has the contract, and we know by deduction that B has the pink slip. Hence, our answer checks out and is correct. A has the contract. Any other answer is wrong.

Wrong answers: At Rice University School for Continuing Studies, where for 17 years the clone taught the course on Mental Gymnastics, there were multiple emails about this envelope problem:

"The company wants to fire you, so both envelopes have a pink slip."

"Both envelopes have the pink slip because envelope B says it doesn't matter which one you take."

"Both envelopes have the contract because envelope B says it doesn't matter which one you take."

"It is a trick, and both envelopes are empty."

"I would have nothing to do with a company that plays games with the workers."

"This doesn't make sense. Who gets the contract and who gets the pink slip should depend on their work record and nothing else."

"Why would the truth of the statement on the envelope depend on what the envelope had inside?"

"The company is testing to see if you can read English."

"The first envelope said it had to have the contract, so it had to have it."

"Why would the company lie on envelope one?"

"The envelope they hand you first has the contract."

"The company was trying to fool you, so envelope one doesn't have the contract."

Comment: Notice how derailed and irrelevant these emails are and how much they reflect confused thinking and, in some cases, failure to even correctly read, much less understand the problem. The truth is there is no company. This is an exercise in logical thinking—nothing more and nothing less.

Problem Three

Using Aristotle's method of comparing and contrasting by analysis of similarities and differences, work your right brain on pattern extraction by completing sequences:

1. 1 3 5 7 __
2. AB CE CD EG EF G_
3. blowhard hardhat hatcheck ____mate
4. toner tone ton __
5. stone tone ton __
6. astray stray tray ___
7. snit in snot on prod or mode ___
8. bib bib ton, not 399 993 pin ___
9. din don fan fen pep pip cod ___
10. 289,735 897,352 973,528 735,289 _____
11. stops ____ top to
12. polygram 12345678 pray 1674 ploy _____
13. gum gun bar bat sun sup lip ___
14. hole pit seed kick punt boat edge shore strengthen hurt _____ clever
15. bird crane stretch sprint run snag lozenge mint new note ____ beak
16. 7,913 992 488 569 72,155 614_
17. Q O M K I _
18. A E I O _
19. JK KJ LM IH NO G_
20. retire rite strafe fart inept pen peruse _____

Norms: Age 20 – 39: 8 – 12 correct = average; 13 – 16 correct = above average; 17 – 18 correct = superior; 19 – 20 correct = gifted

Age 40 – 59: 6 – 10 correct = average; 11 – 15 correct = above average; 16 – 18 correct = superior; 19 – 20 correct = gifted

Age 60 – 79: 4 – 6 correct = average; 7 – 10 correct = above average; 11 – 17 correct = superior; 18 – 20 correct = gifted

OK? Did you actually fill in the blanks with your answers? Did you have a reason for your answers? Did you do some thinking? Thinking is key. The thinking is the thing that makes mental might. It is nice to get the right answers, but more important is to do the actual thinking. Answers are explained in chapter three.

Problem Four

Place bets on this three-horse race the way Lewis Carroll did such that he knew he would win £20 no matter what horse won the race. (Odds are official odds of the London bookmaker at the time of the race.)

Horse A. Odds 2:1

Horse B. Odds 5:1

Horse C. Odds 10:1

Think about the odds. They show how to make an easy profit. To start, you might try some bets on each horse to find out what's what. Let's bet on each horse to win 20 pounds. 10 on horse A gets us 20. 4 on B gets us 20, and 2 on horse C gets us 20. But we only bet 10 + 4 + 2 = 16. Therefore, this scene gives a profit of 4. To get a profit of 20 pounds, we just have to multiple our bets by 5. Betting 50 on A gets 100. 20 on B gets 100, and 10 on C gets 100. Each horse will pay 100, but our total bets are just 80 pounds. Therefore, our profit is 20 pounds no matter which horse wins.

Problem Five

Consider the conditional syllogism A ⊠ B (A entails B). Determine which of the following arguments are valid or invalid: Note A is the antecedent and B is the consequence.

A	~B	~A	B
/∴B	/∴~A	/∴ ~B	/∴ A

How does this analysis set show that successful testing does not prove a hypothesis true, for that is the fallacy of affirming the consequent? How does this analysis set show that unsuccessful tests can defeat a hypothesis for denying the consequent does deny the antecedent? A, therefore B and not B, therefore not A are the only valid arguments. Not A, therefore not B is wrong because B could be caused by something other than A. B, therefore A is wrong because B could be caused by something other than A.

Now apply this reasoning to a real-life situation: If you take cyanide, you will die. Cyanide entails death.

Case 1. You take cyanide. Therefore, you die

Case 2. You didn't die. Therefore, you didn't take cyanide.

Case 3. You didn't take cyanide. Therefore, you didn't die? Wrong. There are many other causes of death.

Case 4. You died. Did you take cyanide? Not necessary. You will die sooner or later from something. And most of us will not die from taking cyanide.

Answer: Case 1. affirms the antecedent and is true in all cases as that is the premise. If you take cyanide, you will die. That is also true in real life. Affirming the antecedent is correct logic.

Case 2. As you are alive, you didn't take cyanide. This is negating the consequent, which automatically negates the antecedent. If cyanide always causes death and you are still alive, it follows that you did not take cyanide. Correct logic.

Case 3. Negating the antecedent does not mean you won't die, as there are many causes of death.

Case 4. Affirming the consequence does not affirm the antecedent. Not taking cyanide does not prevent you from death from some other cause. This is the error of affirming the consequence and is the logical reason a positive experimental result does not prove the antecedent. Affirming the consequence is an error in logic and not correct thinking.

Problem Six

Road Signs: There are three roads, A, B, and C. Only one road is safe. The others have dragons at the end that will eat the traveler who does not know how to think. Each road has a sign. Not much is known about how truthful the signs are, except at least one sign is false. What road is safe? How do you know?

Sign A: Signs B and C are true.

Sign B: Road A is the one to take, or else C is the correct road.

Sign C: Road B is not the one to take.

Answer: Assume A is true, then B and C are true. This violates the premise as there must be at least one false sign. Therefore A is false, and that makes B and C false. If B is false, then B is the road to take. Sign C says don't take B. If that is false, B is the road to take.

Conclusion: All signs are false. Assuming any one sign is false will always lead to B as the road to take.

Problem Seven

A Stradivarius was stolen. Four people are suspects. One of them is the culprit. Each makes one statement. The guilty one's statement is false. The statements of the innocent are true. Who stole the violin?

A.   I was not in town at the time of the theft.
B.   C is the culprit.
C.   B's statement is false.
D.   C's statement is true.

Assume A is the culprit, then the other statements would be true. But B says C is the culprit, and that is false if A is the culprit. C and A can't both be culprits. Therefore, A is innocent, and A's statement has to be true. The premise says only the guilty person makes a false statement.

Assume B is the culprit. Then, his statement is false, and that would be correct. C is not the culprit if B is the culprit. Now let's look at C's statement. It says B's statement is false, and it is if B is the culprit. Now look at D's statement. It says C's statement is true, and that is true if B's statement is false, and that is correct again if B is the culprit. Therefore, B is the culprit.

You can check this by assuming C makes the false statement. And you can check by assuming D makes the false statement.

Answer:
A.   True
B.   False
C.   True
D.   True

Problem Eight

Make up a peg list from 1 to 10 using rhymes to suggest the images. Example: 1. is one and one reminds me of ton, and I see a ton of coal in a truck.

How did you do?
Some suggestions:
One is ton
Two is shoe
Three is tree
Four is core
Five is hive

Six is fix

Seven is heaven

Eight is gate

Nine is sign

Ten is hen

You can also use rhyme to link items, and for some people, that works well. Try it to see if you like it and to see if it likes you.

This way of making a peg list helps some people. Very young children have no trouble making images, and in fact, they think it is fun. For very young children, a word-rhyming peg list works best. The rhyme reminds the kid of the image that is on the peg.

Problem Eight True or False

a.   Don't be inapposite.

b.   Solve the face-name problem by making associations that help recall the name.

c.   The statement (All whales are mammals) is logically equivalent to the statement (No whale is not a mammal) and entails that some whales are mammals and that a few whales are mammals.

d.   Pleonasm and supererogation should alert us to the possibility of exaggeration.

e.   Multiply 225 x 235 mentally by adding 40,000 + 10,000 + 2,000 + 600 + 250 + 25 = 52,875

f.   "By the way," "Before I forget" and "Incidentally" are flag words that alert us to the possibility that an important message will follow—usually a message that the speaker doesn't want us to regard as important.

g.   To subtract 17 from 100, it is easier to think of what number added to 17 makes 100.

h.   The statement ("Bankruptcy for Global Crossing is not possible at all") is not likely to be true because it claims that the possible is not possible at all.

i.   "This is the lowest price I can do for you" might mean that someone else can get a lower price.

j.   If someone was born in 1872 and died in 1932, the shortcut to calculate how old they were when they died would involve taking 2 from 1,872 and 2 from 1,932 and then adding 30 to 30 to get 60.

Answer—all are true.

a.   true and good advice. b. true c. true, and this whale washed up on the beach is also a mammal. The statement is the universal categorical affirmative. d. true e. true, but using a calculator will be faster f. true g. true h. true i. true j. true.

Problem Nine

Poaching has become a problem on the King's hunting lands because hunting is a source of food for the people. Four suspects have been identified; each makes three statements. Not much is known about their truthfulness except that the culprit makes only one true statement. Who is the poacher?

A.   1. D is innocent.

       2. I am not the poacher.

       3. Hunting is a source of food in these parts.

B.   1. C being a suspect is a case of mistaken identity.

       2. A's second statement is true.

       3. Not all of my statements are true.

C.   1. I am not the poacher.

       2. D is the poacher.

       3. My being a suspect is not a case of mistaken identity.

D.   1. A's statements are not all true.

       2. At least one of C's statements is true.

       3. I do not like to eat game.

Take note of the important items in the premise, for they control the answer.

1.   Hunting is a source of food.

2.   Suspects have been identified.

3.   The poacher makes only one true statement.

Answer: C is the poacher.

Assume A is the poacher. Statement 1 would be true. Two would be false. Three is true because it is given in the premises. Therefore, A has two true statements if we assume he is the poacher. But the poacher makes only one true statement. A must be innocent.

Assume B is the poacher. Statement 1 would be false as all suspects have been identified. Statement 2 is true. If B is the poacher, A is not the poacher. Statement 3 is true because his statement 1 is false. So, B has two true statements if we assume he was the poacher. As the poacher makes only one true statement, B is innocent.

Assume C is the poacher. Statement 1 is false if he is the poacher. Statement 2 is false if C is the poacher. Statement 3 is true as all suspects have been identified. So, C is the poacher because he made only one true statement. We can check by assuming D is the poacher.

Assume D is the poacher. Then statement 1 is true because of A's statement that D is innocent. Statement 2 is also true because C says he is not the poacher. Statement 3 is either true or false, but that would not change the fact that if D were the poacher, he would be making two true statements. That contradicts the premise. D is innocent.

Problem Ten

Discuss this passage from *Alice's Adventures in Wonderland:*

"She took down a jar from one of the shelves as she passed: it was labeled "ORANGE MARMALADE," but to her great disappointment, it was empty..."

Answer: Alice was disappointed because she assumed the label was true. But she deserves credit for opening the jar. She probably opened to get some marmalade. But still, opening the jar was an act of verification, what Shakespeare called ocular proof. Before accepting anything important as fact, we should verify. Note that orange marmalade is ambivalent. It could mean marmalade made from oranges, in which case, it would be a kind of dull brown, or it could be marmalade which was colored orange. Or it could mean both made from oranges and colored orange. The problem comes from the double meaning of the word *orange*—a fruit or a color.

Problem Eleven

A notorious robber has made a lucrative living by robbing travelers in the forest. Three suspects are identified. Their statements follow. One makes two true statements; one makes one true and one false statement; one makes two false statements. Which one is the robber?

A.   1. I am not the robber.

        2. C is the robber.

B.   1. C is innocent.

        2. A is the robber.

C.   1. I am not the robber.

        2. B is innocent.

Hint: Get the premises straight. Among the suspects, there have to be two true statements, two false statements, and one true and one false.

Answer: C is the robber

Assume A is the robber. Then A1 is F and A2 is F. And B1 is T, B2 is T, but C1 is T and C2 is T. Therefore, A can't be the robber as the premises are not satisfied if he were.

Assuming B is the robber gives TF TF TF for A, B, and C. Therefore, B is innocent.

Assuming C is the robber gives A1T A2T B1F B2F C1F C2T. This is the exact distribution of truth in the premises and the only correct answer. Only if C is the robber do we get the correct specified distribution of truth

Note: Did you see this problem before. Did you solve it then? Did you solve it now?

Problem Twelve

What are the relative merits of the following "explanations" of rain in Clear Lake City, Texas:

a.   "It rained because the confluence of cold air moving southeastward from Alberta and moist air moving northward from the Gulf of Mexico caused the ambient temperature of the atmosphere over Clear Lake City to drop below the dew point."
b.   "It rained because the Chickahominy elders performed a rain dance."
c.   "It rained because the pastor of the Saint Luke's Catholic Church in Pearland offered up a mass for rain."

Answer: a. is the scientific method applied to weather. If the temperatures are known and the wind and other data available, like the dew point, not only will it rain but also the rain can be reasonably predicted. The other two explanations are mere assertions with no support from science and no evidence of effectiveness. Rain dances have no effect on rain. That fact has been proven time and time again. Because of the failure of dances to cause rain, human sacrifice was tried by the Mayans. That didn't work either.

Whoa! Doctor Patten is jumping up and down. He has something to add about the Mayans.

Sidebar by Doctor Patten

Friends, the ancient Mayans believed their great God Chaac controlled the rain. They recognized how dependent on rain the corn crop was. Repeated observations showed when there was little rain, there was little corn. When there was no rain, there was no corn. What's the solution? That's the question. How can we make it rain?

The real solution was to pump underground water to the surface and water the corn. That solution was beyond Mayan capabilities at the time. They were too busy thinking about something else, a fake solution. The Mayan solution was human sacrifice. Eventually, they did stumble on a real solution that worked for them.

That solution was to move elsewhere where it does rain. But until they arrived at that solution, the priests experimented with human sacrifice. Whenever a drought took hold, volunteers were drowned in the cenotes at Uxmal and Chichen Itza and elsewhere throughout the Mayan kingdom. Besides humans, many valuable objects were thrown into the cenote. The idea was to appease Chaac to get Chaac to have his maidens, those of the heavens, pour water down on those beneath using their special water jars.

We know this was the motivation behind the sacrifices because the hieroglyphics written in stone left by the priests as well as the sacred Mayan books tell us it was. The evidence recovered from the cenotes, including human skeletons adorned with gems, confirms the sacrifices.

So, what happened?

After some sacrifices, it rained. Conclusion: Sacrifice worked! When it doesn't rain, kill people.

All this sounds silly to modern ears. But the point is it happened. A whole civilization went haywire because it was concluded that when one event (the rain) followed another (the sacrifice), the two were related as cause and effect. Sadly, once this idea caught on, the solution became generally applicable to other problems. There was no stopping the Mayan theocracy from finding lots and lots of reasons for human sacrifice. In fact, there is a reasonable theory of the destruction of Mayan society based on the extreme need for sacrificial victims. We know from the records that toward the end, wars were organized to get human victims for sacrifice. Think about all those young men and women killed for a simple error in logic, post hoc propter hoc. Think about them and weep.

Problem Thirteen

Unpack, evaluate, and defeat the following argument:

"All of the scientists are telling us that global warming will destroy us. Aren't they the same scientists preaching evolution? If they believe in evolution, then everything will change to match the environment, so what are they worried about?"

Unsigned letter to the editor of the Delaware Times, January 31, 2006

Answer: A statement is a sentence that makes a definite claim. A set of statements makes an argument. And a set of arguments makes a case. A statement is either true or false at a given time and place. If I say it is raining and it is raining, then my statement is true. If it is not raining, it is false. Let's look at her statements to appraise the truth value.

"All of the scientists are telling us that global warming will destroy us."

Is that a true statement? *All* means all, so if we can find a single counter-example, we can prove the statement wrong. The fact is I am a scientist, and I am not telling any such thing. Therefore, the statement is an overgeneralization and wrong. The overwhelming majority of scientists are warning us about the effects of warming. They are predicting difficult times, but they are not saying warming will destroy us. They have correctly predicted the increase in strong storms, wildfires, descent of the polar vortex, and droughts.

Here is the official position of the American Chemical Society (Chemical & Engineering News, November 9, 2020, page 5): "While some still doubt the merits of a global green-power agenda, it is clear to most that climate change is a real and significant threat to the global economy, health, and environmental welfare. The American Chemical Society's public policy on climate change is unequivocal, noting that climate change is real, serious, and has been influenced by anthropogenic activity. Unmitigated climate change will lead to increases in extreme weather events and will cause significant sea level rise, causing property damage and population displacement. It also will continue to degrade ecosystems and natural resources, affecting food and water availability and human health, further burdening economies and societies."

Notice how specific the predictions are and how they are backed by evidence. No one is saying global warming will destroy us.

The official position of the American Society for the Advancement of Science is the same as that of the American Chemical Society.

"Aren't they the same scientists preaching evolution?"

Ho ho ho. Scientists don't preach. And scientists, therefore, do not preach evolution. Evolution is a fact. Whether the correspondent likes it or not. My Jesuit friend Father Meyers (professor at Fordham University) said, "You're a fool if you don't believe in evolution. The only question is did God have anything to do with it?"

Religious people are sometimes anti-science because they don't like the fact that science has proven evolution. Most modern religions, including that of the Roman Catholic Church, recognize evolution as fact.

"If they believe in evolution, then everything will change to match the environment, so what are they worried about?"

The editors of the Delaware Times answered this last question thusly:

"Go ask the dinosaurs."

Problem Fourteen

Memorize the following definitions, for they will serve you well for the rest of your life:

Truth: What is as opposed to what is **not.**

Knowledge: A justified belief that what is true is true.

Bullshit or BS: A statement made for effect without regard to whether it is true or not.

Statement: A sentence that makes a definite claim.

A set is a collection of things.

Argument: A set of statements.

Case: A set of arguments.

Liar: He who represents something as true when he knows it is not true or he who represents something as false when he knows it is true.

Problem Fifteen

Compare and contrast the answers of two candidates for a United States Coast Guard Captain's license:

Question: What should be done to safeguard your vessel & SOB (SOB = souls on board, meaning crew and passengers) in the event of a severe storm at sea?

Candidate One's answer: "I would pray to the Virgin Mary."

Candidate Two's answer: "Batten down the hatches. Call all crew and passengers to put on their Type I lifejackets, slow to steering way, quarter into the wind and waves to prevent breaching, broaching, and pooping. If needed, deploy the anchors, fish oil, and sea dredge. If taking on water, activate the bilge pumps. If sinking, call "mayday" on the radio, giving the exact GPS position. If the radio were not working, launch the distress rockets and shoot the emergency flares. If sinking, abandon ship to the lifeboats while the ship is still under command and making way.

Answer: Candidate two has a reality-based approach to the problem. Candidate one has a supernatural approach to the problem. Which candidate do you think failed the examination? Which candidate would you trust as your sea captain?

Problem Sixteen

- This amusement park has three rides. It also has three gates with signs that identify the ride to which they lead. But the architect forgot the layout of the connecting paths. Please help. Draw three paths (straight or curved) that connect the rides to their gates. The paths can't meet or cross, nor can they travel outside the walls of the park.

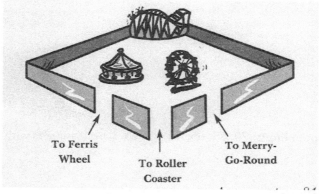

Fig7.1

Answer: Think about this problem for at least 20 minutes. If you can't solve it, look at it before you go to sleep. If you awake and still don't get it, then, and only then, read the answer.

Go from the Ferris Wheel gate directly to the Ferris Wheel. Go to the Merry-Go-Round by circling to the right of the Ferris Wheel and hitting the Merry-Go-Round directly. Go to the Roller Coaster by circling inside of the Merry-Go-Round path and looping left and then right around the Merry-Go-Round. Thus, the Roller Coaster path goes right, then left around the distal Ferris Wheel, then left toward the Ferris Wheel entrance, and then right to the Roller Coaster. Remember, the answer is not important. The mental work to try to get the answer is what builds mental might.

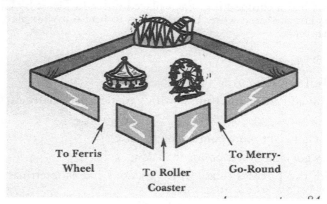

Fig7.2

Problem Seventeen

Memorize the times tables up to 12 x 12. Be able to recall the correct result instantly. Test yourself on the following:

6 x 7 =
8 x 6 =
9 x 7 =
7 x 3 =
12 x 11 =
8 x 9 =
4 x 6 =
9 x 10 =

Square the speed limits: 70, 85, 65, 40, 45, 25. Check answers with a calculator.

Problem Eighteen

Explain the protocol and results of the ACTIVE study. Write your answer and be as specific and as factual as you can. Then review your work by rereading the section in Chapter one. Grade your answer: Five facts recalled A, four B, three C, two D, just a general idea, and no specifics or facts recalled F. Extra credit if you explained CIT.

Problem Nineteen

Music Logic Puzzle (adapted from Piano Explorer November 2020)

Four students had a competition. Each played different pieces by Clementi. No two students got the same score. Use the clues to find out who played what and who got what score.

Scores: 65, 73, 84, 92
Players: Felix, Lucy, John, Ava
Pieces: Gradus ad Parnassum, Fantasy with Variations, Monferrinas, Capriccios
Hints:
1. John got eight more points than Felix.
2. Lucy got eight fewer points than Ava.
3. With two pieces, Fantasy with Variations and Monferrinas, one got 73, and Ava played the other one.

4. Monferrinas scored higher than Gradus ad Parnassum.
5. Gradus ad Parnassum got 84 points.

Note: The problem will not solve itself. You have to solve it. Work it out mentally.

Answer: Two scores are eight over. Those are 73 and 92 because 73 is eight more than 65 and 92 is eight more than 84. Therefore, either John or Ava has the 73, OR either John or Ava has the 92. Summary: John is either 73 or 92. Ava is either 73 or 92.

According to hint three, someone got 73, and Ava played another piece. Therefore, Ava is not 73. She is, therefore, 92, which makes John the 73. Once we know the positions of Ava and John, we also know Lucy and Felix. So the order has to be

65 Felix
73 John
84 Lucy
92 Ava

According to hint 4, Manferrinas scored higher than Gradus ad Parnassum, but hint 5. Says Gradus received 84. Therefore, the only available higher score is 92, which has to belong to Ava. So, Ava played Monferrinas. Lucy played Gradus because she is the 84.

Since Ava played Monferrinas, 73 must have played Fantasy, and that was John. Only one piece is left (Capriccios), so that would belong to Felix.

65 Felix Capriccios
73 John Fantasy
84 Lucy Gradus
92 Ava Monferrinas

Checking this set against the hints: John got eight more than Felix—check. Lucy got 8 points less than Ava—check. Fantasy got 73, and Ava played Monferrinas—check. Monferrinas scored higher than Gradus—check. Gradus got 84—check.

Lightning Source UK Ltd.
Milton Keynes UK
UKHW020711270223
417728UK00015B/1042